Successes and Failures of Health Policy in Europe

Four decades of divergent trends and converging challenges

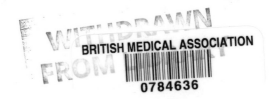

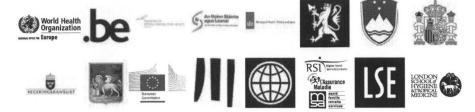

The European Observatory on Health Systems and Policies supports and promotes evidence-based health policy-making through comprehensive and rigorous analysis of health systems in Europe. It brings together a wide range of policy-makers, academics and practitioners to analyse trends in health reform, drawing on experience from across Europe to illuminate policy issues.

The European Observatory on Health Systems and Policies is a partnership between the World Health Organization Regional Office for Europe, the Governments of Belgium, Finland, Ireland, the Netherlands, Norway, Slovenia, Spain, Sweden and the Veneto Region of Italy, the European Commission, the European Investment Bank, the World Bank, UNCAM (French National Union of Health Insurance Funds), the London School of Economics and Political Science, and the London School of Hygiene & Tropical Medicine.

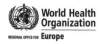 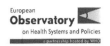

Successes and Failures of Health Policy in Europe

Four decades of divergent trends and converging challenges

Edited by

Johan P. Mackenbach and Martin McKee

 Open University Press

Open University Press
McGraw-Hill Education
McGraw-Hill House
Shoppenhangers Road
Maidenhead
Berkshire
England
SL6 2QL

email: enquiries@openup.co.uk
world wide web: www.openup.co.uk

and Two Penn Plaza, New York, NY 10121-2289, USA

First published 2013

A catalogue record of this book is available from the British Library

ISBN-13: 978-0-33-524751-6 (pb)
ISBN-10: 0-33-524751-2
eISBN: 978-0-33-524752-3

Library of Congress Cataloging-in-Publication Data
CIP data applied for

Typesetting and e-book compilations by
RefineCatch Limited, Bungay, Suffolk
Printed and bound in the UK by Bell & Bain Ltd, Glasgow

European Observatory on Health Systems and Policies Series

The European Observatory on Health Systems and Policies is a unique project that builds on the commitment of all its partners to improving health systems:

- World Health Organization Regional Office for Europe
- Government of Belgium
- Government of Finland
- Government of Ireland
- Government of the Netherlands
- Government of Norway
- Government of Slovenia
- Government of Spain
- Government of Sweden
- Veneto Region of Italy
- European Commission
- European Investment Bank
- World Bank
- UNCAM
- London School of Economics and Political Science
- London School of Hygiene & Tropical Medicine

The series

The volumes in this series focus on key issues for health policy-making in Europe. Each study explores the conceptual background, outcomes and lessons learned about the development of more equitable, more efficient and more effective health systems in Europe. With this focus, the series seeks to contribute to the evolution of a more evidence based approach to policy formulation in the health sector.

These studies will be important to all those involved in formulating or evaluating national health policies and, in particular, will be of use to health policy-makers and advisers, who are under increasing pressure to rationalize the structure and funding of their health system. Academics and students in the field of health policy will also find this series valuable in seeking to understand better the complex choices that confront the health systems of Europe.

The Observatory supports and promotes evidence-based health policy-making through comprehensive and rigorous analysis of the dynamics of health care systems in Europe.

Series Editors

Josep Figueras is the Director of the European Observatory on Health Systems and Policies, and Head of the European Centre for Health Policy, World Health Organization Regional Office for Europe.

Martin McKee is Director of Research Policy and Head of the London Hub of the European Observatory on Health Systems and Policies. He is Professor of European Public Health at the London School of Hygiene & Tropical Medicine as well as a co-director of the School's European Centre on Health of Societies in Transition.

Elias Mossialos is the Co-director of the European Observatory on Health Systems and Policies. He is Brian Abel-Smith Professor in Health Policy, Department of Social Policy, London School of Economics and Political Science and Director of LSE Health.

Richard B. Saltman is Associate Head of Research Policy and Head of the Atlanta Hub of the European Observatory on Health Systems and Policies. He is Professor of Health Policy and Management at the Rollins School of Public Health, Emory University in Atlanta, Georgia.

Reinhard Busse is Associate Head of Research Policy and Head of the Berlin Hub of the European Observatory on Health Systems and Policies. He is Professor of Health Care Management at the Berlin University of Technology.

European Observatory on Health Systems and Policies Series

Series Editors: Josep Figueras, Martin McKee, Elias Mossialos, Richard B. Saltman and Reinhard Busse

Published titles

Regulating entrepreneurial behaviour in European health care systems
Richard B. Saltman, Reinhard Busse and Elias Mossialos (eds)

Hospitals in a changing Europe
Martin McKee and Judith Healy (eds)

Health care in central Asia
Martin McKee, Judith Healy and Jane Falkingham (eds)

Funding health care: options for Europe
Elias Mossialos, Anna Dixon, Josep Figueras and Joe Kutzin (eds)

Health policy and European Union enlargement
Martin McKee, Laura MacLehose and Ellen Nolte (eds)

Regulating pharmaceuticals in Europe: striving for efficiency, equity and quality
Elias Mossialos, Monique Mrazek and Tom Walley (eds)

Social health insurance systems in western Europe
Richard B. Saltman, Reinhard Busse and Josep Figueras (eds)

Purchasing to improve health systems performance
Josep Figueras, Ray Robinson and Elke Jakubowski (eds)

Human resources for health in Europe
Carl-Ardy Dubois, Martin McKee and Ellen Nolte (eds)

Primary care in the driver's seat
Richard B. Saltman, Ana Rico and Wienke Boerma (eds)

Mental health policy and practice across Europe: the future direction of mental health care
Martin Knapp, David McDaid, Elias Mossialos and Graham Thornicroft (eds)

Decentralization in health care
Richard B. Saltman, Vaida Bankauskaite and Karsten Vrangbæk (eds)

Health systems and the challenge of communicable diseases: experiences from Europe and Latin America
Richard Coker, Rifat Atun and Martin McKee (eds)

Caring for people with chronic conditions: a health system perspective
Ellen Nolte and Martin McKee (eds)

Nordic health care systems: recent reforms and current policy challenges
Jon Magnussen, Karsten Vrangbæk and Richard B. Saltman (eds)

Diagnosis-related groups in Europe: moving towards transparency, efficiency and quality in hospitals
Reinhard Busse, Alexander Geissler, Wilm Quentin and Miriam Wiley (eds)

Migration and health in the European Union
Bernd Rechel, Philipa Mladovsky, Walter Devillé, Barbara Rijks, Roumyana Petrova-Benedict and Martin McKee (eds)

Health Systems, health, wealth and societal well-being: assessing the case for investing in health systems
Josep Figueras and Martin McKee

Contents

List of contributors

Peter Anderson
Professor, Substance Use, Policy and Practice, Institute of Health and Society, Newcastle University, UK and Professor, Alcohol and Health, Faculty of Health, Medicine and Life Sciences, Maastricht University, Netherlands

Ahti Anttila
Director of Research of the Mass Screening Registry, Finnish Cancer Registry, Helsinki, Finland

Béatrice Blondel
Senior Research Scientist, Epidemiological Research Unit on Perinatal Health and Women's and Children's Health, INSERM, National Institute of Health and Medical Research, Paris, France

Caroline Bollars
Technical officer, World Health Organization Regional Office for Europe, Copenhagen, Denmark

Laura Currie
PhD student, Health Services Research, Division of Population Health Sciences, Royal College of Surgeons, Dublin, Ireland

Liselotte Schäfer Elinder
Associate Professor, Department of Public Health Sciences, Karolinska Institutet, Stockholm, Sweden

Anna B. Gilmore
Professor of Public Health, University of Bath and UK Centre of Tobacco Control Studies, United Kingdom

Patrick Goodman
Professor, Dublin Institute of Technology, Dublin, Ireland

Susann Henschel
PhD student, "Air pollution & Health", FOCAS Institute, School of Physics, Dublin Institute of Technology, Dublin, Ireland

Marina Karanikolos
Research Fellow at the European Observatory on Health Systems and Policies and the London School of Hygiene and Tropical Medicine, London, United Kingdom

Babak Khoshnood
Senior Research Scientist Epidemiological Research Unit on Perinatal Health and Women's and Children's Health, INSERM, National Institute of Health and Medical Research, Paris, France

Johan P. Mackenbach
Professor and Chair, Department of Public Health, Erasmus MC, Rotterdam, the Netherlands and honorary Professor, London School of Hygiene & Tropical Medicine

Jose M. Martin-Moreno
Professor of Preventive Medicine and Public Health at the University of Valencia, Spain and Director of Programme Management at the World Health Organization Regional Office for Europe, Copenhagen, Denmark

Andrew McCulloch
Chief Executive, The Mental Health Foundation, United Kingdom

Martin McKee
Professor of European Public Health at the London School of Hygiene & Tropical Medicine, United Kingdom, and Research Director at the European Observatory on Health Systems and Policies, London, United Kingdom

Sylvia Medina
Coordinator, European and International Activities, and Coordinator, Apheis and Aphekom Projects on Air Pollution and Health in Europe, Department of Environmental Health, French Institute for Public Health Surveillance (InVS), Saint Maurice, France

Francesco Mitis
Technical officer, World Health Organization Regional Office for Europe, Copenhagen, Denmark

Ionela Petrea
Head, Department of International Development Mental Health, Trimbos Institute, Netherlands and Institute of Mental Health and Addiction, Utrecht, Netherlands

Ralf Reintjes
Professor of Epidemiology and Public Health Surveillance, Hamburg University of Applied Sciences, Germany and Adjunct Professor for Infectious Disease Epidemiology, University of Tampere, Finland

Dinesh Sethi
Programme Manager, World Health Organization Regional Office for Europe, Copenhagen, Denmark

Ingrid Wolfe
Child Health Research Fellow, ECOHOST and Child Public Health Consultant, Guys' and St Thomas's NHS Trust, London and Paediatrician, Whittington NHS Trust, London, United Kingdom

Jennifer Zeitlin
Senior Research Scientist Epidemiological Research Unit on Perinatal Health and Women's and Children's Health, INSERM, National Institute of Health and Medical Research, Paris, France and Adjunct Associate Professor Department of Health Evidence and Policy, Mount Sinai School of Medicine, New York, United States of America

List of tables, figures and boxes

Tables

Figures

Boxes

Foreword

The diversity of Europe offers a remarkable natural laboratory for health policy. There are many examples of how countries have learnt from the experiences of others, with innovations first tried in one, and subsequently being adopted in others, such as compulsory seat-belt wearing, bans on smoking in public places, and the use of taxation to reduce hazardous drinking. However, there are also many examples of policies that, although shown to be successful, have not been taken up elsewhere. What can explain these differences? This book brings together a wealth of evidence on the adoption of evidence-based policies in Europe. It begins by reviewing the evidence on what works to reduce the burden of disease from many of the common risk factors, providing what is, in effect, a guide to evidence-based health policy. However it goes much further, identifying those countries that have taken the lead in implementing evidence-based health policies as well as those that have lagged behind. Then, in a truly innovative set of analyses, it seeks to explain these differences. As expected, resources are important but this is not the only factor. Governments are, to a large extent, reflecting the values held by their people. This is as it should be, but it also begs a question. Should political leaders be following the public mood or should they be leading it, setting out a vision for what could be done to improve health and well-being? The Member States of the European Region of WHO have made their views clear, endorsing the health strategy Health 2020, with its call for political leadership for health. This book should help and encourage them to turn their commitments into action.

Zsuzsanna Jakab
Regional Director, WHO Regional Office for Europe

Acknowledgements

This volume is one of a series of books produced by the European Observatory on Health Systems and Policies. We are especially grateful to the Rockefeller Foundation, which awarded us residencies at its centre in Bellagio, Italy, where the book was completed, to Pilar Palacia, the Director of the Bellagio Centre, and to her staff. The other residents provided advice, encouragement and stimulating conversation during our four weeks there. We are also grateful to the chapter authors for their effort and enthusiasm, as well as their patience as we went through a number of iterations of their papers. We would like to make special mention of Marina Karanikolos, who did a remarkable job in assembling data that informed our work and that of the chapter authors. Initial drafts of the papers were presented at a workshop at the European Public Health Association Scientific Conference in Copenhagen, and we are grateful to those who participated there. Johan Mackenbach would like to thank Andrea Madarisova Geckova (Kosice), Janos Sandor (Debrecen), Roza Adany (Debrecen) and Radoran Chereches (Cluj) for their help in understanding recent population health patterns in central and eastern Europe. As always, we received excellent support from the Secretariat of the Observatory, in particular Josep Figueras and Suzy Lessof. Despoina Xenikaki provided invaluable administrative support for our work. The publishing process was managed with the usual efficiency by the Observatory's publishing team, headed by Jonathan North, ably assisted by Caroline White and with copy editing by Jane Ward. Finally, we are grateful to our families for their patience and forbearance as we undertook this task.

List of abbreviations

AIDS	acquired immunodeficiency syndrome
ASH	Action on Smoking and Health
BSE	bovine spongiform encephalopathy
CIS	Commonwealth of Independent States
DALY	disability-adjusted life-years
EU	European Union
EU25	countries belonging to the EU after January 2004
EU27	countries belonging to the EU after January 2007
FSID	Foundation for the Study of Infant Deaths
GDP	gross domestic product
HIV	human immunodeficiency virus
MMR	measles, mumps and rubella
MRSA	methicillin-resistant *Staphylococcus aureus*
OECD	Organisation for Economic Co-operation and Development
PYLL	potential years of life lost
RTI	road traffic injury
SARS	severe acute respiratory syndrome
SHS	second-hand smoke
SIDS	sudden infant death syndrome
TCS	Tobacco Control Scale
TFA	*trans*-fatty acids
UNICEF	United Nations Children's Fund
WHO	World Health Organization

chapter one

Introduction

Johan Mackenbach and Martin McKee

A natural laboratory

Whatever way one looks at it, Europe is a continent of enormous diversity. Despite the powerful forces of globalization, there are still significant differences in attitudes, beliefs and lifestyles among the people of Norway in the north, Portugal in the west, Malta in the south, the Russian Federation in the east and all those in between. These differences are apparent in many ways, from their national cuisine, poetry and music, to their health and their wealth. Their governments are equally diverse, most obviously in terms of how they see the responsibilities of the state and the individual. However, they are, at least formally, united in the pursuit of certain shared goals relating to the well-being of their people, even if they differ in the means to achieve them.

And they do differ, often quite widely. This is apparent in the choices they have made in many policies of direct relevance to health. Some have acted resolutely to tackle the enormous toll of disability and premature death from tobacco while others have left it to individuals. Some have put in place organized systems to detect cancer early and to treat it, while others have left it to opportunistic encounters between individuals and their physicians. Some have invested in measures to make their roads safe while others have not.

This book is about the impact of these differences in health policy on population health in Europe since the early 1970s. During these years, the health of Europeans overall has improved markedly. Yet that progress has been very uneven. While western European countries have experienced gains in life expectancy at birth of 7 to 12 years, some in the former USSR have yet to recover to the levels reached in 1970. Moreover, within the different parts of Europe, countries have varied greatly in what they have achieved.

These variations are even more striking when trends in mortality from specific conditions, such as cardiovascular diseases, lung and cervical cancer or road traffic injuries (RTIs) are analysed, and they raise important questions about whether some countries have been more successful in their health policies than others. Do between-country differences in rates of smoking-related diseases reflect differences in the strictness of tobacco control efforts? Do differences in screening policies explain why some countries have higher cervical cancer mortality? Are lower rates of RTIs wholly or partly a reflection of more comprehensive road safety programmes?

These questions have never been systematically addressed, and because Europe provides a unique 'natural laboratory' in which to investigate them, this book fills an important gap. A comparative analysis of the successes and failures of health policy in different European countries is important for several reasons. First, it will identify 'best practices' from which other countries can learn, and which could be implemented more widely in order to improve population health throughout Europe. Second, it will make it possible to quantify what these policies have achieved and, more importantly, what they might achieve in the future. Third, it will be a basis for understanding why some countries have succeeded while others have failed to tackle the determinants of health among their people, so that others can learn from their experiences.

In the remainder of this introductory chapter we will first provide a broader context for our comparative analysis of the successes and failures of health policy in Europe by briefly describing recent trends and current patterns of health in Europe. We will summarize previous attempts to understand what role, if any, purposeful actions by governments and others have played in determining the variation. We will then set out the areas of health policy that are covered in this book and how the rest of the book will be structured.

The unequal health of Europeans

The epidemiological transition

The broader canvas against which we should study the health trends that we describe and analyse in this book is the epidemiological transition that European populations have undergone during the 20th century. The term 'epidemiological transition' was first coined in 1971 by Omran, and subsequently modified (Omran 1983; Olshansky and Ault 1986; Mackenbach 1994; Vallin and Meslé 2004), but it still provides a useful framework for characterizing changes in population health.

During this transition, which in different parts of Europe began between 1850 and 1920 (Riley 2001), mortality declined precipitously and life expectancy rose in a truly spectacular manner. Originally, three stages were distinguished. In the first stage, which Omran called the age of 'pestilence and famine', mortality was still high, particularly among children, and was mainly caused by infectious diseases. In the second stage, which he termed the age of 'receding pandemics', deaths from infectious diseases declined rapidly and life expectancy started to rise. In the third stage, the age of 'degenerative and man-made diseases', life expectancy continued to rise as a result of further declines in mortality among the young but ultimately reached a plateau because of the simultaneous increase in cardiovascular diseases, cancers and RTIs (Omran 1971).

This long-term trend in life expectancy, which extends far beyond the period that we are covering in this book, can also clearly be observed in European data.

Figure 1.1 illustrates the situation in a few exemplary countries, and also shows some of the temporary setbacks in life expectancy coinciding with two World Wars and other dramatic historical events.

In the first decades of the 20th century, life expectancy at birth was already on the rise in countries in the western part of the European region, such as Sweden, England and Wales, Austria, and Italy, so that by 1930 their life expectancy surpassed 50 years or, in the case of Sweden, 60 years. In the eastern part of the European region, by comparison, the rise of life expectancy at birth started much later, but then rose more steeply during the 1940s and 1950s so that by 1965 male life expectancy at birth in European countries clustered in a narrow range around the age of 70. In a later extension of his theory, Omran (1983) described the more rapid declines of mortality in the eastern parts of the European region as representing an 'accelerated model', as opposed to the 'classical model' seen in the western parts of the region.

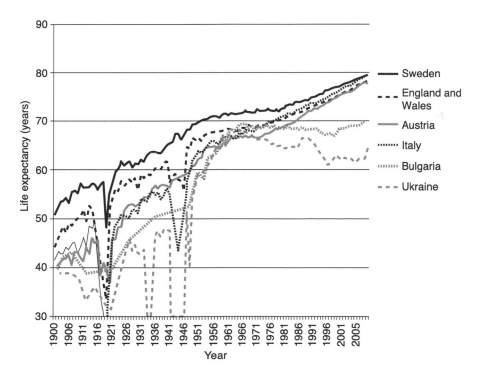

Figure 1.1 Trends in male life expectancy at birth in Sweden, England and Wales, Austria, Italy, Bulgaria and Ukraine, 1900–2008

Source: Human Life-Table Database (2012) except Ukraine (Vallin et al. 2002)

Figure 1.1 also shows that the period of stagnation of life expectancy that corresponds with Omran's third stage did not last long in the western part of the European region and was succeeded by a period of renewed mortality decline that started around 1970, justifying the date selected for the analyses in this book. This renewed increase of life expectancy resulted from declines in mortality from cardiovascular diseases, injury and several other causes; it has been called a 'fourth stage' of the epidemiological transition in which mortality gradually shifts to higher ages (Olshansky and Ault 1986). Others prefer to distinguish different transitions (Mackenbach 1994) and to call this an entirely new transition, in which cardiovascular diseases may gradually be replaced as main causes of death by health conditions of old age such as mental and neurological diseases and 'frailty' (Vallin and Meslé 2004; Meslé and Vallin 2006).

What is certain is that this renewed increase of life expectancy has not been shared equally between countries, and that life expectancy has diverged again. While life expectancy at birth increased during the 1970s and 1980s in the western parts of the European Region, it stagnated and even declined somewhat in the eastern part of the region, until it finally started to rise again in the 1990s (Central and Eastern Europe) or even later (the former USSR). As a result of these diverging developments, life expectancy varies tremendously within Europe (Fig. 1.2).

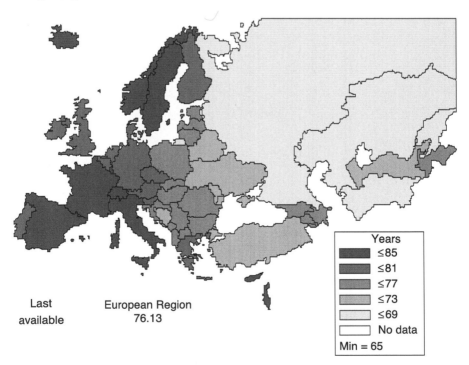

Figure 1.2   Geographical variations in life expectancy at birth in Europe, both genders, in quintiles ca. 2008

Source: WHO Regional Office for Europe 2012

Disease-specific patterns

Chronic diseases are now the main cause of death in Europe, the most significant among them being ischaemic heart disease, cerebrovascular disease and cancer. Over the period 1970–2010, standardized mortality rates for ischaemic heart disease and cerebrovascular disease have fallen uniformly in many but not all European countries.

There are a number of reasons for this fall in mortality rates, not all fully understood. They include reductions in risk factors, such as better diets and lower rates of smoking, as well as better treatment and, particularly for cerebrovascular disease, control of hypertension. Cerebrovascular disease was a condition for which there was no effective treatment until the late 1950s. An additional factor, most prominent in the former USSR but likely to play some role in vulnerable populations in other countries, is hazardous alcohol consumption, now recognized as an important cause of sudden cardiac death (Tomkins et al. 2012). However, the precise contribution of these factors varies over time and from place to place (Ford and Capewell 2011). As a result of these disparate developments, current levels of mortality from ischaemic heart disease and cerebrovascular disease now differ widely within Europe (Fig. 1.3).

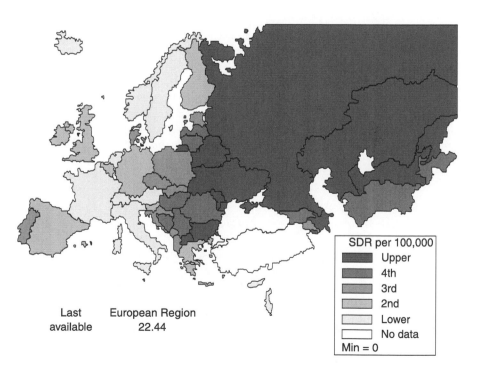

Figure 1.3   Geographical variation in mortality from cerebrovascular disease in Europe, both genders aged 0–64 years, in quintiles, ca. 2008

Source: WHO Regional Office for Europe 2012
Note: SDR, standardized mortality rate

Cancer gives rise to a much more complex picture. Although cancer is often treated as a single disease, it is in reality simply a description of a biological process affecting many different parts of the body, in many different ways, all differing greatly in their aetiology and susceptibility to treatment. Like ischaemic heart disease and cerebrovascular disease, death rates overall are falling, but this conceals some very different trends among men and women in different parts of Europe.

Much of this variation results from differing timing of the smoking epidemic (Thun et al. 2012). The industrial production of cigarettes, accompanied by progressively sophisticated marketing, encouraged a situation in which, by the middle of the 20th century, smoking among men in many parts of Europe was ubiquitous. Women in western Europe followed this trend, but only after a delay of several decades, while cultural norms meant that, until the late 1980s, smoking among women in what was then the USSR remained rare. This has since changed dramatically with the entry of the transnational tobacco companies (Gilmore and McKee 2004). The consequences have been successive waves of smoking-related cancers across Europe, now fortunately declining among men in most countries as the smoking epidemic has begun to recede, but still rising among women. These cancers arise not only in the lungs but also in the larynx, oesophagus, kidney and bladder, while smoking also increases the risk of cancers at other sites, including the cervix.

In contrast, there has been a steady decline in deaths from stomach cancer across Europe throughout the past century, reflecting at least in part improvements in hygiene and, specifically, a decline in infection with the bacterium *Helicobacter pylori* (Sonnenberg 2010). However, some cancers are steadily increasing in incidence, such as cancer of the breast, now the most common in women in most countries (except where it is displaced by lung cancer). The reasons are thought to include better nutrition and, therefore, more rapid growth before puberty (Berkey et al. 2011), changes in patterns of child bearing (Hirte et al. 2007), and increased consumption of alcohol among women (Seitz et al. 2012).

Given the diversity in causes of cancer, patterns vary markedly. Death rates from lung cancer remain high in some western European countries compared with the eastern regions, a consequence of the still low rates among women in the east, while deaths from cervical cancer are much higher in the east (Figs 1.4 and 1.5).

Other non-communicable diseases are of major importance in many parts of Europe. They include diabetes mellitus, with increases in both type 1, believed to result from an infection with a virus in genetically susceptible individuals (Patterson et al. 2009), and type 2, caused primarily by increased levels of obesity (Gonzalez et al. 2009). Death rates from chronic obstructive pulmonary disease are generally declining, but in western Europe they still vary by a factor of more than 10, with the highest rates in Denmark, a country where smoking rates remain high.

Death rates from cirrhosis also vary greatly. There is a band of countries in south-eastern Europe with particularly high rates, stretching from Slovenia through Hungary and Romania to the Republic of Moldova and Ukraine (Fig. 1.6). However, overall, rates are declining, although in some cases only in

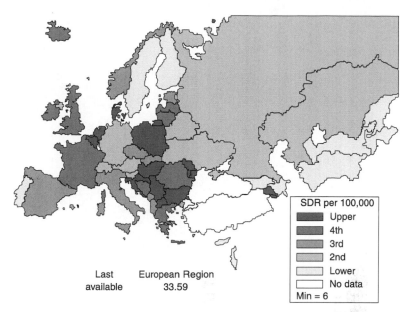

Figure 1.4 Geographical variation in mortality from trachea/bronchus/lung cancer in Europe, both genders, all ages, in quintiles ca. 2008

Source: WHO Regional Office for Europe 2012
Note: SDR, standardized mortality rate

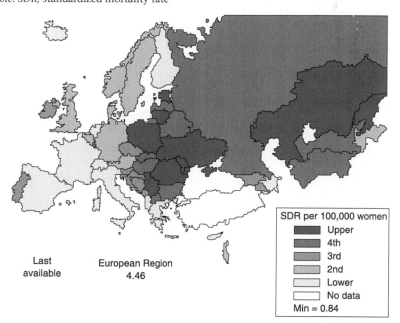

Figure 1.5 Geographical variation in female mortality from cervical cancer in Europe, all ages, in quintiles, ca. 2008

Source: WHO Regional Office for Europe 2012
Note: SDR, standardized mortality rate

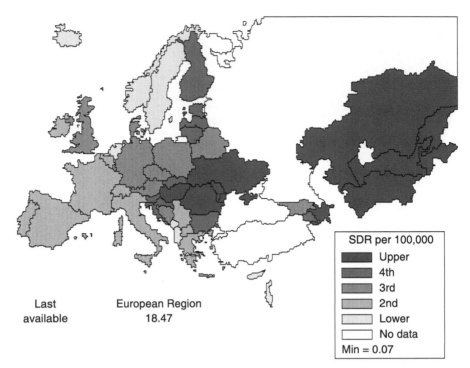

Figure 1.6 Geographical variation in mortality from chronic liver disease and cirrhosis in Europe, both genders, all ages, in quintiles ca. 2008

Source: WHO Regional Office for Europe 2012
Note: SDR, standardized mortality rate

the very recent past, and there have been some sustained declines in countries where rates were once high, such as France.

So far, this description has focused on mortality, largely because of the limited amount of data on disability. Yet this gives only a partial picture of the overall burden of disease. In particular, it underemphasizes the toll of ill health caused by mental illness, even though this is estimated to account for 20% of the total burden of disease in Europe. The one measure of mental illness that is available in most countries is the death rate from suicide, although, as will be discussed later in this book, this is subject to a number of limitations, often arising from the stigma that is attached to suicide in many societies. Notwithstanding these limitations, there are wide variations within Europe in death rates from suicide (Fig. 1.7), as for other causes of death, with the highest rates in the countries of the former USSR.

Injuries are the fourth most common cause of death in Europe and one of the leading causes of death in childhood. Indeed deaths from injury in childhood display one of the steepest gradients between east and west of any cause of death. All of these deaths are entirely preventable. Many deaths from injury occur on the roads. As we will see later in this book, some countries have made enormous progress in reducing these deaths, through a combination of improved transport

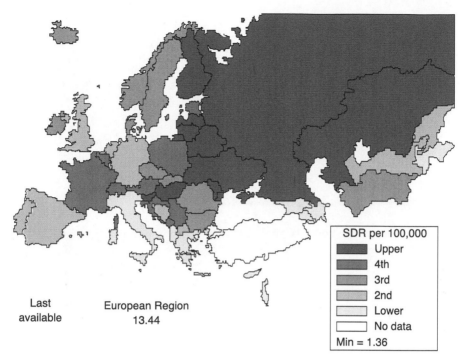

Figure 1.7 Geographical variation in mortality from suicide and self-inflicted injuries in Europe, both genders, all ages, in quintiles, ca. 2008

Source: WHO Regional Office for Europe 2012
Note: SDR, standardized mortality rate

infrastructure, safer vehicles and enforcement of legislation on speed and drunk driving. Others, for a variety of reasons, have failed to do so (McKee et al. 2000; van Beeck et al. 2000). The east–west divide in injury mortality is stark, but some countries in western Europe also have relatively high rates (Fig. 1.8).

Most unintentional injuries occur around the home. Again, substantial gains have been made in recent decades in improving safety. Dangerous toys, such as those with sharp edges or parts that can be swallowed easily, have been withdrawn from sale in most countries. Yet many dangers remain, such as those from unguarded play areas, unsafe electrical installations and inadequate lighting. As with injuries on the roads, there is still a wide geographical variation.

Although the epidemiological transition has seen remarkable declines in infectious diseases over the past century, the struggle between humans and microorganisms continues. On several occasions in recent decades, bacteria, viruses and the vectors that transmit them have taken advantage of opportunities that have arisen. These include the wars in the Balkans in the 1990s and the social and economic turmoil that accompanied the dissolution of the USSR (Suhrcke et al. 2011), as well as the creation of incubators for tuberculosis in overcrowded and poorly maintained prisons (Stuckler et al. 2008). These events allowed diseases once considered defeated, such as diphtheria, to re-emerge.

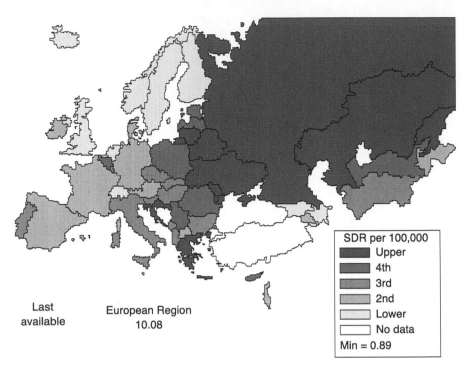

Figure 1.8   Geographical variation in mortality from road traffic accidents in Europe, both genders, all ages, in quintiles, ca. 2008

Source: WHO Regional Office for Europe 2012
Note: SDR, standardized mortality rate

They also include the failure to manage the use of antibiotics in health care facilities, leading to the emergence of antibiotic resistance.

So far, this analysis has looked at deaths from specific causes. It is also informative to look at deaths associated with the processes of giving birth and being born. Historically, this was an extremely dangerous process. Much can go wrong, and a failure to recognize complications and to deal with them swiftly can easily lead to the death of the mother and the child (Richardus et al. 2003). Once again, Europe has seen great successes in recent decades. Maternal death in some countries is now extremely rare, particularly when compared with the still very high rates in many other parts of the world. However, in some parts of Europe, there is still considerable room for improvement. This is most obviously the case in the countries of the former USSR, but there are also unacceptably high rates in some western European countries. Similar variations can be seen with neonatal mortality (Fig. 1.9), although the available data may underestimate the scale of the problem in some countries of the former USSR because of weaknesses in birth registration (Badurashvili et al. 2001).

In the next section we examine some of the reasons that have been proposed to explain why some countries enjoy better health than others.

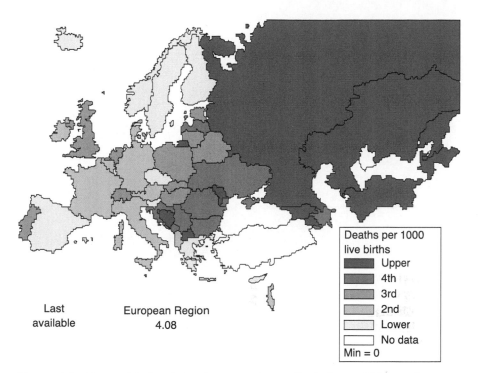

Last available   European Region 4.08

Deaths per 1000 live births
Upper
4th
3rd
2nd
Lower
No data
Min = 0

Figure 1.9   Geographical variation in neonatal mortality in Europe, both genders, in quintiles ca. 2008

Source: WHO Regional Office for Europe 2012

Explaining European health patterns

Economic factors

Research that has sought to explain between-country differences in life expectancy or mortality from specific causes often starts from the observation that aggregate health outcomes tend to be closely correlated with national income, typically measured by gross domestic product (GDP). This was first described systematically by Preston, who in a seminal paper showed that during the 20th century there has always been a strong cross-sectional relationship between GDP and life expectancy (Preston 1975). In global comparisons, the relationship is steeper at lower than at higher levels of GDP, and this can also be observed in Europe in 2008, although even a straight line would do reasonably well in summarizing this relationship (Fig. 1.10). Moreover, studies on the evolution of mortality over time have shown an association between economic growth and mortality from many different causes, such as cardiovascular diseases, cerebrovascular disease, cancers, disorders of infancy and motor vehicle injuries (Brenner 1987).

Some of the trends and variations in mortality described earlier in this chapter were undoubtedly driven by economic development. The western

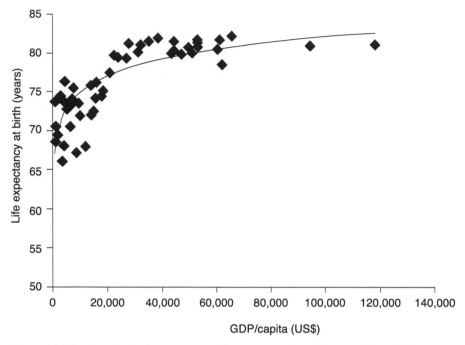

Figure 1.10 Association between gross domestic product (GDP in US$) and life expectancy at birth in Europe, 2008

Source: WHO Regional Office for Europe 2012

part of the European region experienced almost continuous economic growth, while many countries in the eastern part experienced economic stagnation in the 1980s, a result of the failure of the communist economic model and outright economic decline in the 1990s, exacerbated by forced restructuring of the economy (Stuckler et al. 2009).

This relationship between national income and life expectancy must, however, be an indirect one, because as Preston already showed, the relationship has shifted upwards over time. At a given level of national income, life expectancy was higher in 1960 than in 1930, implying that only part of the rise in national life expectancies between 1930 and 1960 could be explained by the rise of national incomes (Preston 1975). Similar upward shifts have been seen more recently (Bloom and Canning 2007).

The explanation is that the mechanisms that link economic development to improved health outcomes are only partly dependent on average income levels. Sanitary measures that were at one time attainable only for countries with the highest levels of development have spread to other countries even before these countries reached the same income levels, because the knowledge was freely available and the required technical equipment became cheaper over time (Preston 1975; Mackenbach 2007). The same is likely to be true for the health policies of today.

As this book focuses on the role of collective human agency in explaining health variations within Europe, we will now briefly review some of the previous studies looking at the impact of policy variations on health outcomes. These studies can be divided in two groups: studies that focus on specific health outcomes from which policy impacts are inferred indirectly, and studies that directly relate policy exposures to health outcomes. We will limit ourselves to studies that have looked at a broad range of health outcomes; where relevant, disease-specific studies will be reviewed in subsequent chapters.

Indirect studies

If one can identify specific health outcomes that are likely to be influenced mainly by a particular policy, then one can use trends or geographical variations in these outcomes to infer the contribution of a particular policy even without explicitly linking outcomes to policy exposures.

One example of this approach can be found in the area of 'amenable mortality'. Several decades ago it was proposed that rates of mortality from certain causes that are amenable to medical care could be used as indicators of the effectiveness of health care. This gave rise to the concept of 'avoidable' or 'amenable' mortality, originally developed by Rutstein et al. (1976) for application in a clinical context, and operationalized for application at the population level by Holland and colleagues (Charlton et al. 1983; Charlton et al. 1987; Holland 1990). Causes of death that are often used in these analyses include tuberculosis, other infectious diseases, Hodgkin's disease, testicular cancer, cervical cancer, cerebrovascular disease, appendicitis and maternal and perinatal mortality. Some of these causes are amenable to prevention, others to treatment.

In advanced industrialized countries, including those in the western part of the European region, mortality from most of these conditions has declined strongly over time in the period covered by this book (Nolte and McKee 2003, 2004, 2008). The declines have also been used to estimate the contribution of improvements in health care to total mortality decline during the 20th century (Mackenbach 1996).

Similarly, variations between countries in rates of mortality from amenable conditions have been interpreted as indicating differences between countries in the performance of their health systems (Nolte and McKee 2003, 2004, 2008). However, they show only weak relationships with health care supply or expenditure (Mackenbach et al. 1990; Mackenback 1991; OECD 2010). Nevertheless, they do suggest that some of the observed variations in mortality within Europe result from variations in the performance of health care systems.

Declines in amenable mortality have been much smaller in the eastern part of the region, and current levels of amenable mortality are considerably higher, suggesting that part of the health disadvantage in that part of Europe is a reflection of deficiencies in health care (Jozan and Prokhorskas 1997; Andreev et al. 2003).

Another example of an indirect approach can be found in a range of studies looking at the contribution of specific risk factors to trends in mortality or variations in mortality across countries. Because some of these variations in risk factors reflect the success or failure of policies to tackle them, such analyses can be used to generate hypotheses on the population health impact of these policies.

One of the earliest attempts to do this used data from the World Health Organization (WHO) MONICA study, undertaken in 38 populations from 21 countries between the mid-1980s and 1990s. Although this was the most exhaustive survey of the risk factors for cardiovascular diseases to date, it contained limited information on treatment. Nonetheless, it concluded that preventive measures to reduce exposure to risk factors had made a substantial contribution to the observed decline in cardiovascular mortality over the period of the study. Subsequent work has used increasingly sophisticated models with much more detailed data (Capewell et al. 1999). Examples involve work using the IMPACT model (Ainsworth et al. 2011) and, more recently, the DYNAMO model (Kulik et al. 2012). The IMPACT model has now been applied to data from many countries worldwide. Although the relative contribution varies, it identifies both reduction in risk factors and expansion of effective treatment as playing important roles (Unal et al. 2003; Aspelund et al. 2010; Bandosz et al. 2012). An example of a study of geographical variation is the Intersalt study, showing an association between salt intake and blood pressure, both among individuals and across countries (Elliott et al. 1996). Collectively, these studies suggest that part of the variation in mortality in Europe results from risk factors amenable to health policy.

Direct studies

Studies that have sought to examine the relationship between policies and population health outcomes directly have largely focused on three different policy areas: political regimes, social policies and health care policies. Research on political regimes has looked primarily at two different aspects: democratic versus authoritarian rule and the political composition of governments.

Democracy may be important for health for several reasons, for example because a democratic government is held accountable for its actions and there may be stronger mechanisms for selecting competent and honest people (Besley and Kudamatsu 2006). A recent overview of 20 studies of the effect of democratic government on population health outcomes shows that most, but not all, found a positive association, with various controls for other determinants (Klomp and de Haan 2009). As many of these studies include a wide range of countries with a similarly wide range of political regimes, including many low-income countries, it is unclear whether the smaller variation in degrees of democracy observed in Europe today may actually contribute to the observed differences in health.

Political composition of governments may be equally relevant. It is often thought that social democratic governments are more committed to the expansion of the welfare state and to other social policies that are conducive to health (Borrell et al. 2007). One analysis did indeed find a correlation between cumulative years of government by 'pro-redistributive parties' on the one hand and infant mortality and life expectancy on the other hand, but this study did not control for confounding factors (Navarro et al. 2003, 2006). Another has found an association between the proportionality of the electoral system and both infant mortality and life expectancy, suggesting that, as proportional voting systems encouraged the election of coalitions, the resulting governments are more likely to represent the interests of all members of society and not just one section (Wigley and Akkoyunlu-Wigley 2011). It is unclear, at the current state of our knowledge, whether one should expect an important contribution of political composition of governments to the explanation of inequalities in health within the European region.

Other research has looked at the effectiveness of governments, often captured in a range of measures of the quality of governance. For example, one study has demonstrated a positive association between good governance and health outcomes in a sample of 101 countries, but it used structural equation modelling to show that this is mediated through the effect of governance on income and the quality of the health system (Klomp and de Haan 2008).

An area of policy that has attracted a lot of interest recently is that of social or welfare policies. Within Europe, countries differ significantly in their approach to these policies. The differences have been summarized in the form of three (sometimes four) different 'welfare regimes': a Nordic or social democratic, an Anglo-Saxon or liberal, and a continental or Christian-democratic regime (Esping-Andersen 1990); to these three a Mediterranean or family-based regime has sometimes been added (Ferrera 1996).

The Nordic welfare states can be characterized by three common features: they are comprehensive, institutionalized and universalistic. As most Nordic countries also have high life expectancy, researchers have asked whether the two are indeed related. A recent analysis of 17 countries, including many in Europe, found that social spending and universalism, controlling for GDP, were related positively to life expectancy. In more detailed analyses, they found that generosity in family policies was associated with lower infant mortality, and that generosity in basic pensions lowers old age mortality (Lundberg et al. 2008; Kangas 2010). While these and similar analyses of aggregate health measures such as total mortality provide indications of potentially relevant relationships, they do not elucidate the mechanisms underlying them, and it, therefore, remains unclear whether the associations represent causal effects.

The most frequently investigated relationship, however, is that between health care and population health indicators. One of the earliest studies, by Cochrane and colleagues (1978), sought associations between health system 'outputs', such as mortality at different ages and maternal deaths, and 'inputs', grouped into social and economic factors, lifestyle factors and health system inputs. They found some intuitive results, such as more nurses per head of population being associated with lower maternal and infant mortality, but also some counterintuitive ones, such as more doctors being associated with higher mortality at younger ages.

Since then, many similar studies have been undertaken. However, many include samples of countries worldwide and, given the lack of data on adult mortality outside developed countries, they have used measures of infant, maternal and under-five mortality as their measures of health outcome. These analyses also include countries with a much larger range of variation in resources than is seen in Europe. The studies also vary considerably in terms of the sophistication with which they have taken account of data limitations and methodological challenges. Many show a strong association between the density of qualified health workers and health outcomes, typically showing a closer association with maternal mortality than with child mortality (Anand and Barnighausen 2004).

Fewer studies have looked for associations in developed countries. Hitiris and Posnett (1992) found a small negative association between health expenditure and crude mortality rates, but they controlled for few other factors. A more detailed study found that higher health expenditures in western European countries were associated with lower infant and female mortality and, at any given level of expenditure, countries with tax-based health systems achieved lower infant mortality rates than those with social insurance (Elola et al. 1995). Other studies in individual countries also found associations between health expenditure and health outcomes (Collins and Klein 1980; Forbes and McGregor 1984). However, all these studies had limitations, including a failure to account for what expenditure could buy in terms of health system inputs. A more complex analysis, undertaken by the Organisation for Economic Co-operation and Development (OECD), disentangled many of the determinants of health and, while finding that sociodemographic factors such as education levels and national income were the most important drivers of potential years of life lost (PYLLs), it also found a significant association with health expenditure, but only for females (Or 2000). It was suggested that this reflected the differing pattern of causes of death between men and women, with the former being dominated by injuries and violence that were less amenable to medical care.

Collectively, these studies suggest that some of the differences between European countries in population health indicators may be related to varying political conditions, social policies and levels of health care expenditure. As these may all be associated with the health policies that are the focus of this book, they should be taken into account when we search for the health impact of these policies.

The scope of this book

The variations in health trends described earlier in this chapter raise important questions. Many countries in Europe have seen their health situation improve dramatically over the past decades, but to what extent did this result from purposeful action to improve health, or was it a side-effect of improvements in living conditions and health behaviours that came about spontaneously? Some countries have seen equally dramatic setbacks. To what extent were these the result of deteriorating living conditions or health behaviours, or a breakdown of previously successful programmes to tackle health risks? And to the extent that these favourable or unfavourable health trends reflect the success or failure of health-related policies, why do some countries perform better than others?

These are the types of question that this book has addressed. More systematically, this book has the following aims, to:

• assess the extent to which different European countries vary in the implementation of health policies that are known to be effective

- assess the extent to which differences between European countries in implementation of health policies have had an impact on trends and levels of relevant health outcomes
- identify 'best practices' of health policy, and indicate opportunities for further health gains by implementing these 'best practice' policies throughout Europe
- identify determinants of successes and failures of health policy, and derive guidance for policy-makers on how to achieve optimal results.

We define health policies as 'decisions, plans and actions that are undertaken to achieve specific health goals within a society'. It is irrelevant whether these policies originate within or outside the health care sector, or whether they are initiated by public or private institutions. The defining characteristics of the 'decisions, plans and actions' are that they explicitly aim to prevent or ameliorate health problems, or to reduce exposure to well-known health risks, and that they are taken on a population-wide basis ('within a society').

Importantly, unlike the often cited definition of the WHO ('decisions, plans, and actions that are undertaken to achieve specific health care goals within a society' (World Health Organization 2012)), our definition does not limit health policy to actions that imply initiation by, or delivery of, health care. We conceptualize health policy as including policies on health care but having a much broader scope.

In this book we have limited ourselves to health policies that are based on primary or secondary prevention. We considered that there is already an abundance of international comparisons of health care policy, focusing on differences between countries in how health care systems are organized and how health care is financed, to which we have ourselves contributed a substantial amount. Readers seeking more information on this topic may find the web site of the European Observatory on Health Systems and Policies (2012) a useful starting point. We believe that it will be more useful to focus on how countries differ in policies that aim at preventing health problems, because this is an area that is studied much less often and yet may be of equal or greater relevance for improving population health outcomes.

We will deal with both methods of primary prevention (aiming to avoid the occurrence of disease by reducing exposure to health risks or by strengthening individuals' ability to cope with these health risks) and methods of secondary prevention (aiming to avoid the progression of disease to a symptomatic stage, by diagnosing and treating disease in early stages before it causes significant morbidity). Other terms that we will sometimes use to distinguish between different approaches of prevention are health protection (methods that provide passive protection against health risks and do not involve individuals' active participation) and health promotion (methods that enable people to increase control over their health and its determinants).

This book will cover 11 areas of health policy that have been identified in preliminary analyses as having contributed to major population health gains in at least some European countries. These are tobacco; alcohol; food and nutrition; fertility, pregnancy and childbirth; child health; infectious diseases;

hypertension detection and treatment; cancer screening; mental health; road safety; and air pollution.

For each of these areas, similar analyses have been carried out using the following general approach. First, reviews were carried out to search and grade scientific evidence on the effectiveness of potentially relevant policies. Second, data were collected on the actual implementation of these policies in different European countries, and analyses were made of the impact of these policies on health outcomes. Sometimes these analyses could cover a range of countries and allowed an assessment of the statistical association between policy implementation and policy outcomes. At other times, these analyses were conducted in the form of case studies covering single countries. Third, the possible determinants of between-country differences in implementation of effective health policies were explored. All analyses were limited to health policies that may have affected population health in the period 1970–2010.

The final part of the analysis consisted of a systematic between-country analysis. The evidence collected in the 11 area-specific analyses was synthesized to provide an overview of the generic effectiveness of national health policies, seeking to identify countries whose overall success was better than might be expected given other factors known to influence health policies. Using these 'best practices', the potential population health impacts of implementing 'best practices' throughout Europe were estimated. An exploration was then carried out to identify the governance conditions that are associated with successful health policy. Finally, implications for policy-makers were formulated. The results of these syntheses are presented in the final five chapters of this book.

The area-specific analyses were commissioned from experts in the field. Outlines for these chapters were discussed during an author workshop hosted by the European Public Health Conference in Copenhagen in November 2011. Draft versions of chapters were edited into the final versions appearing in this book during a residency by the editors at the Rockefeller Foundation's Bellagio Centre in April/May 2012. This residency also allowed the editors to write the introduction and final five chapters of this book.

A final word is needed about the boundaries of Europe as applied in this book. It is far from obvious how Europe should be defined. It is part of the Eurasian land mass, with the border with Asia a question of culture and history as much as of physical geography. This was already noted dismissively by Metternich, who suggested that Asia began on the outskirts of Vienna. Two partly European countries, Turkey and the Russian Federation, have the largest parts of their land masses in Asia, and both simultaneously draw on cultural traditions from east and west. The European Region of the WHO stretches from western Greenland to Vladivostok and includes a number of countries that are unambiguously in Asia, such as Kazakhstan, Uzbekistan, Kyrgyzstan, Tajikistan and Israel. For the purposes of this book, we have taken a pragmatic approach, defining Europe as those countries that are part of the WHO's European Region, minus Kazakhstan, Uzbekistan, Kyrgyzstan, Tajikistan, Israel and Turkey. When we further exclude the mini-states of Andorra, Liechtenstein, Monaco, San Marino and the Vatican City, this gives us 43 nations to consider in this book.

Notwithstanding our European focus, we hope and expect that this book will be useful for public health practitioners, health policy-makers and public health scientists both in Europe and elsewhere.

References

Ainsworth, J.D., Carruthers, E., Couch, P. et al. (2011) IMPACT: a generic tool for modelling and simulating public health policy, *Methods in Information Medicine*, 50(5):454–63.

Anand, S. and Barnighausen, T. (2004) Human resources and health outcomes: cross-country econometric study, *Lancet*, 364(9445):1603–9.

Andreev, E.M., Nolte, E., Shkolnikov, V.M. et al. (2003) The evolving pattern of avoidable mortality in Russia, *International Journal of Epidemiology*, 32(3):437–46.

Aspelund, T., Gudnason, V., Magnusdottir, B.T. et al. (2010) Analysing the large decline in coronary heart disease mortality in the Icelandic population aged 25–74 between the years 1981 and 2006, *PLoS One*, 5(11):e13957.

Badurashvili, I., McKee, M., Tsuladze, G. et al. (2001) Where there are no data: what has happened to life expectancy in Georgia since 1990? *Public Health*, 115(6):394–400.

Bandosz, P., O'Flaherty, M., Drygas, W. et al. (2012) Decline in mortality from coronary heart disease in Poland after socioeconomic transformation: modelling study, *British Medical Journal*, 344:d8136.

van Beeck, E.F., Borsboom, G.J. and Mackenbach, J.P. (2000) Economic development and traffic accident mortality in the industrialized world, 1962–1990, *International Journal of Epidemiology*, 29(3):503–9.

Berkey, C.S., Willett, W.C., Frazier, A.L. et al. (2011) Prospective study of growth and development in older girls and risk of benign breast disease in young women, *Cancer*, 117(8):1612–20.

Besley, T. and Kudamatsu, M. (2006) Health and democracy, *Political Economy*, 96(2):313–18.

Bloom, D.E. and Canning, D. (2007) Commentary: the Preston curve 30 years on: still sparking fires, *International Journal of Epidemiology*, 36:498–9; discussion 502–3.

Borrell, C., Espelt, A. and Rodriguez-Sanz, M. (2007) Politics and health, *Journal of Epidemiology and Community Health*, 61(8):658–9.

Brenner, M.H. (1987) Relation of economic change to Swedish health and social well-being, 1950–1980, *Social Science and Medicine*, 25(2):183–95.

Capewell, S., Pell, J.P., Morrison, C. and McMurray, J. (1999) Increasing the impact of cardiological treatments. How best to reduce deaths, *European Heart Journal*, 20(19):1386–92.

Charlton, J.R., Hartley, R.M., Silver, R. and Holland, W.W. (1983) Geographical variation in mortality from conditions amenable to medical intervention in England and Wales, *Lancet*, i(8326):691–6.

Charlton, J.R., Holland, W.W., Lakhani, A. and Paul, E.A. (1987) Variations in avoidable mortality and variations in health care, *Lancet*, i(8537):858.

Cochrane, A.L., St Leger, A.S. and Moore, F. (1978) Health service 'input' and mortality 'output' in developed countries, *Journal of Epidemiology and Community Health*, 32(3):200–5.

Collins, E. and Klein, R. (1980) Equity and the NHS: self-reported morbidity, access, and primary care, *British Medical Journal*, 281(6248):1111–15.

Elliott, P., Stamler, J., Nichols, R. et al. (1996) Intersalt revisited: further analyses of 24 hour sodium excretion and blood pressure within and across populations. Intersalt Cooperative Research Group, *British Medical Journal*, 312(7041):1249–53.

Elola, J., Daponte, A. and Navarro, V. (1995) Health indicators and the organization of health care systems in western Europe, *American Journal of Public Health*, 85(10):1397–1401.

Esping-Andersen, G. (1990) *The Three Worlds of Welfare Capitalism*. Cambridge, UK: Polity Press.

European Observatory on Health Systems and Policies (2012) Website. London: European Observatory on Health Systems and Policies, http://www.euro.who.int/en/who-we-are/partners/observatory (accessed 4 June 2012).

Ferrera, M. (1996) Southern model of welfare in social Europe, *Journal of European Social Policy*, 6/1:17–37.

Forbes, J.F. and McGregor, A. (1984) Unemployment and mortality in post-war Scotland, *Journal of Health Economics*, 3(3):239–57.

Ford, E.S. and Capewell, S. (2011) Proportion of the decline in cardiovascular mortality disease due to prevention versus treatment: public health versus clinical care, *Annual Review of Public Health*, 32:5–22.

Gilmore, A.B. and McKee, M. (2004) Moving east: how the transnational tobacco industry gained entry to the emerging markets of the former Soviet Union. Part I: establishing cigarette imports, *Tobacco Control*, 13(2):143–50.

Gonzalez, E.L., Johansson, S., Wallander, M.A. and Rodríguez, L.A. (2009) Trends in the prevalence and incidence of diabetes in the UK: 1996–2005, *Journal of Epidemiology and Community Health*, 63(4):332–6.

Hirte, L., Nolte, C. Bain, E., and McKee, M. (2007) Breast cancer mortality in Russia and Ukraine 1963–2002: an age-period cohort analysis, *International Journal of Epidemiology*, 36(4):900–6.

Hitiris, T. and Posnett, J. (1992) The determinants and effects of health expenditure in developed countries, *Journal of Health Economics*, 11(2):173–81.

Holland, W. (1990) Avoidable death as a measure of quality, *Quality Assurance in Health Care*, 2(3–4):227–33.

Human Life-Table Database (2012) website. Munich: Max-Planck-Gesellschaft, http://www.lifetable.de (accessed 4 June 2012).

Jozan, P. and Prokhorskas, R. (1997) *Atlas of Leading and 'Avoidable' Cause of Death in Countries of Central and Eastern Europe*. Budapest: Hungarian Central Statistical Office Publishing.

Kangas, O. (2010) One hundred years of money, welfare and death: mortality, economic growth and the development of the welfare state in 17 OECD countries 1900–2000, *International Journal of Social Welfare*, 19:S42–S59.

Klomp, J. and de Haan, J. (2008) Effects of governance on health: a cross-national analysis of 101 countries, *Kyklos*, 61:599–614.

Klomp, J. and de Haan, J. (2009) Is the political system really related to health? *Social Science and Medicine*, 69(1):36–46.

Kulik, M.C., Nusselder, W.J., Boshuizen, H.C. et al. (2012) Comparison of tobacco control scenarios: quantifying estimates of long-term health impact using the DYNAMO-HIA modeling tool, *PLoS One*, 7(2):e32363.

Lundberg, O., Yngwe, M.A., Stjärne, M.K. et al. (2008) The role of welfare state principles and generosity in social policy programmes for public health: an international comparative study, *Lancet*, 372(9650):1633–40.

Mackenbach, J.P. (1991) Health care expenditure and mortality from amenable conditions in the European Community, *Health Policy*, 19(2–3):245–55.

Mackenbach, J.P. (1994) The epidemiologic transition theory, *Journal of Epidemiology and Community Health*, 48(4):329–31.

Mackenbach, J.P. (1996) The contribution of medical care to mortality decline: McKeown revisited, *Journal of Clinical Epidemiology*, 49(11):1207–13.

Mackenbach, J.P. (2007) Commentary: did Preston underestimate the effect of economic development on mortality? *International Journal of Epidemiology*, 36(3):496–7; discussion 498–502.

Mackenbach, J.P., Bouvier-Colle, M.H. and Jougla, E. (1990) Avoidable mortality and health services: a review of aggregate data studies, *Journal of Epidemiology and Community Health*, 44(2):106–11.

McKee, M., Zwi, A., Koupilova, I., Sethi, D. and Leon, D. (2000) Health policy-making in central and eastern Europe: lessons from the inaction on injuries? *Health Policy Plan*, 15(3):263–9.

Meslé, F. and Vallin, J. (2006) Diverging trends in female old-age mortality: the United States and the Netherlands versus France and Japan, *Population and Development Review*, 32(1):123–45.

Navarro, V., Borrell, C., Benach, J. et al. (2003) The importance of the political and the social in explaining mortality differentials among the countries of the OECD, 1950–1998, *International Journal of Health Services*, 33(3):419–94.

Navarro, V., Muntaner, C., Borrell, C. et al. (2006) Politics and health outcomes, *Lancet*, 368(9540):1033–7.

Nolte, C.M. and McKee, M. (2003) Measuring the health of nations: analysis of mortality amenable to health care, *British Medical Journal*, 327(7424):1129.

Nolte, C.M. and McKee, M. (2004) *Does Health Care Save Lives? Avoidable Mortality Revisited*. London: Nuffield Trust.

Nolte, C.M. and McKee, M. (2008) Measuring the health of nations: updating an earlier analysis, *Health Affairs (Millwood)*, 27(1):58–71.

OECD (2010) *Health Care Systems: Efficiency and Policy Settings*. Paris: Organisation for Economic Co-operation and Development.

Olshansky, S.J. and Ault, A.B. (1986) The fourth stage of the epidemiologic transition: the age of delayed degenerative diseases, *Milbank Quarterly*, 64(3):355–91.

Omran, A.R. (1971) The epidemiologic transition. A theory of the epidemiology of population change, *Milbank Quarterly*, 49(4):509–38.

Omran, A.R. (1983) The epidemiologic transition theory. A preliminary update, *Journal of Tropical Pediatrics*, 29(6):305–16.

Or, Z. (2000) *Determinants of Health Outcomes in Industrialised Countries: A Pooled, Cross-country, Time-series Analysis*. [*OECD Economic Studies 30*.] Paris: Organisation for Economic Co-operation and Development.

Patterson, C.C., Dahlquist, G.G. and Gyürüs, E., for the EURODIAB Study Group (2009) Incidence trends for childhood type 1 diabetes in Europe during 1989–2003 and predicted new cases 2005–20: a multicentre prospective registration study, *Lancet*, 373(9680):2027–33.

Preston, S.H. (1975) The changing relation between mortality and level of economic development, *Population Studies*, 29(2):231–48.

Richardus, J.H., Graafmans, W.C., Verloove-Vanhorick, S.P. and Mackenbach, J.P. (2003) Differences in perinatal mortality and suboptimal care between 10 European regions: results of an international audit. *BJOG: An International Journal of Obstetrics and Gynaecology*, 110(2):97–105.

Riley, J.C. (2001) *Rising Life Expectancy. A Global History*. Cambridge, UK: Cambridge University Press.

Rutstein, D.D., Berenberg, W., Chalmers, T.C. et al. (1976) Measuring the quality of medical care. A clinical method, *New England Journal of Medicine*, 294(11): 582–8.

Seitz, H.K., Pelucchi, C., Bagnardi, V. and La Vecchia, C. (2012) Epidemiology and pathophysiology of alcohol and breast cancer: update 2012, *Alcohol and Alcoholism*, 47(3):204–12.

Sonnenberg, A. (2010) Differences in the birth-cohort patterns of gastric cancer and peptic ulcer, *Gut*, 59(6):736–43.

Stuckler, D., Basu, S., McKee, M. and King, L. (2008) Mass incarceration can explain population increases in TB and multi-drug resistant TB in European and central Asian countries, *Proceedings of the National Academy of Sciences USA*, 105(36):13280–5.

Stuckler, D., King, L. and McKee, M. (2009) Mass privatisation and the post-communist mortality crisis: a cross-national analysis, *Lancet*, 373(9661):399–407.

Suhrcke, M., Stuckler, D., Suk, J.E. et al. (2011) The impact of economic crises on communicable disease transmission and control: a systematic review of the evidence, *PLoS One*, 6(6):e20724.

Thun, M., Peto, R., Boreham, J. and Lopez, A.D. (2012) Stages of the cigarette epidemic on entering its second century, *Tobacco Control*, 21(2):96–101.

Tomkins, S., Collier, T., Oralov, A. et al. (2012) Hazardous alcohol consumption is a major factor in male premature mortality in a typical Russian city: prospective cohort study 2003–2009, *PLoS One*, 7(2):e30274.

Unal, B., Critchley, J. and Capewell, S. (2003) Impact of smoking reduction on coronary heart disease mortality trends during 1981–2000 in England and Wales, *Tobacco Induced Disease*, 1(3):185.

Vallin, J. and Meslé, F. (2004) Convergences and divergences in mortality. A new approach to health transition. *Demographic Research*, Special Collection 2(Article 2):11–44, http://www.demographic-research.org/special/2/2/ (accessed 4 June 2012).

Vallin, J., Meslé, F., Adamets, S. and Pyrozhkov, S. (2002) A new estimate of Ukrainian population losses during the crises of the 1930s and 1940s, *Population Studies (Camb)*, 56(3):249–63.

Wigley, S. and Akkoyunlu-Wigley, A. (2011) Do electoral institutions have an impact on population health? *Public Choice*, 148:595–610.

WHO Regional Office for Europe (2012) *European Health for All Database (HFA-DB)*. Copenhagen: WHO Regional Office for Europe, http://data.euro.who.int/hfadb/ (accessed 4 June 2012).

World Health Organization (2012) [website]. Geneva: World Health Organization, http://www.who.int/topics/health_policy/en/ (accessed 4 June 2012).

chapter two

Tobacco

Laura Currie and Anna B. Gilmore

Introduction

Smoking is the largest single cause of death and disease in the European Union (EU), accounting for over 650,000 premature deaths annually (Peto et al. 2006). Tobacco use is estimated to have cost the economy between €98 and €130 billion, or between 1.0% and 1.4% of the EU's GDP in 2000 (ASPECT Consortium 2004). Despite widespread awareness of the harms of smoking and the proliferation of policies within EU Member States to discourage it, a third of all citizens in the EU over the age of 15 years currently smoke tobacco products (European Commission 2009). While the prevalence of current smoking across the EU and consumption levels in both western and eastern Europe have shown a decline in recent years, smoking rates remain alarmingly high and continue to rise among females in some Member States.

To curb tobacco use, governments have implemented increasingly stringent tobacco control regulations over the last two decades. Action at the national level has been reinforced and reinvigorated by the WHO's Framework Convention on Tobacco Control – a widely embraced public health treaty that obligates parties to implement a wide range of evidence-based tobacco control measures (World Health Organization 2003). In support of this implementation, the WHO has established the MPOWER policy package, highlighting priority interventions (Box 2.1).

This chapter will examine successes and failures of tobacco control policy in Europe. It starts by examining the evidence base for the MPOWER tobacco control policies. It then identifies European countries that have successfully implemented these policies and examines the extent to which policy implementation and enforcement have impacted on health outcomes in these countries. It concludes by examining some of the reasons that underlie success and failure in tobacco control policy.

Box 2.1 The MPOWER package

M: monitoring tobacco use and prevention policies
P: protecting people from tobacco smoke through comprehensive bans on smoking in public places
O: offering assistance to smokers to help them to quit tobacco use
W: warning about the dangers of tobacco use through mass media campaigns and health warnings on tobacco product packages
E: enforcing bans on tobacco advertising, promotion and sponsorship
R: raising tobacco taxes to discourage consumption.

Source: World Health Organization 2008.

Evidence for the effectiveness of tobacco control policies

Protecting people from second-hand smoke

Second-hand smoke (SHS) is made up of the smoke emitted from the burning end of a cigarette or other tobacco product, in combination with smoke exhaled by the smoker. Evidence from a range of studies accumulated over many years has shown that exposure to SHS causes death, disease and disability in adults and children (Royal College of Physicians 2005, 2010), and that exposure to smoking behaviour is a driver of uptake of smoking among young people.

Policies that make public places and workplaces smoke-free will protect workers and the general public from the harmful effects of SHS. Substantial evidence suggests that the implementation of smoke-free legislation is associated with reductions in exposure to SHS by 80–90% among those with the highest rates of prelegislation exposure, and by up to 40% in the general population (IARC 2009).

Importantly and contrary to what is often argued by the opponents of comprehensive smoke-free policies, they do not lead to increased exposure to SHS in the home (IARC 2009). The prevalence of smokers who have introduced a smoke-free policy at home has increased over time (Borland et al. 2006), and there is a downward trend in SHS exposure rates at home among children (IARC 2009). Furthermore, there is substantial evidence that smoke-free workplace policies reduce smokers' average consumption by two to four cigarettes per day, with comprehensive restrictions showing stronger association with decreased consumption than partial restrictions.

Offering smoking cessation treatment and support

Even if there were no new smokers, appreciable reductions in smoking-related mortality and morbidity would not be seen for some decades unless current smokers quit (Kulik et al. 2012). While most tobacco users who quit do so without assistance, quit rates can be improved greatly with smoking cessation interventions.

Smoking cessation interventions that have a potential for population-level impact include smoking cessation counselling or brief advice provided by health care professionals, and the availability of pharmacotherapy, quitlines and other technology-based interventions (Internet, mobile phone support). Brief advice to quit smoking from a doctor can increase the likelihood that smokers will successfully quit and stay abstinent (Stead et al. 2008a), while offering more intensive support (behavioural counselling or prescription for pharmacotherapy) can increase quit rates (Aveyard et al. 2012). The use of pharmacotherapy increases the odds of successful cessation; recent meta-analyses found average odds ratios of 1.58 with nicotine replacement therapies (Stead et al. 2008b), 1.69 for bupropion (Hughes et al. 2007) and 2.31 for varenicline (Cahill et al. 2011; Zhu et al. 2012). Use of pharmacotherapy is influenced by the extent to which health care providers recommend it, how widely it is otherwise marketed, and its cost. Smokers' quitlines provide an accessible behavioural counselling service; however, their uptake is also dependent on how effectively they are promoted.

Warning about the dangers of tobacco use

Mass media campaigns reach large numbers of people through print and broadcast media with anti-tobacco messages that discourage tobacco use. Before the widespread implementation of bans on tobacco advertising, the primary aim of mass media campaigns was to counter industry advertising and change smoking behaviour by discouraging smoking. Campaigns aimed to discourage initiation among young people and encourage smoking cessation among adults, often promoting available cessation services. More recently, campaigns also aim to change social norms and build support for other tobacco control policies.

Reviews suggest that well-funded and implemented mass media campaigns, as part of comprehensive tobacco control programmes, are associated with reductions in smoking rates among both adults and youths (Friend and Levy 2002; Bala et al. 2008; Durkin et al. 2012). Youths who are exposed to anti-tobacco mass media campaigns are less than half as likely to become established smokers (Siegel and Biener 2000), and adults are more likely to quit (Durkin et al. 2012). The intensity and duration of campaigns is important as higher exposure is associated with less smoking (Emery et al. 2012).

Tobacco product warning labels communicate the risks associated with tobacco use and reach all tobacco users (Hammond et al. 2006). The extent to which smokers understand the risks associated with their use of tobacco influences their smoking behaviour; those who perceive greater health risk from smoking are more likely to intend to quit and to quit successfully (Hammond et al. 2006).

Enforcing bans on advertising, promotion and sponsorship

While the tobacco industry claims that their advertising activities are designed to maintain or increase relative market shares of individual brands among adult consumers rather than to increase overall consumption, evidence from analysis of industry documents shows that these campaigns are targeted towards young people to attract new 'replacement' smokers (Pollay 2000; Cummings et al. 2002; Ling and Glantz 2002). Advertising and promotions have been identified as a causal determinant of tobacco consumption, and exposure to these activities increases the likelihood that adolescents will start to smoke (Lovato et al. 2011).

Comprehensive bans on tobacco advertising, promotion and sponsorship are highly effective in reducing smoking (Saffer and Chaloupka 2000; Blecher 2008), while partial bans have little or no effect as advertising shifts from mediums that are restricted to those that are not restricted (Saffer 2000; Saffer and Chaloupka 2000).

Raising tobacco prices through taxation

Governments can discourage tobacco consumption by increasing tobacco prices through taxation. A recent comprehensive review of the vast literature on the effectiveness of tobacco taxation (Chaloupka et al. 2011; IARC 2011) concluded that increasing tobacco prices through increased taxation reduces overall consumption and prevalence of tobacco use among adults and young people and has a greater impact on younger people, who are particularly price responsive. It also induces current users to quit, reduces initiation and uptake among young people, with a greater impact on the transition to regular use, and lowers tobacco use among continuing users. Recent analysis of demand for tobacco products in 11 European countries (Austria, Finland, France, Germany, Ireland, Italy, the Netherlands, Portugal, Spain, Sweden, United Kingdom) using time-series data spanning over 50 years found that, on average, a 10% increase in the real price of cigarettes reduces tobacco consumption by 3–4% (Nguyen et al. 2012). However, this same study suggested that a 10% increase in income increases consumption by 3–4%, suggesting the importance of regular tax increases that outpace inflation and growth in incomes.

Successes and failures of tobacco control policy in Europe

Tobacco control policy and population health outcomes

Success of tobacco control policy can be defined in three ways: (1) implementing (and enforcing) evidence-based tobacco control policies; (2) achieving improvements in intermediate outcomes, such as reductions in smoking prevalence (through reduced initiation and/or increased cessation), reductions in consumption of cigarettes or, in the case of smoke-free policies, reductions in exposure to SHS through the implementation of such policies; and (3) achieving improvements in distal health outcomes from both active smoking (e.g. reductions in lung cancer or smoking-related mortality and morbidity) and passive smoking (e.g. reductions in hospital admissions from heart attacks or asthma).

Measuring the success of tobacco control policies in terms of distal health outcomes is complex because the timing between the onset of smoking and development of disease, and in turn between quitting and reduction in disease risk, varies among the numerous diseases linked to tobacco use. With lung cancer, health effects are not generally apparent until 20 to 30 years after smoking becomes widespread in a population, and they do not reach their peak until 30 to 40 years after the peak in prevalence, whereas the impact on cardiovascular diseases is apparent sooner. Likewise, the reversal of risk after quitting smoking occurs more quickly for coronary heart disease than for lung cancer. This can make interpretation of trends in disease outcomes complex, particularly the interpretation of how they reflect the impact of tobacco control policies implemented in the past.

A four-stage model of the smoking epidemic has been described, based on observations of trends in cigarette consumption and tobacco-related diseases (Lopez et al. 1994). Early on, smoking prevalence among men is relatively low but increasing, while prevalence among women is very low and there is no apparent difference in patterns of mortality by smoking status. As the epidemic progresses, male smoking prevalence increases rapidly and peaks at 50–80% of the population, while the prevalence of ex-smokers is relatively low. By the end of this phase, mortality among male smokers begins to rise. Meanwhile, there are slight increases among women, but these increases lag behind those in men. In the next phase, tobacco control policies are implemented and strengthened and smoking becomes less socially acceptable. Male smoking prevalence reaches a plateau at a high level and then starts to decline, with declines faster among the most highly educated. Female rates plateau at a lower level than men, but for a more prolonged period. Higher rates of smoking are seen among younger women and declines in prevalence are faster among more educated women. In the last phase, smoking prevalence among both males and females continues to decline slowly and social differences persist. Male smoking-related mortality peaks at 30–35% of all deaths and begins to decline about ten years later, while for women smoking-related mortality peaks at around 20–25% of all deaths and begins to decline 10 to 20 years after the decline for men.

Trends in lung cancer mortality across Europe since the early 1970s mirror these patterns, although different countries are in different phases of this epidemic, and the interval between peaks in male and female smoking prevalence is shorter in some countries. An examination of lung cancer mortality data from the WHO Mortality Databank by age, sex and year of death from 1970 to 2007 for 36 countries in Europe shows that, by 2003, the highest lung cancer mortality rates were seen among men in Hungary, Poland and Estonia, with lowest rates in Sweden, Iceland and Portugal (Bray and Weiderpass 2010). For women, the highest rates were in Denmark, Iceland and Hungary and the lowest in Spain and the Ukraine (Bray and Weiderpass 2010). Lung cancer mortality rates in men have shown decline in most European countries since the early 1990s, particularly in the Nordic countries, in Britain and Ireland (United Kingdom and Eire) and in the continental region; however, overall male rates are still increasing in parts of the southern region (Portugal), the western Balkans (the former Yugoslav Republic of Macedonia), the central and eastern region (Bulgaria and Romania) and the former USSR (Republic of Moldova) (Bray and Weiderpass 2010). For women, overall lung cancer mortality rates are still increasing in most countries, although rates are beginning to stabilize in some countries in the central and eastern region (Hungary, Poland, Czech Republic), the Nordic countries and Britain and Ireland (Denmark, Iceland and the United Kingdom) (Bray and Weiderpass 2010). Lower lung cancer mortality rates seen among more recent birth cohorts may reflect recent changes in smoking habits partly attributable to policies introduced in the last two decades and suggest that a plateau may be on the horizon for some of those countries where rates are still on the rise (Bray and Weiderpass 2010).

Given the complexity of interpreting the impact of tobacco control policy implementation on distal health outcomes, such as reductions in smoking-related mortality, the focus here is largely on intermediate outcomes, notably reductions in smoking prevalence and cigarette consumption, although the impact of smoke-free policies on heart attacks is discussed in Box 2.2. First, how European countries differ in the implementation of tobacco control policies is considered, and then the impact of tobacco control on smoking prevalence and cigarette consumption is analysed.

Implementation of tobacco control in Europe

As noted above, MPOWER recommends completely smoke-free environments in all health care and educational facilities and indoor public places, including workplaces, bars and restaurants. European countries differ significantly, however, in the degree to which they have implemented this (Fig. 2.1), with Hungary, Bulgaria, the Czech Republic, Romania and Austria lagging behind most other European countries, and Ireland and the United Kingdom being the European front-runners. This figure also shows the relationship between the percentage of residents in each European country who report never (or almost never) being exposed to tobacco smoke in their workplace (European Commission 2009) and the smoke-free policy in their country (Joossens and Raw 2011). There is a positive association between protection from workplace tobacco smoke exposure and smoke-free policy scores, suggesting that citizens in countries with more comprehensive smoke-free policies tend to be more adequately protected from workplace exposure.

Large variations between countries are also found in the availability of quit-line services, free or low-cost pharmacological treatment and smoking cessation support through primary health care services, as shown by a study of the availability of measures to help dependent smokers to quit in 31 European countries. The measures were ranked according to (1) the provision of financial incentives for recording patients' smoking status in medical notes, (2) reimbursement for providing brief advice in primary care, (3) the geographical coverage of the network of cessation support, (4) the cost of accessing these services, (5) the presence of a national quitline, and (6) whether pharmacotherapy was freely available or partially reimbursed. The United Kingdom had the most comprehensive smoking cessation services in Europe, followed by Denmark, Romania, Poland and Luxembourg, while treatment in Latvia, Bulgaria, Iceland and Lithuania were ranked lowest (Joossens and Raw 2011).

MPOWER recommends highly visible and sustained anti-tobacco campaigns in the mass media (World Health Organization 2008). Monitoring of MPOWER policies in 2011 by WHO indicates that many European countries did not

Box 2.2 Smoke-free policies and distal health outcomes: myocardial infarctions

Passive smoking, or exposure to second-hand smoke, increases the risk of coronary heart disease by as much as 60% (Glantz and Parmley 1991, 1995; He et al. 1999; Thun et al. 1999; Whincup et al. 2004; Barnoya and Glantz 2005; Institute of Medicine 2010). The observed increase is higher in more recent studies that have used more accurate measures of exposure. Successfully implemented and enforced smoke-free air laws reduce population-level exposure to second-hand smoke considerably (IARC 2009). Consequently, smoke-free air laws could be expected to reduce the incidence of acute coronary events, including myocardial infarction, with almost immediate effect.

A large body of evidence supports a reduction in acute coronary events following the implementation of comprehensive smoke-free legislation (Glantz 2008; Meyers et al. 2009; Mackay et al. 2010; Sims et al. 2010; Cronin et al. 2012), with some indication that the effects increase over time (Mackay et al. 2010; Cronin et al. 2012). A recent meta-analysis of the effect of comprehensive smoke-free legislation suggests that acute coronary events fall by around 10% following the implementation of legislation (Mackay et al. 2010). While earlier studies, finding larger effects, may not have adequately controlled for other factors that might influence the incidence of acute coronary events, Sims et al. (2010) found a small but significant reduction in the number of emergency admissions for myocardial infarction following the implementation of comprehensive legislation in England, using a more robust study design accounting for potential confounders and secular trends. The smaller effect size found in this study may be partly explained by the relatively low levels of exposure resulting from the partial smoke-free restrictions in place prior to the introduction of the comprehensive law in 2007.

Even conservative estimates of the declines in hospital admissions for acute coronary syndromes following the implementation of smoke-free air laws suggest important public health implications of this intervention given the scale of the cardiovascular disease burden in the population (Sims et al. 2010).

implement even one national mass media campaign during 2009 or 2010 (defining a national mass media campaign as a communication activity lasting at least one 3-week period during a year and that utilizes television, radio, print, outdoor billboards or the Internet to inform and educate the public about tobacco control issues). Countries which did not have such a campaign included Armenia, Austria, Azerbaijan, Belarus, Belgium, Bosnia and Herzegovina, Bulgaria, Croatia, Iceland, Kyrgyzstan, Latvia, Lithuania, Montenegro, Norway, Portugal, Slovakia, Slovenia, Spain, Tajikistan, Ukraine and Uzbekistan. Only 9 of the 53 European countries implemented a mass media campaign that fully met MPOWER standards: Denmark, Greece, Ireland, the Netherlands, the Russian Federation, Serbia, Sweden, Turkey and the United Kingdom (World Health Organization 2011).

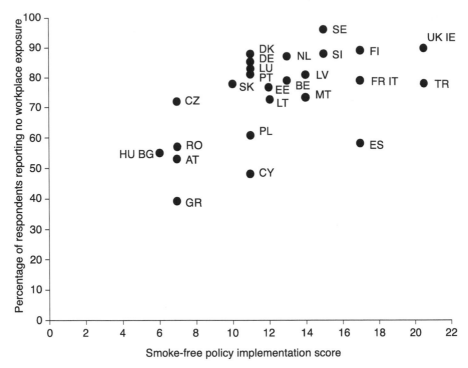

Figure 2.1   Protection from workplace tobacco smoke exposure and smoke-free policy score in 28 European countries

Sources: Self reported exposure (European Commission 2009), Smoke-free policy implementation score (Joossens and Raw 2011)
Notes: Smoke-free policies are scored from 0 to 22, according to the places covered by the legislation (workplaces; cafes, bars and restaurants; public transport; educational and health facilities) and the degree of coverage (complete ban with no smoking rooms, partial ban with allowance for smoking rooms, or meaningful restrictions). AT, Austria; BE, Belgium; BG, Bulgaria; CZ, Czech Republic; DK, Denmark; DE, Germany; EE, Estonia; IE, Ireland; GR, Greece; ES, Spain; FR, France; IT, Italy; CY, Cyprus; LV, Latvia; LT, Lithuania; LU, Luxembourg; HU, Hungary; MT, Malta; NL, Netherlands; PL, Poland; PT, Portugal; RO, Romania; SI, Slovenia; SK, Slovakia; FI, Finland; SE, Sweden; TR, Turkey; UK, the United Kingdom

MPOWER recommends legislatively mandated clear, visible health warnings covering at least half of the principal display area of tobacco product packages, with specific and rotating warnings regarding the health risks of smoking including graphic images. While all European countries require rotating health warnings on tobacco product packages with content, print and language specifications, only ten countries have implemented graphic health warnings: Belgium, France, Georgia, Latvia, Romania, Spain, Switzerland, the former Yugoslav Republic of Macedonia, Turkey and the United Kingdom (World Health Organization 2011).

MPOWER recommends comprehensive bans on tobacco advertising with sufficient penalties to deter circumvention. Most European countries have a ban on national television, radio and print media as well as on some but not all other forms of direct and indirect advertising, with moderate to high compliance (World Health Organization 2011). Notable exceptions are

Andorra, Armenia, Austria, Azerbaijan, Georgia, Monaco, the Russian Federation and Switzerland, which have failed to implement a ban that extends to at least national television, radio and print media (World Health Organization 2011).

Finally, MPOWER recommends that excise tax should constitute at least 70% of the final retail price of tobacco, that incentives for trading down to cheaper tobacco products be minimized and that tobacco tax increases exceed increases in inflation to prevent tobacco from becoming more affordable (World Health Organization 2008). Figure 2.2 shows the weighted average retail sales price for a pack of 20 cigarettes and the tax as a percentage of this price across the EU. Few countries have reached the MPOWER target and the weighted average retail price for a pack of cigarettes varies from as low as €2.14 in Lithuania to as high as €8.50 in Ireland (as of March 2011).

The ratification of the Framework Convention on Tobacco Control by almost all European countries (notable exceptions being Andorra, the Czech Republic, Monaco and Switzerland) has brought some degree of convergence of tobacco control policies across the EU (Studlar et al. 2011). However, as noted above, there is still considerable variation between European countries in the implementation of policies. A study by Joossens and Raw (2006) quantified the implementation of the six key tobacco control policies at country level using a comprehensive Tobacco Control Scale (TCS), which ranked 30 countries by their total score on a 100-point scale. Policies included are cigarette prices (maximum of 30 points), smoke-free workplaces and public places including

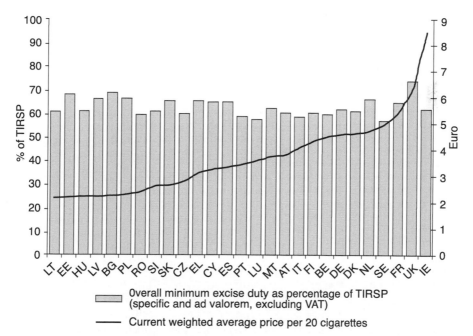

Overall minimum excise duty as percentage of TIRSP (specific and ad valorem, excluding VAT)

Current weighted average price per 20 cigarettes

Figure 2.2 Overall excise duty as a percentage of total price and current weighted average price for 20 cigarettes in the European Union

Source: Joossens and Raw 2011

Notes: TIRSP, tax inclusive retail sales price; see Fig. 2.1 for country abbreviations bars and restaurants and public transport (22), spending on public information campaigns (15), comprehensive bans on advertising and promotion (13), large direct health warning labels (10) and cessation treatment including the operation of a national quitline and reimbursement of pharmaceutical treatment products (10).

In 2005, only four countries scored 70 or more (Ireland, United Kingdom, Norway and Iceland); two countries scored above 60 (Malta and Sweden); seven scored above 50 (Finland, Italy, France, the Netherlands, Cyprus, Poland and Belgium), and the rest scored 49 or below (Joossens and Raw 2006). By 2007, the average score on the scale increased by 5%, suggesting some improvement in the implementation of measures across the region. States in the central and eastern region and the former USSR continued to be well represented among the countries scoring lowest on this scale in 2007. When repeated in 2010, the United Kingdom, Ireland and Norway were among the leaders, while the Czech Republic, Luxembourg, Austria and Greece were among the laggards. Slovenia has made good progress, rising in the rankings, but Bulgaria has fallen. Country rankings and the contribution of each policy to the overall score are shown in Fig. 2.3 (Joossens and Raw 2011).

Impact of tobacco control on smoking

Martínez-Sánchez et al. (2010) examined the correlation between implementation of tobacco control policies as measured by the TCS in 2007 and smoking prevalence from the Eurobarometer survey in 2008 in the countries belonging to the EU after January 2007 (EU27). They found that high TCS scores, reflecting more tobacco control policies having been implemented, were significantly associated with a lower population prevalence of smokers; however, while there was also an association with self-reported exposure to SHS at home and at work, it fell short of statistical significance. Using a sample of almost 60,000 non-smokers from across the EU27 in 2006–2007, Tual et al. (2010) examined the relationship between tobacco control policy implementation and SHS exposure using exhaled carbon monoxide – a more objective measure of exposure to tobacco smoke than the self-reported data used by Martínez-Sánchez et al. (2010) – adjusting for age, gender and survey setting. They found that the concentration of exhaled carbon monoxide decreased with the strength of tobacco control policies implemented, indicating that countries with a higher degree of tobacco control policy implementation as measured by the TCS have lower exposure to SHS.

The impact of policies on smoking prevalence acts through reducing initiation among young people and increasing cessation among adults. Hublet et al. (2009) examined the association between the implementation of four tobacco control policies (tobacco price, smoke-free air laws, bans on advertising, and youth access restrictions including bans on vending machine sales) using policy-specific subscales of the TCS and self-reported smoking prevalence among 15 year olds, using data from the WHO Health Behaviour in School-aged Children survey undertaken in 29 European countries. They found that higher real prices were associated with less regular smoking in

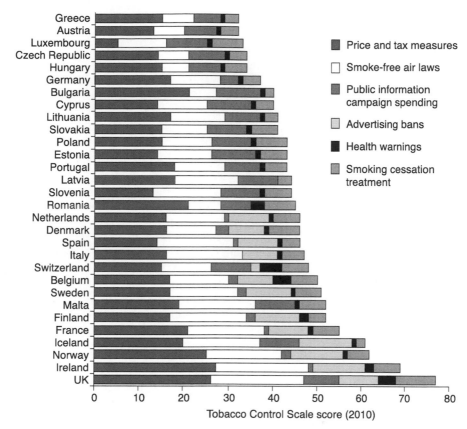

Figure 2.3 Tobacco Control Scale scores for 31 European countries, 2010

Source: Created from data of Joossens and Raw (2011)
Note: Countries missing data on public information campaign spending and given a 0 score in this domain include Turkey, Malta, Italy, Romania, Slovenia, Latvia, Portugal, Estonia, Poland, Slovakia, Lithuania, Cyprus, Bulgaria, Germany, Hungary, Czech Republic, Luxembourg, Austria and Greece

boys but not girls, and that a restrictive policy on vending machine sales is significantly associated with less smoking in boys and girls, although reaching only borderline significance among girls. A statistically significant association was not found between the other policies examined and smoking among young people in this study. Schaap et al. (2008) examined the impact of policies on smoking cessation by age and education level using cross-sectional data from national health surveys. They found a positive association between TCS scores and quit ratios in all age groups, but consistent differences by education group were not seen. These findings suggest that countries with more developed tobacco control policies have higher quit ratios than countries with less developed tobacco control policies.

Gallus et al. (2012) examined the association between TCS score in 2010, which by then incorporated measures of policy enforcement, and the prevalence of current smokers and former smokers and the ratios of male-to-female smoking prevalence and current-to-former-smoking prevalence. The analysis used comparable primary data from the Pricing Policies and Control of Tobacco in Europe (PPACTE) survey conducted in the same year in 16 European countries. They found that implementation of tobacco control policy was inversely related to the male-to-female and current-to-former-smoking prevalence ratios. The TCS score was also directly related to the prevalence of former smokers and inversely associated with smoking prevalence, although the latter was not statistically significant. These findings indicate that countries that have been more successful in implementing tobacco control policies may have moved further along in the tobacco epidemic, with a higher prevalence of former smokers and higher proportions of female and former smokers relative to male smokers and current smokers.

While these studies generally suggest that greater implementation of tobacco control policies is associated with lower smoking prevalence, lower SHS exposure and a higher proportion of former smokers, the studies all examine policy and outcomes in a cross-sectional manner, precluding causal attribution. It may be that countries that are further along in the tobacco epidemic and, therefore, have a higher proportion of former smokers are more likely to have populations supporting the implementation of tobacco control policies.

The TCS has been expanded to measure policy implementation between 1970 and 2010 in 11 European countries. It used published scores for 2005 and 2007 as a reference and consulted various sources for the following four non-price tobacco control policies: smoke-free air laws, bans on tobacco advertising, health warnings and smoking cessation treatment. Nguyen et al. (2012) used this index, along with separate variables for price and income, in analyses of demand for cigarettes in the 11 European countries. Overall, they found the expected negative relationship between the TCS index and cigarette consumption, with estimates suggesting that each 10% increase in the TCS score would reduce cigarette consumption by 2–3%. The same models provide estimates for price, suggesting that a 10% increase in price would reduce consumption of cigarettes by 3–4%.

Discussion and conclusions

Why have some countries been more successful at implementing tobacco control policies than others?

Successes have been achieved in tobacco control across Europe and worldwide despite tobacco industry attempts to prevent, impede and undermine policy. Interference in policy-making by the tobacco industry is well documented in a now large body of literature analysing previously confidential tobacco company documents (IARC 2011). Transnational tobacco companies have attempted to prevent or dilute proposed regulations by means of traditional lobbying of government decision-makers, creation of front organizations to present industry arguments, mounting legal challenges against proposed (or enacted) legislation, commissioning research designed to mislead and sow confusion, employing consultants or public relations firms to lobby on their behalf, and proposing weaker legislation or voluntary agreements (Clifford et al. 2011, 2012; IARC 2011; Shirane et al. 2011; Skafida et al. 2011). As an example, Box 2.3 summarizes industry efforts to influence and undermine policy on tobacco excise, drawing on recent case studies in the Czech Republic, a country with one of the weakest tobacco control records in the EU (Shirane et al. 2011); Bulgaria, a country whose tobacco control policy ranking fell from bad to worse (Skafida et al. 2011); Poland, an early leader in tobacco control among EU accession states that has since lost momentum (Clifford et al. 2011); and France, a country where large excise increases were achieved despite strong links between industry and state (Clifford et al. 2012).

It is impossible to discuss tobacco control without considering corruption. Across Europe, smoking prevalence tends to be higher in countries with higher levels of corruption (Bogdanovica et al. 2011). Corruption can influence whether tobacco control policies are implemented and observed, and it can undermine the effectiveness of policies in a number of ways. First, tobacco companies are likely to secure greater influence on policy where there is greater corruption in the public sector. Second, corruption may influence compliance with and enforcement of enacted legislation (Bogdanovica et al. 2011). Third, the illicit tobacco trade thrives in countries with higher corruption (Chaloupka et al. 2012) and where law enforcement is undermined (Gounev and Bezlov 2010).

Despite Article 5.3 of the WHO Framework Convention on Tobacco Control, which requires signatories to protect health policy-making from 'commercial or other vested interests of the tobacco industry', recent case studies of industry influence on tobacco excise policy suggest that government officials continue to engage with the tobacco industry, as discussed in Box 2.3. Tobacco control policies, and, therefore, public health suffer when policy-makers maintain connections with the transnational tobacco companies as this provides a direct avenue for policy influence.

The extent to which tobacco industry lobbying exerts influence on policy-making processes depends on the extent to which policy-makers are receptive to their lobbying tactics and, in turn, the extent to which politicians perceive the tobacco industry to be a legitimate stakeholder and/or an economically important industry. Civil society engagement plays a key role in both exposing industry tactics and lobbying for political support. The 'vital importance' of civil society organizations in advocating for tobacco control policies nationally and internationally is acknowledged by the WHO Framework Convention on Tobacco Control Guiding Principle No. 7, which states 'The participation of civil society is essential in achieving the objective of the Convention and its protocols' (World Health Organization 2003). Civil society organizations contribute to successful policy implementation and enforcement by distributing and translating research findings, generating supportive media coverage, lobbying governments directly, exposing industry influences and framing the debates surrounding tobacco control policies. Coalitions of civil society organizations also demonstrate significant support through the breadth of interest groups represented.

Box 2.3 Tobacco industry influence on tobacco excise policy

Tobacco taxation threatens the long-term profitability of the tobacco industry; consequently, transnational tobacco companies have an interest in influencing both excise levels and taxation structures (Shirane et al. 2012). Excise levels affect the retail price that consumers pay and thus the quantities they consume, with implications for sales volumes. The choice of excise regime, whether it is predominately specific (a fixed amount per quantity), *ad valorem* (a proportion of some measure of value such as a weighted average price) or a mixture of both, has implications for the competitiveness of tobacco companies, depending on the market structure and the company brand portfolio (Shirane et al. 2012).

Recent case studies suggest that the transnational tobacco companies have continuously and often successfully sought to influence tobacco excise policy. Philip Morris/Philip Morris International and British American Tobacco lobbied separately on excise structure – each seeking to obtain a structure that advantaged its brand portfolio at the expense of its competitors – and lobbied collaboratively on excise levels in attempts to prevent significant tax increases (Shirane et al. 2012). The companies lobbied indirectly, developing local capacity and forming a National Tobacco Manufacturers Association in Poland (Clifford et al. 2011), establishing the Central Europe Tax Task Force, and working with tobacconists in France (Clifford et al. 2012). They also lobbied directly, establishing relationships with politicians and relevant government ministries, particularly those for finance and trade, offering technical excise expertise and donating money to the Polish Senate (Clifford et al. 2011) and the main political parties in the Czech Republic (Shirane et al. 2011). In Poland and France, senior politicians and officials had close ties with or were previously employed by the tobacco industry (Clifford et al. 2011, 2012).

Transnational tobacco companies secured influence over tax policy in all four countries. Philip Morris/Philip Morris International and British American Tobacco both successfully influenced tax structures in the Czech Republic and Bulgaria but had less success in France. As previously documented in Hungary (Szilagyi and Chapman 2003), the transnational tobacco companies prevented considerable tobacco tax increases in the countries acceding to the EU in 2004 by ensuring lengthy derogations to the requirement to meet minimum tax levels required by EU Directives (Clifford et al. 2011; Shirane et al. 2011; Skafida et al. 2011). Furthermore, the tobacco industry took advantage of low increases in excise duties to increase their own prices and, therefore, profit at the expense of potential government revenue (Clifford et al. 2011, 2012).

In these ways, the tobacco industry undermines existing tobacco excise policy by ensuring a supply of cheaper products, through pricing strategy, product innovation, exploitation of loopholes in excise policy and involvement in illicit trade.

Conclusions

While the causal links between smoking and morbidity and mortality were established in the 1950s, few countries introduced policies to discourage tobacco smoking for another two decades, thereby allowing smoking rates and associated health consequences to reach epidemic levels. Over the last half century, we have seen a shift from a situation where governments promote tobacco growth and production in the interest of their economies to one of increasingly stringent regulation of tobacco use in the interest of public health. Once considered a legitimate economic entity, the tobacco industry is now more widely perceived as a vector of disease. The widespread implementation of smoke-free policies and voluntary home smoking bans shows that the social acceptability of smoking is decreasing, although to a varying degree across countries. An increasing number of European countries have achieved substantial reductions in rates of tobacco use and will ultimately achieve similar reductions in morbidity and mortality. These successes owe much to the development and implementation of comprehensive national tobacco control strategies.

However, there is still considerable scope to strengthen implementation and enforcement of evidence-based policies fully consistent with the MPOWER recommendations and the Framework Convention for Tobacco Control. Smoking prevalence across the WHO European Region is declining; with full implementation of MPOWER policies this decline could be accelerated (Mendez et al. 2012). Yet, even with full and immediate implementation of all MPOWER policies across the WHO European Region, modelling suggests that it will not be possible to achieve rates of tobacco use across the region of below 10% within a 20-year time horizon (Mendez et al. 2012). While immediate implementation of existing policies has considerable potential to reduce the tobacco disease burden, it is now time to consider new and innovative approaches to regulating supply as a means of reducing demand for tobacco products.

References

ASPECT Consortium (2004) Tobacco or Health in the European Union: past, present and future. Luxembourg: European Commission.

Aveyard, P., Begh, R., Parsons, A. and West, R. (2012) Brief opportunistic smoking cessation interventions: a systematic review and meta-analysis to compare advice to quit and offer of assistance, *Addiction*, 107(6):1066–73.

Bala, M., Strzeszynski, L. and Cahill, K. (2008) Mass media interventions for smoking cessation in adults, *Cochrane Database of Systematic Reviews*, (1):CD004704.

Barnoya, J. and Glantz, S.A. (2005) Cardiovascular effects of secondhand smoke: nearly as large as smoking, *Circulation*, 111:2684–98.

Blecher, E. (2008) The impact of tobacco advertising bans on consumption in developing countries, *Journal of Health Economics*, 27(4):930–42.

Bogdanovica, I., McNeill, A., Murray, R. and Britton, J. (2011) What factors influence smoking prevalence and smoke free policy enactment across the European Union Member States, *PLoS One*, 6(8):e23889.

Borland, R., Yong, H.-H., Cummings, K.M. et al. (2006) Determinants and consequences of smoke-free homes: findings from the International Tobacco Control (ITC) Four Country Survey. *Tobacco Control*, 15(suppl 3):iii42–iii50.

Bray, F.I. and Weiderpass, E. (2010) Lung cancer mortality trends in 36 European countries: secular trends and birth cohort patterns by sex and region 1970–2007, *International Journal of Cancer*, 126(6):1454–66.

Cahill, K., Stead, L.F. and Lancaster, T. (2011) Nicotine receptor partial agonists for smoking cessation, *Cochrane Database of Systematic Reviews*, (2):CD006103.

Chaloupka, F., Leon, M., Straif, K. et al. (2011) Effectiveness of tax and price policies in tobacco control, *Tobacco Control*, 20:235–8.

Chaloupka, F.J., Yurekli, A. and Fong, G.T. (2012) Tobacco taxes as a tobacco control strategy, *Tobacco Control*, 21(2):172–80.

Clifford, D., Silver, K.E. Ciecierski, C. and Gilmore, A. (2011) Our materials will be the basis for the official Polish position during negotiations: tobacco industry influence on Poland's tobacco excise policy and their EU accession negotiations. A Pricing Policy and Control of Tobacco in Europe (PPACTE) Project output. Bath: University of Bath.

Clifford, D., Ratte, S., Silver, K.E., Skafida, V. and Gilmore, A.B. (2012) A dying trade? The impact of a series of major tax increases in France and the tobacco industry's reponse. A Pricing Policy and Control of Tobacco in Europe (PPACTE) Project output. Bath: University of Bath.

Cronin, E.M., Kearney, P.M. and Kearney, P.P. for the Coronary Heart Attack Ireland Registry (CHAIR) Working Group (2012) Impact of a national smoking ban on hospital admission for acute coronary syndromes: a longitudinal study, *Clinical Cardiology*, 35(4):205–9.

Cummings, K.M., Morley, C.P., Horan, J.K., Steger, C. and Leavell, N.R. (2002) Marketing to America's youth: evidence from corporate documents. *Tobacco Control*, 11(suppl 1):15–17.

Durkin, S., Brennan, E. and Wakefield, M. (2012) Mass media campaigns to promote smoking cessation among adults: an integrative review, *Tobacco Control*, 21(2):127–38.

Emery, S., Kim, Y., Choi, Y.K. et al. (2012) The effects of smoking-related television advertising on smoking and intentions to quit among adults in the United States: 1999–2007, *American Journal of Public Health*, 102(4):751–7.

European Commission (2009) *Special Eurobarometer 332/Wave 72.3: Tobacco*. Brussels: TNS Opinion & Social for the Directorate of General Health and Consumers.

Friend, K. and Levy, D.T. (2002) Reductions in smoking prevalence and cigarette consumption associated with mass-media campaigns, *Health Education Research*, 17(1):85–98.

Gallus, S., Lugo, A., La Vecchia, C. et al. (2012) *Pricing Policies and Control of Tobacco in Europe (PPACTE) WP2: European Survey on Smoking*. Dublin: PPACTE Consortium.

Glantz, S.A. (2008) Meta-analysis of the effects of smokefree laws on acute myocardial infarction: an update, *Preventive Medicine*, 47(4):452–3.

Glantz, S.A. and Parmley, W.W. (1991) Passive smoking and heart disease: epidemiology, physiology and biochemistry, *Circulation*, 1991(83):1–12.

Glantz, S.A. and Parmley, W.W. (1995) Passive smoking and heart disease: mechanisms and risk, *Journal of the American Medical Association*, 273:1047–53.

Gounev, P. and Bezlov, T. (2010) *Examining the Links Between Organized Crime and Corruption*. Brussels: Centre for the Study of Democracy for the European Commission Directorate of General Justice, Freedom and Security.

Hammond, D., Fong, G.T., McDonald, P.W., Cameron, R. and Brown, K.S. (2006) Effectiveness of cigarette warning labels in informing smokers about the risks of smoking: findings from the International Tobacco Control (ITC) Four Country Survey, *Tobacco Control*, 15(suppl III):iii19–iii25.

He, J., Vupputuri, S., Allen, K. et al. (1999) Passive smoking and the risk of coronary heart disease: a meta-analysis of epidemiologic studies, *New England Journal of Medicine*, 340:920–6.

Hublet, A., Schmid, H., Clays, E. et al. (2009) Association between tobacco control policies and smoking behaviour among adolescents in 29 European countries, *Addiction*, 104(11):1918–26.

Hughes, J.R., Stead, L.F. and Lancaster, T. (2007) Antidepressants for smoking cessation, *Cochrane Database of Systematic Reviews*, (1):CD000031.

IARC (2009) *IARC Handbooks of Cancer Prevention, Tobacco Control*, Vol. 13: *Evaluating the Effectiveness of Smoke-free Policies*. Lyon, France: International Agency for Research on Cancer.

IARC (2011) *IARC Handbooks of Cancer Prevention, Tobacco Control*, Vol. 14: *Effectiveness of Tax and Price Policies in Tobacco Control*. Lyon, France: International Agency for Research on Cancer.

Institute of Medicine (2010) *Secondhand Smoke Exposure and Cardiovascular Risk: Making Sense of the Evidence*. Washington, DC: National Academies Press.

Joossens, L. and Raw, M. (2006) The Tobacco Control Scale: a new scale to measure country activity, *Tobacco Control*, 15(3):247–53.

Joossens, L. and Raw, M. (2011) *The Tobacco Control Scale 2010 in Europe*. Brussels: Association of European Cancer Leagues.

Kulik, M.C., Nusselder, W.J., Boshuizen, H.C. et al. (2012) Comparison of tobacco control scenarios: quantifying estimates of long-term health impact using the DYNAMO-HIA modeling tool, *PLoS One*, 7(2):e32363.

Ling, P.M. and Glantz, S. (2002) Why and how the tobacco industry sells cigarettes to youth: evidence from industry documents, *American Journal of Public Health*, 92:908–16.

Lopez, A.D., Collishaw, N. and Piha, T. (1994) A descriptive model of the cigarette epidemic in developed countries. *Tobacco Control*, 3:242–7.

Lovato, C., Watts, A. and Stead, L.F. (2011) Impact of tobacco advertising and promotion on increasing adolescent smoking behaviours, *Cochrane Database of Systematic Reviews*, (2):CD003439.

Mackay, D.F., Irfan, M.O., Haw, S. and Pell, J.P. (2010) Meta-analysis of the effect of comprehensive smoke-free legislation on acute coronary events, *Heart*, 96(19):1525–30.

Martínez-Sánchez, J.M., Fernández, E., Fu, M. et al. (2010) Smoking behaviour, involuntary smoking, attitudes towards smoke-free legislation, and tobacco control activities in the European Union, *PLoS One*, 5(11):e13881.

Mendez, D., Alshanqeety, O. and Warner, K.E. (2012) The potential impact of smoking control policies on future global smoking trends. *Tobacco Control*, Epub ahead of print (PMID:22535364).

Meyers, D.G., Neuberger, J.S. and He, J. (2009) Cardiovascular effect of bans on smoking in public places: a systematic review and meta-analysis, *Journal of the American College of Cardiology*, 54(14):1249–55.

Nguyen, L., Rosenqvist, G. and Pekurinen, M. (2012) *Demand for Tobacco in Europe: An Econometric Analysis of 11 Countries for the PPACTE Project*. [Report 6/2012:172.] Helsinki: National Institute for Health and Welfare.

Peto, R., Lopez, A.D., Boreham, J. and Thun, M. (2006) Mortality from smoking in developed countries 1950–2000, 2nd edn. Oxford: Oxford University Press.

Pollay, R.W. (2000) Targeting youth and concerned smokers: evidence from Canadian tobacco industry documents. *Tobacco Control*, 9:136–47.

Royal College of Physicians (2005) *Going Smoke-free: The Medical Case for Clean Air in the Home, at Work and in Other Public Places*. London: Royal College of Physicians.

Royal College of Physicians (2010) *Passive Smoking and Children: A Report of the Tobacco Advisory Group of the Royal College of Physicians*. London: Royal College of Physicians.

Saffer, H. (2000) Tobacco advertising and promotion, in P. Jha and F.J. Chaloupka (eds) *Tobacco Control in Developing Countries*, Ch. 9. New York: Oxford University Press on behalf of WHO and the World Bank.

Saffer, H. and Chaloupka, F. (2000) The effect of tobacco advertising bans on tobacco consumption, *Journal of Health Economics*, 19(6):1117–37.

Schaap, M.M., Kunst, A.E., Leinsalu, M. et al. (2008) Effect of nationwide tobacco control policies on smoking cessation in high and low educated groups in 18 European countries, *Tobacco Control*, 17(4):248–55.

Shirane, R., Smith, K., Ross, H. et al. (2011) *Tobacco Industry Influence in the Czech Republic: Manipulating Tobacco Excise Tax and Tobacco Control Policies in Times of Major Political Change. A Pricing Policy and Control of Tobacco in Europe (PPACTE) Project Output.* Bath: University of Bath.

Shirane, R., Skafida, V., Clifford, D. et al. (2012) *Pricing Policy and Control of Tobacco in Europe: Industry and Market Response Synthesis Report. A Pricing Policy and Control of Tobacco in Europe (PPACTE) Project Output.* Bath: University of Bath.

Siegel, M. and Biener, L. (2000) The impact of an antismoking media campaign on progression to established smoking: results of a longitudinal youth study, *American Journal of Public Health*, 90:380–6.

Sims, M., Maxwell, R., Bauld, L. and Gilmore, A. (2010) Short term impact of smoke-free legislation in England: retrospective analysis of hospital admissions for myocardial infarction, *British Medical Journal*, 340:c2161.

Skafida, V., Silver, K.E., Rechel, B. and Gilmore, A. (2011) *Bulgarian Tobacco and Trans-national Tobacco Company Influence On Tobacco Excise Policy: A Story of Lobbying, Smuggling and Failed Privatisations. A Pricing Policy and Control of Tobacco in Europe (PPACTE) Project Output.* Bath: University of Bath.

Stead, L.F., Bergson, G. and Lancaster, T. (2008a) Physician advice for smoking cessation, *Cochrane Database of Systematic Reviews*, (2):CD000165.

Stead, L.F., Perera, R., Bullen, C., Mant, D. and Lancaster, T. (2008b) Nicotine replacement therapy for smoking cessation, *Cochrane Database of Systematic Reviews*, (1):CD000146.

Studlar, D.T., Christensen, K. and Sitasari, A. (2011) Tobacco control in the EU-15: the role of member states and the European Union, *Journal of European Public Policy*, 18(5):728–45.

Szilagyi, T. and Chapman, S. (2003) Tobacco industry efforts to keep cigarettes affordable: a case study from Hungary. *Central European Journal of Public Health*, 11(4):223–8.

Thun, M., Henley, J. and Apicella, L. (1999) Epidemiological studies of fatal and non-fatal cardiovascular disease and ETS exposure from spousal smoking. *Environmental Health Perspectives*, 107:841–6.

Tual, S., Piau, J.P., Jarvis, M.J., Dautzenberg, B. and Annesi-Maesano, I. (2010) Impact of tobacco control policies on exhaled carbon monoxide in non-smokers, *Journal of Epidemiology and Community Health*, 64:554–6.

Whincup, P.H., Gilg, J.A., Emberson, J.R. et al. (2004) Passive smoking and risk of coronary heart disease and stroke: prospective study with cotinine measurement, *British Medical Journal*, 329:200–5.

WHO Regional Office for Europe (2012) *European Health for All Database (HFA-DB).* Copenhagen: WHO Regional Office for Europe, http://data.euro.who.int/hfadb/ (accessed 4 June 2012).

World Health Organization (2003) *WHO Framework Convention on Tobacco Control.* Geneva: World Health Organization.

World Health Organization (2008) *MPOWER: A Policy Package to Reverse The Tobacco Epidemic.* Geneva: World Health Organization.

World Health Organization (2011) *WHO Report on the Global Tobacco Epidemic 2011: Warning about the Dangers of Tobacco.* Geneva: World Health Organization.

Zhu, S.H., Lee, M., Zhuang, Y.L. and Gamst, A. (2012) Interventions to increase smoking cessation at the population level: how much progress has been made in the last two decades? Tobacco Control, 21: 110–118.

chapter **three**

Alcohol

Peter Anderson

Introduction

There are many reasons for having policies and programmes to reduce the harm done by alcohol. Alcohol itself, as well as heavy drinking and the state of being dependent on alcohol, causes enormous damage to the health, well-being and personal security of individuals, families and communities. This damage can be summarized through alcohol's impact on mortality or through its impact on disability-adjusted life-years (DALYs), a summary measure used by the WHO that captures both impairment resulting from ill health and premature death. Taking the population aged 15–59 years, often core productive years, alcohol is the world's number one risk factor for DALYs, far more important than unsafe sex, tobacco use or diabetes (World Health Organization 2011). In the EU, among people aged 15–64 years, 1 in 7 of all male deaths and 1 in 12 of all female deaths are caused by alcohol (Shield et al. 2012).

Both the volume of lifetime alcohol use and a combination of frequency of drinking and amount drunk per drinking occasion increase the risk of alcohol-related harm, largely in a dose-dependent manner (Anderson 2012). Alcohol affects personal security, individual health, educational attainment, jobs and income; it also has a cost to society and contributes to health inequalities (Box 3.1). At any given level of alcohol consumption, poorer people can be as much as three or four times as likely to die from an alcohol-related condition as richer people (Rehm et al. 2009a). Within the EU, at least one-quarter of the difference in life expectancy between newer and older Member States is linked to alcohol (Zatonski 2008). Moreover, given the persistence of the current economic crisis, it should be noted that economic downturns also increase alcohol-related deaths. In the EU, countries experiencing an increase of more than 3% in unemployment have experienced as much as a 28% increase in deaths from alcohol use disorders (Stuckler et al. 2009a).

The main goal of alcohol policy is to promote public health and social well-being. Alcohol policy addresses market failures by deterring children from using

Box 3.1 The impact of alcohol

Personal security. Alcohol is an intoxicant affecting a wide range of structures and processes in the central nervous system and a causal factor for intentional and unintentional injuries and harm to people other than the drinker, including interpersonal violence, suicide, homicide, crime and drink driving fatalities (Anderson et al. 2009). It is also a causal factor for risky sexual behaviour, spread of sexually transmitted diseases and human immunodeficiency virus (HIV) infection (Rehm et al. 2009a).

Individual health. Alcohol is a dependence-producing drug, similar to other substances under international control (World Health Organization 2004). It is an immunosuppressant, increasing the risk of communicable diseases, including tuberculosis, community-acquired pneumonia, and the acquired immunodeficiency syndrome (AIDS) (Rehm et al. 2010). Alcoholic beverages and the ethanol within them are classified as a carcinogen by the International Agency for Research on Cancer, increasing the risk of cancers of the oral cavity and pharynx, oesophagus, stomach, colon, rectum and breast in a linear dose–response relationship (IARC 2010). Alcohol use is, overall, detrimental to cardiovascular health (Anderson 2012). Although light to moderate drinking has a protective effect against ischaemic heart disease, this only becomes relevant in those at appreciable risk of this disorder (Roerecke and Rehm 2010). Episodic heavy drinking, by comparison, significantly increases the risk of sudden cardiac death (Britton and McKee 2000), acting through acute physiological mechanisms (McKee and Britton 1998) and probably through direct damage to the myocardium (Leon et al. 2010). The absolute risk of dying from an adverse alcohol-related condition increases linearly with the amount of alcohol consumed over a lifetime, with no safe level (National Health and Medical Research Council 2009).

Educational attainment. There is evidence that drinking can impair educational attainment (Lye and Hirschberg 2010). Carrell et al. (2011) exploited the discontinuity in drinking at age 21 years at the United States Air Force Academy, in which the minimum legal drinking age of 21 years is strictly enforced. They found that drinking caused significant reductions in academic performance, particularly for the highest-performing students.

Jobs and income. Heavy drinking increases the risk of unemployment, sickness absenteeism and sickness while present at work (Anderson et al. 2012). The workplace itself can lead to alcohol-related harm through structural factors, such as stress and high effort/low reward work (Anderson et al. 2012). Wide socioeconomic differences in alcohol-related mortality are well documented (Zatonski 2008). Socioeconomic variables act on the collective as well as the individual level (Blomgren et al. 2004), with evidence that social networks influence the drinking behaviour of the individual (Rosenquist et al. 2010).

Societal cost burden. A number of studies across the world have estimated the social cost of alcohol, concluding that the economic costs from alcohol's impact on health, well-being and productivity reaches some US$ 300–400 purchasing power parity per head of population in any one year (Rehm et al. 2009b). Well over one-half to two-thirds of all of these costs are from lost productivity (Anderson and Baumberg 2010).

Health inequalities. There are enormous differences in life expectancy between different parts of Europe, and this has been most comprehensively studied in the EU, where about 25% of the difference in life expectancy between western and eastern Europe for men aged 20–64 years in 2002 is attributed to alcohol, largely as a result of differences in heavy episodic drinking patterns and deaths from cardiovascular diseases and injuries (Zatonski 2008).

alcohol (Anderson 2012), protecting people other than drinkers from the harm done by alcohol (Laslett et al. 2010), counteracting alcohol's power to cheat the brain into feeling reward rather than seeing harms (Anderson et al. 2009) and providing all consumers with information about the effects of alcohol. Given growing commitments to tackling health inequalities (European Parliament 2011), the reduction of inequalities in alcohol-related ill health becomes an additional policy goal. The concept of stewardship emphasizes the obligation of states to provide conditions that allow people to be healthy and, in particular, to take measures to reduce health inequalities (Nuffield Council on Bioethics 2007).

This chapter will provide an overview of evidence-based policies that reduce alcohol-related harm. It will then describe the extent to which different European countries vary in the successfulness of their alcohol policies, and finally consider some of the social, institutional and other determinants of successes and failures of alcohol policy.

Effectiveness of alcohol policies

The evidence base

Alcohol's harm is preventable, as shown by the extensive evidence on effective alcohol policies (Anderson et al. 2009, 2012; WHO Regional Office for Europe 2009; Babor 2010). Table 3.1 summarizes this evidence for the three WHO European subregions (WHO Regional Office for Europe 2009). The table shows that tax increases (of 20% or even 50%) represent the most cost-effective response. In some countries, the effect of alcohol tax increases may be mitigated by illegal production, tax evasion and illegal trading, which accounts for nearly 30% of all consumption globally, just under 50% in low-income countries, and just over 10% in high-income countries. Reducing this unrecorded consumption (by 20–50%) via concerted tax enforcement strategies by law enforcement and excise officers can add to the effect. Specific intervention strategies need not, and indeed do not, get implemented in isolation but should be combined to

Table 3.1 Costs, impact and cost-effectiveness of different alcohol policy options in Europe

Target area specific intervention(s)	Coverage (%)	WHO subregion (exemplar countries)								
		Eur-A (e.g. Spain, Sweden)			Eur-B (e.g. Bulgaria, Poland)			Eur-C (e.g. Russian Federation, Ukraine)		
		Annual cost[a]	Annual effect[b]	Cost-effectiveness ratio[c]	Annual cost[a]	Annual effect[b]	Cost-effectiveness ratio[c]	Annual cost[a]	Annual effect[b]	Cost-effectiveness ratio[c]
School-based education	80	0.84	–	N/A	0.70	–	N/A	0.34	–	N/A
Mass media campaign	80	0.83	–	N/A	0.95	–	N/A	0.79	–	N/A
Brief interventions for heavy drinkers	30	4.20	672	6256	0.77	365	2100	1.78	667	2671
Drink-driving legislation and enforcement (via random breath-testing campaigns)	80	0.77	204	3762	0.74	160	4625	0.72	917	781
Reduced access to retail outlets	80	0.78	316	2475	0.56	414	1360	0.47	828	567
Comprehensive advertising ban	95	0.78	351	2226	0.56	224	2509	0.47	488	961
Increased excise taxation (by 20%)	95	1.09	2301	472	0.92	726	1272	0.67	1759	380
Increased excise taxation (by 50%)	95	1.09	2692	404	0.92	852	1083	0.67	1995	335
Tax enforcement (20% less unrecorded)	95	1.94	2069	939	1.26	706	1780	0.87	1741	498
Tax enforcement (50% less unrecorded)	95	2.21	2137	1034	1.34	790	1692	0.93	1934	480

Source: WHO Regional Office Europe 2012

Notes: N/A, not applicable because there is no effect (the cost-effectiveness ratio would, therefore, approach infinity)

[a]Implementation cost in 2005 international dollars (millions) per million persons

[b]Effect as disability-adjusted life-years (DALYs) saved effect per million persons

[c]Cost-effectiveness expressed in terms of international dollars per DALY saved

maximize possible health gains up to the point where it remains affordable to do so. The optimal mix of interventions at different spending limits will depend on the relative cost and cost-effectiveness of the individual components, as well as the synergies that exist between them.

Best buys for alcohol policy

The three best buys for alcohol policy are price increase, limits on availability and bans on advertising (World Health Organization and World Economic Forum 2011).

When alcohol becomes cheaper, more is consumed and more harm ensues (Wagenaar et al. 2010; Österberg 2012). When it is more expensive, less is consumed and less harm result. Heavy drinkers and people dependent on alcohol also drink less when the price goes up (Österberg 2012). However, managing the price of alcohol can be a little complicated, for a number of reasons.

- It is the affordability of alcohol compared with other goods that matters (Rabinovich et al. 2009a,b). So, if the price of alcohol stays the same, but incomes go up, alcohol consumption goes up. Specific or targeted taxes do not work. This is the case, for example, with the German alcopop tax, which, because of its specificity, simply switched consumption of sprits-based mixed beverages to beer-based mixed beverages (Anderson 2012).
- If the price of legal alcohol goes up, then more people will brew or distil their own alcohol, or try to get hold of illegal alcohol. This is clearly important for many parts of the world, including the former USSR (including the Baltic states (Lang et al. 2006; Parna et al. 2007)) and is causing increasing concern among authorities in western Europe (McKee et al. 2012), although the scale of the problem is contested (Lachenmeir 2012). However, as with tobacco smuggling, the appropriate response is effective enforcement rather than simply regarding it as a problem that is too difficult.
- Alcohol prices differ between neighbouring jurisdictions, which leads to consumers crossing nearby borders to purchase cheaper alcohol (Rabinovich et al. 2009b). This is much less of an issue than imagined, but it is also important to note that some responses can make matters worse. In 2004, when Estonia joined the EU, Finland reduced alcohol taxes by one-third, to act as a disincentive for consumers to buy cheaper alcohol from Estonia. However, the consequence was that sudden alcohol-caused deaths jumped immediately by 17% (government revenue fell by the same amount) (Koski et al. 2007). It was the more deprived who were penalized, with the vast majority of the increase in deaths occurring among poorer as opposed to richer consumers (Herttua et al. 2008). The damaging effects came from Finnish, not Estonian, alcohol.
- A tax increase is not normally followed by an equivalent price increase, with producers and retailers responding in different ways (Rabinovich et al. 2009b). Sometimes the price goes up more than would be expected. Other times, and more commonly, the price goes up less than expected, meaning

that producers and retailers have the capacity to absorb some of the price that would have resulted from a tax increase.

One way to get round some of these issues is to set a minimum price per gram of alcohol sold. This option also has many other advantages in that, even more than tax increases, this targets heavy drinking occasions and heavy drinkers much more than lighter drinkers (Purshouse et al. 2010), and it appears minimally regressive (Ludbrook et al. 2012). Minimum alcohol prices in British Columbia, Canada, have been adjusted intermittently over the years 1989–2010 (Stockwell et al. 2012). Time-series analyses found that a 10% increase in the minimum price of an alcoholic beverage reduced consumption of spirits and liqueurs by 7%, wine by 9%, alcoholic sodas and ciders by 14%, beer by 1.5% and all alcoholic drinks by 3%. In Europe in May 2012, the Scottish Parliament introduced a minimum price per gram of alcohol; the United Kingdom Government launched its alcohol strategy in March 2012, which also calls for a minimum price per unit of alcohol. All the estimates suggest that introducing a minimum price would have immediate and great effect in improving health and well-being, as well as productivity (Purshouse et al. 2010).

When alcohol is easier to get, more alcohol is consumed and more harm results; when alcohol is more difficult to get, less is consumed and less harm results (Bryden et al. 2012; Österberg 2012). So, limits on availability, for example by reducing the number of outlets and the days and hours of sale, save lives.

Commercial communications, particularly through social media and electronic communication outlets, encourage non-drinkers to start drinking and existing drinkers to drink more (de Bruijn 2012). Even simply watching a movie for one hour with a greater number of drinking scenes, or viewing simple advertisements, can double the amount drunk over the hour's viewing period (Engels et al. 2009). In many jurisdictions, much store is put on self-regulation of commercial communications and withdrawal of communications that are found to breach self-regulatory codes. However, these approaches are increasingly irrelevant, since extensive evidence shows that withdrawn commercial communications simply live on, accessible to all, in social media, which is, in any case, heavily financed by global alcohol producers (Anderson 2012). Many of the leading brands are now posting messages on Facebook every single day, thereby reaching a vast audience of predominantly young people.

Successes and failures of alcohol policy in Europe

Epidemiological catastrophe

The Russian Federation provides a dramatic case study of how bad things can get. Figure 3.1 relates all-cause age-standardized mortality (male and female) in the Russian Federation and western Europe since 1980 to significant events in recent Russian history. Mortality had been increasing slowly for many years, decreased suddenly in the mid-1980s as part of the Gorbachev anti-alcohol campaign, and then increased again to reach a maximum in 1994 (McKee

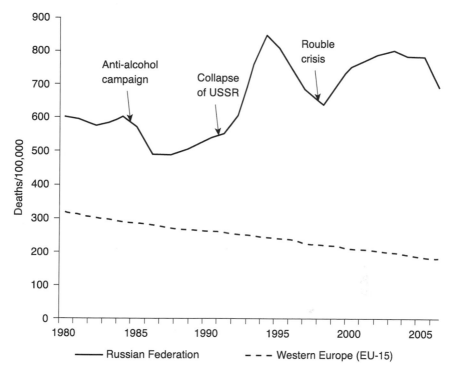

Figure 3.1   Age-standardized mortality (all causes) in the Russian Federation and in western Europe

Source: WHO Regional Office for Europe 2012

1999), coinciding with a rapid programme of mass privatization accompanied by a halving of Russian industrial output and hyperinflation. When the rouble stabilized, mortality went down (1995–1998), but then the rouble collapsed again and mortality went up again as well (1998–1999) (Stuckler et al. 2009b).

These massive fluctuations in all-cause mortality are driven entirely by causes related to alcohol (Leon et al. 1997; Shkolnikov et al. 2001). It is estimated that alcohol was responsible for about three-quarters of all male deaths at ages 15–54 years and about half of all female deaths at these ages during the 1990s in the Russian Federation (Zaridze et al. 2009). A series of detailed studies in one typical Russian city found that two of the most hazardous forms of drinking, consumption of surrogate alcohols such as aftershaves, which typically contain up to 95% ethanol (McKee et al. 2005), and recent experience of *zapoi*, a Russian term for a binge lasting several days, alone accounted for 40% of deaths among working age men (Leon et al. 2007; Tomkins et al. 2012).

Trends in alcohol consumption in Europe

The best indicator of overall volume of alcohol consumption is the sum of recorded and unrecorded adult (age 15+ years) per capita consumption. Using

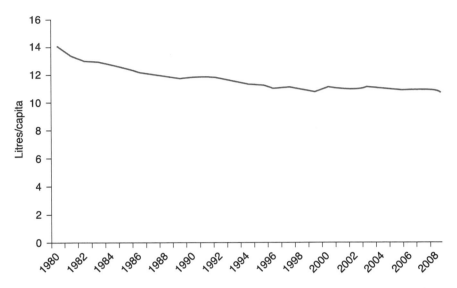

Figure 3.2 Per capita pure alcohol consumption in the European Union among those aged 15+ years, 1980–2009

Source: WHO Regional Office for Europe 2012

this indicator, adult citizens of the EU on average drink 12.5 litres of pure alcohol per year, just under 30 g per day, more than twice the amount of alcohol consumed globally (World Health Organization 2011). Unrecorded consumption makes up about 13% of this consumption, compared with an estimated global average of almost 30%. Just considering recorded consumption derived from sales and tax data, per capita adult consumption has not changed significantly in the EU since the mid-1990s (Fig. 3.2).

However, this overall stability hides wide variation between countries, as illustrated in Fig. 3.3, which demonstrates a harmonization of per capita consumption across Europe, with reductions in southern Europe, increases in north-western Europe, and fluctuations with recent increases in central and eastern Europe.

The variations in patterns of per capita alcohol consumption are accompanied by variations across the EU in the proportion of the total burden of disease (as measured in DALYs) that is attributable to alcohol (Fig. 3.4).

The impact of alcohol policies on alcohol consumption

Some of the most dramatic changes in alcohol consumption have occurred in southern European countries, as illustrated by the examples of France and Italy in Fig. 3.3. This also portrays the increasing consumption in Finland, and the relatively stable but slightly fluctuating pattern of consumption in Sweden. To what extent are these changes in consumption a result of more or less autonomous social changes or of alcohol policy?

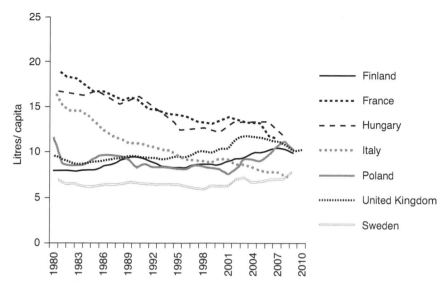

Figure 3.3   Per capita alcohol consumption among those aged 15+ years in selected European Union Member States

Source: WHO Regional Office for Europe 2012

This has been studied by Allamani et al. (2012), who analysed the relative impact of social changes and alcohol policies on alcohol consumption in 12 European countries during the years 1961–2006. Considering the 12 countries as a whole, out only two of a whole range of social factors studied consistently impacted on alcohol consumption: greater urbanization, which was associated with greater alcohol consumption; and later age of first childbirth, which was associated with lower alcohol consumption. Of a range of alcohol policies studied that did not include affordability, restricting availability and increasing purchase age were both associated with lower alcohol consumption. Elsewhere, Rabinovich et al. (2009a) have shown that, across the EU as a whole, the affordability of alcohol, a composite measure of the net effect of alcohol price and income, is positively associated with per capita alcohol consumption. The more affordable alcohol is, the more it is consumed.

For four of the individual countries portrayed in Fig. 3.3, the following results were found.

Finland.   The main policy change impacting on per capita alcohol consumption was the 1969 Act that reduced the legal age of purchase and allowed the sale of medium-strength beer in stores and cafes. This was associated with an increase in alcohol consumption.

France.   The 1977 excise duty increases on beer, the 1987 total advertising ban on TV, the 1991 introduction of a minimum purchase age of 16 years, and the 1995 reduction of the legal blood alcohol concentration for driving from 0.8 g/L to 0.5 g/L were associated with reductions in per capita alcohol consumption.

Spain.   The 1982 introduction of a legal minimum purchase age of 16 years, the 1988 ban on advertising of spirits, the 1989 ban on selling alcohol in

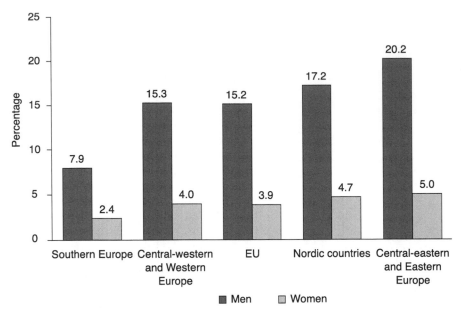

Figure 3.4 Regional variation in the percentage of the total burden of disease (as measured by disability-adjusted life-years) that is attributable to alcohol in those aged 15–64 years, 2004

Source: Mathers et al. 2008 (*Global Burden of Disease, 2004 Update*)
Notes: Southern Europe, the southern region; Central-western and western Europe, Ireland, the United Kingdom and the continental region; Central-eastern and eastern Europe, the central and eastern region and the former USSR

public education places, and the 1990 ban on alcohol in sports events were associated with reductions in per capita alcohol consumption.

Sweden. The 1977 prohibition of the sale of medium-strength beer in grocery stores, the 1982 closure of state-owned retail monopoly stores on Saturdays and the 1990 reduction of the legal blood alcohol concentration for driving from 0.5 g/L to 0.2 g/L were associated with reductions in per capita alcohol consumption. The 2001 opening of state-owned retail monopoly stores and the 2004 abolition of travel allowances from other EU Member States were associated with increases in per capita alcohol consumption.

These results suggest while social changes do impact on levels of alcohol consumption, policies also matter.

Comprehensiveness of policies and alcohol consumption

A number of studies have attempted to score and scale the strictness and comprehensiveness of a country's alcohol policy.

● The European Comparative Alcohol Study developed a scale to measure the strictness and comprehensiveness of alcohol control policy in ten year intervals from 1950 to 2000 for all 15 EU Member States as of 1995, with the exception of Luxembourg, plus Norway (Karlsson and Österberg 2006). The scale omitted alcohol taxation because of data deficiencies. The maximum 20 point scale covered the domains of control of production and wholesale, control of distribution, personal control, control of marketing, social and environmental controls and public policy. The mean score across the ten northern European countries increased from 11 in 1970 to 13 in 1990, before falling to 12 in 2000; in the five southern European countries it increased from 4 in 1970 to 10 in 2000.

• As an extension of their previous work, Karlsson and Österberg (2006) rated alcohol policies across 28 European countries in 2005, using a scale ranging from 0 to 40. This new scale included a country's level of alcohol taxation, and they were now also able to include central and eastern European countries. The mean score was 19 in northern, 9 in southern, and 11 in central and eastern European countries.

• Brand et al. (2007) assessed alcohol policies across 22 European countries in 2003, with a scale ranging from 0 to 100. Compared with the scale used by Karlsson and Österberg (2006), it gives less weight to alcohol taxation and much more weight to drink driving controls. The mean score was 41 in northern, 31 in southern and 54 in central and eastern European countries. While this study confirms the difference in strictness and comprehensiveness of alcohol policy between northern and southern European countries, as found by Karlsson and Österberg (2006), it gives a different view of the relative position of central and eastern European countries.

For all three scales, associations are seen with alcohol consumption. As an example, we show the correlation between a country's score on the scale devised by Brand et al. (2007) and alcohol consumption in 2003 (Fig. 3.5).

Taking the score of Karlsson and Österberg (2006), the main relationship found was when the policy score was higher than the mean, in which case the higher the score the lower the alcohol consumption in the studied year (2005). This suggests a threshold effect, in which little effect is seen until a certain level of strictness and comprehensiveness has been reached. The authors also showed that once the mean score was exceeded the higher score was associated with deaths from cirrhosis and a range of alcohol-related conditions (Karlsson and Österberg 2006).

Discussion and conclusions

There appears to be a dissonance between the health burden attributable to alcohol, on the one hand, and the adequacy of the policy response on the other. In the EU, alcohol is responsible for more than one in eight of all deaths in the working age population, with adult per capita alcohol consumption being stable at more than double the world's average for the past ten years (Shield et al. 2012). According to a 2012 WHO report, *Alcohol in the European Union* (Anderson et al. 2012), areas of policy that were strengthened over the five years between 2006 and 2010 were, primarily, better education and more community action; areas

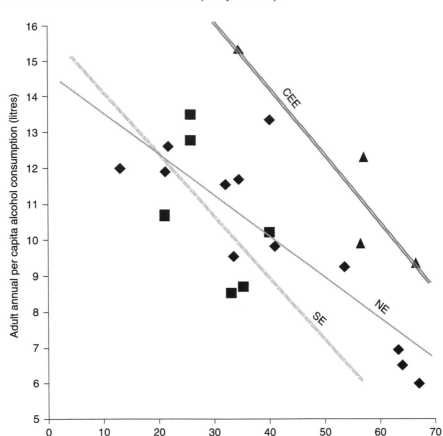

Figure 3.5 Relationship between a country's strictness and comprehensiveness of alcohol policy and adult annual per capita alcohol consumption in 2003, by European region

Source: Data taken from Brand et al. (2007)
Notes: NE, northern European countries; SE, southern European countries; CEE, central and eastern European countries

that did not get stronger or got weaker were pricing and advertising, precisely the opposite from what might have made most difference.

There are, potentially, several reasons for this dissonance. They include lack of adequate alcohol policy infrastructures, lack of knowledge of the harms done by alcohol, an overemphasis in public discourse of the presumed benefits of alcohol, and scepticism among the public of the impact of policy measures, in particular, the impact of tax increases (WHO Regional Office for Europe 2009). But, overriding all of these, and probably contributing to them, is too close a relationship between governments and the alcohol industry, and lack of proper regulation of the industry.

As commented by Crook (2005) in the *Economist*, 'it is the job of elected politicians to set goals for regulators, to deal with externalities, to mediate among different interests, to attend to the demands of social justice, to provide public goods and collect the taxes to pay for them, to establish collective priorities where that is necessary and appropriate, and to organize resources accordingly'. Many commentators and politicians place great emphasis on corporate social responsibility by the alcohol industry to promote joined-up actions with health bodies to reduce the harm done by alcohol. Unfortunately, the incentives are for producers and retailers to be irresponsible rather than responsible. Managing consumer demand is counterproductive for producers and retailers, since most alcohol is drunk in heavy drinking occasions. For example, in the United Kingdom, 82% of all alcohol is consumed by men who drink over 32 g/day and women over 24 g/day, and 55% of all alcohol is consumed by men who drink 64 g/day and by women who drink more than 48 g/day (Baumberg 2009). This is unfortunate, since such consumption increases all risks. Another motivation for self-regulation would be moral, but here collective action is either weak (self-regulation does not work) or illegal (the industry itself introducing a minimum price per gram of alcohol would be considered anti-competitive).

The evidence shows that the alcohol industry has been very effective in avoiding legislation (Anderson et al. 2012). Many countries have, of course, simply followed the advice they were given: the European Commission's *Communication on Alcohol* had a lot to say about the importance of more education but virtually nothing about the importance of price (Gordon and Anderson 2011). One suggested reason for this has been the influence of the alcohol industry itself, the *Communication* being well-aligned to the industry's views on alcohol policy (Anderson 2009). Further, the body invited to broker discussion between the industry and public health, the European Policy Centre, had industry's views at heart, having been employed, for example, by the tobacco industry to lobby the European Commission in favour of its commercial interests (Smith et al. 2010). The Commission's corner stone for the implementation of its strategy is the European Alcohol and Health Forum, set up to provide a common platform at the EU level for stakeholders to collaborate and commit to action to reduce alcohol-related harm.

Unfortunately, analyses of the commitments by the alcohol industry showed them not to be based on evidence, over-reliant on self-regulation and trivial at best (Celia et al. 2010). Moreover, perhaps as a result of learning from the tobacco industry, alcohol trade bodies are engaging in activities to obfuscate the evidence and thus sow confusion (McKee 2006).

To date, the evidence suggests that the alcohol industry, both the production and retail sectors, are not engaged in any meaningful way. Too often the industry is engaged at too low a level, or expectations for industry engagement are too trivial. A frank discussion needs to take place as to how the industry can meet the needs of their shareholders, while producing products that result in less alcohol consumption. The industries themselves cannot legally set a minimum price per gram of alcohol; this is why governments need to act. But the industry can do other things, for example reduce bottle and can sizes or reduce the number of grams of alcohol in a range of popular products – this is something that some parts of the industry are actually doing (HM Government

2012) and is akin to salt and sugar reduction initiatives being led by the food industry (Anderson et al. 2011a). Governments can help to set incentives here, for example by ensuring that taxes are set per gram of alcohol (Anderson et al. 2011b).

This is exactly what the United Kingdom Government has done in its alcohol strategy (HM Government 2012). As paragraph 4.4 of the strategy notes, 'the alcohol industry has a direct and powerful connection and influence on consumer behaviours. We know that: people consume more when prices are lower; marketing and advertising affect drinking behaviour; and store layout and product location affect the type and volume of sales.' The strategy proposes to, 'take one billion units (8 billion grams of alcohol) out of the market by 2015. This will bring significant benefits for public health, reduce crime and demonstrates the positive contribution that industry can make.' The strategy will put into place the correct incentives to support this initiative by introducing a new higher rate of duty for higher-strength beer and a new lower rate of duty for lower-strength beer. The aim is that these 1 billion units are simply no longer drunk, by anyone, and this strategy sets a good example for all other European countries.

References

Allamani, A., Voller, F. Pepe, P. et al. (2011) Balance of power in alcohol policy. Balance across different groups and as a whole between societal changes and alcohol policy. In: Anderson P. et al. eds (2012) Alcohol Policy in Europe Evidence from AMPHORA (see also http://amphoraproject.net/view.php?id_cont=45).

Anderson, P. (2009) Global alcohol policy and the alcohol industry, *Current Opinion Psychiatry*, 22(3):253–7.

Anderson, P. (2012) Alcohol and the workplace, in P. Anderson, L. Møller and G. Galea (eds) *Alcohol in the European Union: Consumption, Harm and Policy Approaches*. Copenhagen: WHO Regional Office for Europe, pp. 69–82.

Anderson, P. and Baumberg, B. (2010) *Cost Benefit Analyses of Alcohol Policy: A Primer*. Warsaw: Institute of Psychiatry and Neurology.

Anderson, P., Chisholm, D. and Fuhr, D.C. (2009) Effectiveness and cost-effectiveness of policies and programmes to reduce the harm caused by alcohol, *Lancet*, 373(9682):2234–46.

Anderson, P., Harrison, O., Cooper, C. and Jane-Llopis, E. (2011a) Incentives for health, *Journal of Health Communication*, 16(suppl 2):107–33.

Anderson, P., Amaral-Sabadini, M.B., Baumberg, B., Jarl, J. and Stuckler, D. (2011b) Communicating alcohol narratives: creating a healthier relationship with alcohol, *Journal of Health Communication*, 16(suppl 2):27–36.

Anderson, P., Møller, L. and Galea, G. (eds) (2012) *Alcohol in the European Union: Consumption, Harm and Policy Approaches*. Copenhagen: WHO Regional Office for Europe.

Babor, T. (2010) *Alcohol – No Ordinary Commodity: Research and Public Policy*. Oxford: Oxford University Press.

Baumberg, B. (2009) How will alcohol sales in the UK be affected if drinkers follow government guidelines? *Alcohol Alcoholism*, 44(5):523–8.

Blomgren, J., Martikainen, P., Makela, P. and Valkonen, T. (2004) The effects of regional characteristics on alcohol-related mortality: a register-based multilevel analysis of 1.1 million men, *Social Science and Medicine*, 58(12):2523–35.

Brand, D.A., Saisana, M., Rynn, L.A., Pennoni, F. and Lowenfels, A.B. (2007) Comparative analysis of alcohol control policies in 30 countries, *PLoS Medicine*, 4(4):e151.

Britton, A. and McKee, M. (2000) The relation between alcohol and cardiovascular disease in Eastern Europe: explaining the paradox, *Journal of Epidemiology and Community Health*, 54(5):328–32.

de Bruijn, A. (2012) The impact of alcohol marketing, in P. Anderson, L. Møller and G. Galea (eds) *Alcohol in the European Union: Consumption, Harm and Policy Approaches*. Copenhagen: WHO Regional Office for Europe, pp. 89–95.

Bryden, A., Roberts, B., McKee, M. and Petticrew, M. (2012) A systematic review of the influence on alcohol use of community level availability and marketing of alcohol, *Health Place*, 18(2):349–57.

Carrell, S.E., Hoekstra, M. and West, J.E. (2011) Does drinking impair college performance? Evidence from a regression discontinuity approach, *Journal of Public Economics*, 95(1–2):54–62.

Celia, C., Diepeveen, S. and Ling, T. (2010) *The European Alcohol and Health Forum: First Monitoring Progress Report*. Cambridge, MA: RAND Europe.

Crook, C. (2005) The good company. *Economist* 22 January.

Engels, R.C., Hermans, R., van Baaren, R.B., Hollenstein, T. and Bot, S.M. (2009) Alcohol portrayal on television affects actual drinking behaviour, *Alcohol and Alcoholism*, 44(3):244–9.

European Parliament (2011) *European Parliament Resolution of 8 March 2011 on Reducing Health Inequalities in the EU (2010/2089(INI)*. Strasbourg: European Parliament.

Gordon, R. and Anderson, P. (2011) Science and alcohol policy: a case study of the EU Strategy on Alcohol, *Addiction*, 106(suppl 1):55–66.

Herttua, K., Makela, P. and Martikainen, P. (2008) Changes in alcohol-related mortality and its socioeconomic differences after a large reduction in alcohol prices: a natural experiment based on register data, *American Journal of Epidemiology*, 168(10):1110–18; discussion 1126–31.

HM Government (2012) *The Government's Alcohol Strategy*. London: The Stationery Office.

IARC (2010) *Alcohol Consumption and Ethyl Carbamate*. Lyon, France: International Agency for Research on Cancer.

Karlsson, T. and Österberg, E. (2006) *Eurocare Bridging the Gap (BtG) Project, Third Meeting of Network: Country Reports and Country Profiles*, May, Barcelona.

Koski, A., Siren, R., Vuori, E. and Poikolainen, K. (2007) Alcohol tax cuts and increase in alcohol-positive sudden deaths: a time-series intervention analysis, *Addiction*, 102(3):362–8.

Lachenmeir, D. (2012) Unrecorded and illict alcohol, in P. Anderson, L. Møller and G. Galea (eds) *Alcohol in the European Union: Consumption, Harm and Policy Approaches*. Copenhagen: WHO Regional Office for Europe, pp. 29–34.

Lang, K., Vali, M., Szucs, S., Adany, R. and McKee, M. (2006) The composition of surrogate and illegal alcohol products in Estonia, *Alcohol and Alcoholism*, 41(4):446–50.

Laslett, A.-M., Catalano, P., Chikritzhs, Y. et al. (2010) *The Range and Magnitude of Alcohol's Harm to Others*. Fitzroy, Australia: AER Centre for Alcohol Policy Research, Turning Point Alcohol and Drug Centre, Eastern Health.

Leon, D.A., Chenet, L., Shkolnikov, V.M. et al. (1997) Huge variation in Russian mortality rates 1984–94: artefact, alcohol, or what? *Lancet*, 350(9075):383–8.

Leon, D.A., Saburova, L., Tomkins, S. et al. (2007) Hazardous alcohol drinking and premature mortality in Russia: a population based case-control study, *Lancet*, 369(9578):2001–9.

Leon, D.A., Shkolnikov, V.M., McKee, M. et al. (2010) Alcohol increases circulatory disease mortality in Russia: acute and chronic effects or misattribution of cause? *International Journal of Epidemiology*, 39(5):1279–90.

Ludbrook, A., Petrie, D., McKenzie, L. and Farrar, S. (2012) Tackling alcohol misuse: purchasing patterns affected by minimum pricing for alcohol, *Applied Health Economics and Health Policy*, 10(1):51–63.

Lye, J. and Hirschberg, J. (2010) Alcohol consumption and human capital: a retrospective study of the literature, *Journal of Economic Surveys*, 24(2):309–38.

Mathers, C., Boerma, T. and Fat, D.M. (2008) *The Global Burden of Disease 2004 Update*. Geneva: World Health Organization.

McKee, M. (1999) Alcohol in Russia, *Alcohol and Alcoholism*, 34(6):824–9.

McKee, M. (2006) A European alcohol strategy, *British Medical Journal*, 333(7574):871–2.

McKee, M. and Britton, A. (1998) The positive relationship between alcohol and heart disease in eastern Europe: potential physiological mechanisms, *Journal of the Royal Society of Medicine*, 91(8):402–7.

McKee, M., Suzcs, S., Sarvary, A. et al. (2005) The composition of surrogate alcohols consumed in Russia. *Alcohol and Clinical Experimental Research*, 29(10):1884–8.

McKee, M., Adany, R. and Leon, D. (2012) Illegally produced alcohol, *British Medical Journal*, 344:e1146.

National Health and Medical Research Council (2009) *Australian Guidelines to Reduce Health Risks from Drinking Alcohol*. Canberra: Commonwealth of Australia.

Nuffield Council on Bioethics (2007) *Public Health: Ethical Issues*. London: Nuffield Council on Bioethics.

Österberg, E. (2012) Pricing of alcohol, in P. Anderson, L. Møller and G. Galea (eds) *Alcohol in the European Union: Consumption, Harm and Policy Approaches*. Copenhagen: WHO Regional Office for Europe, pp. 96–102.

Parna, K., Lang, K., Raju, K., Vali, M. and McKee, M. (2007) A rapid situation assessment of the market for surrogate and illegal alcohols in Tallinn, Estonia, *International Journal of Public Health*, 52(6):402–10.

Purshouse, R.C., Meier, P.S., Brennan, A., Taylor, K.B. and Rafia, R. (2010) Estimated effect of alcohol pricing policies on health and health economic outcomes in England: an epidemiological model, *Lancet*, 375(9723):1355–64.

Rabinovich, L., Brutscher, P.-B., Vries, H. et al. (2009a) *The Affordability of Alcoholic Beverages in the European Union: Understanding the Link Between Alcohol Affordability, Consumption and Harms*. Cambridge, MA: RAND Corporation.

Rabinovich, L., Hunt, P., Staetsky, L. et al. (2009b) *Further Study on the Affordability of Alcoholic Beverages in the EU. A Focus on Excise Duty Pass-through, On- and Off-trade Sales, Price Promotions and Pricing Regulations*. Cambridge, MA: RAND Corporation.

Rehm, J., Anderson, P., Kanteres, F. et al. (2009a) *Alcohol, Social Development and Infectious Disease*. Toronto, ON: Centre for Addiction and Mental Health.

Rehm, J., Mathers, C., Popova, S. et al. (2009b) Global burden of disease and injury and economic cost attributable to alcohol use and alcohol-use disorders, *Lancet*, 373(9682):2223–33.

Rehm, J., Baliunas, D., Borges, G.L. et al. (2010) The relation between different dimensions of alcohol consumption and burden of disease: an overview, *Addiction*, 105(5):817–43.

Roerecke, M. and Rehm, J. (2010) Irregular heavy drinking occasions and risk of ischemic heart disease: a systematic review and meta-analysis, *American Journal of Epidemiology*, 171(6):633–44.

Rosenquist, J.N., Murabito, J., Fowler, J.H. and Christakis, N.A. (2010) The spread of alcohol consumption behavior in a large social network. *Annals in Internal Medicine*, 152(7):426–33, W141.

Shield, K.D., Kehoe, T., Shield, K.D. et al. (2012) Societal burden of alcohol, in P. Anderson, L. Møller and G. Galea (eds) *Alcohol in the European Union: Consumption, Harm and Policy Approaches*. Copenhagen: WHO Regional Office for Europe, pp. 10–28.

Shkolnikov, V., McKee, M. and Leon, D.A. (2001) Changes in life expectancy in Russia in the mid-1990s, *Lancet*, 357(9260):917–21.

Smith, K.E., Fooks, G., Collin, J., Weishaar, H., Mandal, S. and Gilmore, A.B. (2010) Working the system: British American Tobacco's influence on the European Union Treaty and its implications for policy – an analysis of internal tobacco industry documents, *PLoS Medicine*, 7(1):e1000202.

Stockwell, T., Auld, M.C., Zhao, J. and Martin, G. (2012) Does minimum pricing reduce alcohol consumption? The experience of a Canadian province, *Addiction*, 107(5):912–20.

Stuckler, D., Basu, S., Suhrcke, M., Coutts, A. and McKee, M. (2009a) The public health effect of economic crises and alternative policy responses in Europe: an empirical analysis, *Lancet*, 374(9686):315–23.

Stuckler, D., King, L. and McKee, M. (2009b) Mass privatisation and the post-communist mortality crisis: a cross-national analysis, *Lancet*, 373(9661):399–407.

Tomkins, S., Collier, T., Oralov, A. et al. (2012) Hazardous alcohol consumption is a major factor in male premature mortality in a typical Russian city: prospective cohort study 2003–2009, *PLoS One*, 7(2):e30274.

Wagenaar, A.C., Tobler, A.L. et al. (2010) Effects of alcohol tax and price policies on morbidity and mortality: a systematic review, *American Journal of Public Health*, 100(11):2270–8.

WHO Regional Office for Europe (2009) *Evidence for the Effectiveness and Cost–Effectiveness of Interventions to Reduce Alcohol-related Harm*. Copenhagen: WHO Regional Office for Europe.

WHO Regional Office for Europe (2012) *Health for All Database*. Copenhagen: WHO Regional Office for Europe.

World Health Organization (2004) *Neuroscience of Psychoactive Substance Use and Dependence*. Geneva: World Health Organization.

World Health Organization (2011) *Global Status Report on Alcohol and Health*. Geneva: World Health Organization.

World Health Organization and World Economic Forum (2011) *From Burden to Best Buys: Reducing the Economic Impact of Non-Communicable Diseases in Low- and Middle-Income Countries*. Geneva: World Health Organization and World Economic Forum.

Zaridze, D., Brennan, P., Boreham, J. et al. (2009) Alcohol and cause-specific mortality in Russia: a retrospective case–control study of 48,557 adult deaths, *Lancet*, 373(9682):2201–14.

Zatonski, W. (ed.) (2008) *Closing the Health Gap in European Union*. Warsaw: Maria-Sklodowska-Curie Memorial Cancer Center and Institute of Oncology.

chapter four

Food and nutrition

Liselotte Schäfer Elinder and
Caroline Bollars

Introduction

The first survey of food and nutrition policies was published by the League of Nations, a predecessor of the United Nations, in 1937–1938 (League of Nations 1938). It was proposed that every country should form a national nutrition committee and report annually on the state of nutrition in their country. The main focus at that time was nutritional adequacy and diseases associated with nutritional deficiencies. Since then much has changed, but the need for food and nutrition policies is undiminished.

With rising prosperity and the associated abundance of food, nutrition-related health risks have changed considerably (World Health Organization 2009). Traditional risks such as undernutrition or unsafe food and water have largely been replaced by problems related to unbalanced diets and inadequate physical activity, which are important contributors to the chronic diseases, such as ischaemic heart disease and diabetes, that currently dominate morbidity and mortality patterns in Europe. The major food-related risk factors for chronic diseases in Europe today are high blood pressure, overweight and obesity, high blood cholesterol, high blood glucose and low intake of fruit and vegetables (World Health Organization 2009). If physical inactivity is also included, these risk factors together explain 57% of all cardiovascular deaths, 25% of all premature deaths and 12.6% of the total disease burden in Europe, all of which is preventable. Table 4.1 summarizes the food- and nutrition-related burden of mortality in Europe, and shows that these risk factors are important across Europe, not only in the high-income countries.

For several decades, governments have been engaged in defining nutritional recommendations and formulating food and nutrition policies in response to these health challenges, a process continuously supported and monitored by the WHO (WHO Regional Office for Europe 2000, 2006a, 2008; World Health Organization 2004; Andersson et al. 2007). A food and nutrition policy may

Table 4.1 Attributable mortality by nutrition-related risk factor in Europe, 2004

Risk factor	Deaths (in 1000s)		
	Total	High income	Low and middle income
High blood glucose	748	258	490
High blood pressure	2491	740	1752
High cholesterol	926	242	684
Iron deficiency	8	4	4
Low fruit and vegetable intake	423	77	346
Overweight and obesity	1081	318	763
Physical inactivity	992	301	691
Suboptimal breastfeeding	36	2	33
Underweight	28	0	27
Vitamin A deficiency	10	0	10
Zinc deficiency	5	0	5
Total deaths (all causes)	**9493**	**3809**	**5683**

Source: World Health Organization 2009

be defined as a 'specific set of decisions with related actions, established by a government and often supported by special legislation, which addresses a food or nutrition problem or set of problems' (Johns Hopkins Bloomberg School of Public Health 2012).The terms 'food' and 'nutrition' have slightly different meanings, with food referring to the substances that we eat, and nutrition to the actual provision of nutrients needed for life. We will use the general term 'food and nutrition policies' to refer both to policies dealing with the supply of food, and to policies seeking to modify the demand for specific foods. In general, available instruments in health policy are education, legislation/regulation and fiscal measures, which may be used to a varying extent depending on the political context and the scientific evidence.

Up until the 1970s, the focus of European food and nutrition policies was to ensure nutritional adequacy. Concurrently with the rise in food availability and knowledge on the links between diet, health and disease, the focus of nutrition and food policies started to change during the 1970s. A striking development in Europe after the Second World War has been the initial rise in cardiovascular morbidity and mortality followed by a dramatic decline in most European countries during the period 1970–2010 (see Chapter 1). In recent times there has also been a steady rise in obesity. Formulation of food and nutrition policies has occurred in response to these changing disease patterns, defining the policy objectives in relation to the risk factors such as unhealthy diet and physical inactivity. However, policies on paper are not always implemented as intended and an adequate evaluation of policy implementation is lacking in most countries. Furthermore, policy implementation often is a 'natural experiment' without control groups and, therefore, cause and effect cannot easily be established.

Nevertheless, favourable changes in people's diets have occurred during the past four decades. This chapter will start by looking at iodine deficiency, an old problem that has never been completely eradicated in spite of knowledge of how to do so. Efforts to tackle nutrition-related risk factors for cardiovascular diseases will then be considered. A general overview of food and nutrition policies, by country, is presented in Appendix table 4.A1.

Tackling iodine deficiency

The European continent has a long history of iodine deficiency because of its iodine-deficient soils, with endemic goitre as its main clinical manifestation. Brain damage and irreversible intellectual impairment have been and still are major health consequences of this micronutrient deficiency, which all European countries except Iceland have experienced to a greater or lesser degree (World Health Organization 2007).While cretinism, the most extreme expression of iodine deficiency disorders, has become very rare, more subtle degrees of intellectual impairment associated with iodine deficiency are of considerable concern, leading to poor school performance and impaired work capacity (Hetzel 2004). Iodine deficiency remains a major threat to health and development around the world, particularly among preschool children and pregnant women, and it is the greatest single cause of preventable brain damage (de Benoist et al. 2008). Worldwide it is estimated that 2 billion people suffer from iodine deficiency, of which 20% are in Europe.

The most cost-effective and sustainable strategy to reduce iodine deficiency is iodization of salt. The first country to apply this countermeasure was Switzerland, which succeeded in completely eliminating goitre through sustained implementation and monitoring of a programme of salt iodization. After this remarkable success, legislation on iodized salt was passed in many European countries, and iodine deficiency was no longer considered to be an important public health problem (Delange 2002). However, in the 1980s, it gradually became clear that iodine deficiency had reappeared in many European countries where it was thought to have been eliminated (Vitti et al. 2003; World Health Organization 2007).

Four factors have led to this situation. First, in some countries political and social changes have interrupted the salt iodization process and quality control measures that had previously been in place. Second, the formation of common markets along with increasing globalization have led to increased movement of foods across national borders, some processed with iodized salt but some not. Third, a diminishing amount of salt is consumed as table salt while a greater proportion is 'hidden' in processed foods, which are not covered by legislation in many countries. Finally, partly because of concern about hypertension, salt consumption has gradually declined, although it remains high (World Health Organization 2007).

In the 1990s the situation became particularly serious in eastern Europe. In 1997, a meeting held in Munich revealed the recurrence of goitre, and occasionally of endemic cretinism, in some countries in eastern Europe after the interruption of their salt iodization programmes. Many had good salt iodization coverage prior to 1990 but saw a drastic drop in iodine status during the 1990s after the break-up of the USSR. The former USSR began iodizing salt in the 1950s, and by 1970 most of the iodine deficiency disorders had been eliminated. However, as a result of relaxation of monitoring and less stringent enforcement, non-iodized salt started to reappear, again increasing the prevalence of iodine deficiency disorders in the region. For example, cases of goitre increased dramatically in certain *oblasts* in Ukraine and Belarus (Rokx 2003). Since then, an improvement in the availability of iodized salt has been brought about through partnerships formed by United Nations Children's Fund (UNICEF), with the help of other organizations. Unfortunately, the two major salt-producing countries in the region, the Russian Federation and Ukraine, have been slow in achieving universal salt iodization. Only 12 and 37%, respectively, of salt is iodized in these countries. Major challenges in the region include reintroducing the iodization technology in the now private salt producers, engaging with small salt producers, introducing and enforcing existing regulations and controlling the trade in illegal salt (Rokx 2003).

The problem is not limited, however, to eastern Europe. In 2002, only 28% of households in Europe as a whole used iodized salt (Delange 2002), and iodine deficiency is still common throughout Europe. Until 1990, goitre prevalence was used as an indicator of iodine deficiency, but today urinary iodine is used (de Benoist et al. 2008). Iodine deficiency is considered a public health problem in countries where the median urinary iodine concentration is <100 µg/L. Estimations from 2010 show that, of all the WHO regions, the European Region has the highest proportion of insufficient iodine intake. This affects 44% of all schoolchildren and 44% of the general population (Table 4.2).

The number of countries with insufficient iodine intake in the WHO European Region has decreased from 23 in 2003 to 14 in 2010, among them several central and eastern European countries. The list of countries that still have insufficient iodine intake includes Albania, Belgium, Estonia, France, Hungary, Ireland, Latvia, Lithuania, the Republic of Moldova, Norway, Portugal, the Russian Federation and Ukraine; this shows that the problem affects countries throughout the region (Zimmermann and Andersson 2011).

This long list of countries that still have insufficient iodine intake is an indication that the problem is not taken seriously enough, perhaps because governments still equate iodine deficiency with goitre and are unaware of the

Table 4.2 Prevalence of iodine deficiency in the WHO European Region, 2003–2007

Year	Countries with insufficient intake	Total number, millions (%)	
		School-age children	*General population*
2010	14	28.6 (43.6)	359.9 (43.9)
2007	19	38.7 (52.4)	459.7 (52.0)
2003	23	42.2 (59.9)	435.5 (56.9)

Source: Zimmermann and Andersson 2011

adverse effects of iodine deficiency on reproduction and brain development (Zimmermann and Andersson 2011). Even though most countries in the region monitor urinary iodine and/or total goitre prevalence in the population at irregular intervals, much more needs to be done to eradicate iodine deficiency disorders in Europe. The WHO recommends implementation of effective control and surveillance programmes, public information campaigns, and legislation or regulation on universal salt iodization. The last is particularly important for processed foods, which constitute a growing proportion of people's diets. Until universal iodization is achieved, iodine supplementation for the most vulnerable groups, such as pregnant women and young infants, should be considered in regions where there is insufficient iodized salt (Andersson et al. 2010).

Tackling nutrition-related risk factors for cardiovascular diseases

Effectiveness of food and nutrition policies

As noted in the introduction, the rise of cardiovascular diseases after the Second World War has bought new nutrition-related risk factors into focus. In the 1970s, the Seven Countries Study reported positive correlations between deaths from ischaemic heart disease and total fat intake, and later between ischaemic heart disease mortality and saturated fat intake (Keys et al. 1986). Other nutrition-related risk factors for ischaemic heart disease that have been identified include high blood pressure (which partly reflects high salt content of foods), low intake of fruit and vegetables, and intake of *trans*-fatty acids (TFAs; Mente et al. 2009). In the 1990s, overweight, obesity and diabetes type 2 emerged as serious public health threats in Europe and elsewhere, caused by a rising consumption of an energy-dense diet high in added sugar and fat and low in fruit and vegetables, in combination with a sedentary lifestyle.

The recognition of these risk factors has led to a range of dietary intervention studies in the community and in the workplace (James et al. 1997). The main dietary components targeted were fat quality, fruit and vegetable intake and salt. The results have been summarized in systematic reviews showing that it is possible to modify nutrition-related risk factors, and that modifying these risk factors reduces the risk of cardiovascular diseases. Intensive support and encouragement to reduce salt intake has led to a reduction in the amount of salt eaten, and also to lower blood pressure, although with mixed success (Hooper et al. 2004). Replacing some saturated (animal) fats with plant oils and unsaturated spreads reduced the risk of cardiovascular events (Hooper et al. 2011). Dietary advice on the reduction of salt and fat intake and an increase in the intake of fruit, vegetables and fibre lead to modest improvements in cardiovascular risk factors, such as blood pressure and cholesterol levels (Brunner et al. 2007). Obesity prevention programmes, however, often lack effectiveness. For example, programmes to improve physical activity and nutrition in children do improve these behaviours, but only some of these studies show an effect on children's body weight (Waters et al. 2011).

Several international agreements have been drawn up in the field of nutrition with the aim of strengthening national policy action, such as the *Global Strategy on Diet, Physical Activity and Health* (World Health Organization 2004), the *European Charter on Counteracting Obesity* (WHO Regional Office for Europe 2006b), the *European Action Plan for Food and Nutrition Policy 2007–2012* (WHO Regional Office for Europe 2008), and the *2008–2013 Action Plan for the Global Strategy for the Prevention and Control of Non-communicable Diseases* (World Health Organization 2008). Following these initiatives, a monitoring mechanism has been set up by the WHO Regional Office for Europe to help countries to evaluate progress towards their commitments in the international agreements. A 2006 survey on food and nutrition policies revealed that 48 out of 53 countries in the WHO European Region had established national policies. The latest survey in 2011 showed that all 27 EU Member States had a national food and/or nutrition policy either as a stand-alone policy or included in the public health policy (Bollars 2011). These data are reported to the WHO Regional Office for Europe by national focal points. On the basis of the country data, an overview of the policy development stage in the WHO European Region has been produced (Appendix 4.1). However, in order to draw conclusions about policy implementation, more in-depth assessment at country level is needed, and this is not yet available. Consequently, for this chapter, three case studies are presented first that are well documented in the scientific literature and illustrate how governments have committed themselves, on the basis of evidence, to improving diets in the population and the effects on health. Trends in nutrition-related risk factors and ischaemic heart disease mortality in Europe will then be reviewed.

Finland's comprehensive nutrition policy

In the 1960s, Finland had the highest death rate from ischaemic heart disease in the world (Pietinen et al. 2001) and was one of the first countries to take action by reducing risk factors. The Finnish diet at that time was characterized by a high fat intake (40–45% of energy intake), particularly a high saturated fat intake (>20% of energy intake), and salt intake (15 g/day), plus a low intake of fruit and vegetables (Prattala 2003). A comprehensive community health promotion intervention, the North Karelia Project, was initiated by Finnish researchers in 1972. The aim was to reduce mortality and morbidity from cardiovascular diseases by reducing established risk factors, such as smoking, high serum cholesterol and blood pressure, and improving the diet (Vartiainen et al. 1994). The main dietary targets were saturated fat, salt and fruit and vegetables.

Activities included media campaigns, health education, primary health care measures, environmental measures, collaboration with the food industry and the agricultural sector to develop healthier products, collaboration with non-governmental organizations, legislation and community activities in supermarkets and catering services, among others. A large detection and treatment programme for high blood pressure was also started in 1972. After the first five years, the programme was extended to the rest of Finland and the goals were broadened to prevention of all chronic diseases. Concurrently, a comprehensive monitoring system was developed, including regular population surveys on risk factors for cardiovascular diseases, including diet, every five years (Pietinen et al. 2001).

As a result, full-fat milk was to a large extent replaced by low-fat milk. Butter was replaced by margarines based on vegetable oils, and the percentage of Finnish men using butter decreased from 90% in 1972 to < 5% in 2009 (Puska 2009). This resulted in a substantial increase in the ratio of polyunsaturated to saturated fats, leading to lowering of serum cholesterol in the population (Vartiainen et al. 1994). This trend has been sustained and, in 2009, the mean intake of saturated fat in Finland in the working population was 12.9% of energy intake, which is at the lower end of the European range (8.8% in Portugal to 26.3% in Romania; Elmadfa 2009). Daily vegetable consumption among men went up from 16 to 28% during the same period (Prattala 2003), corresponding to a three-fold increase between 1972 and 2001, made possible through increased availability, mainly through the workplace and schools, and lower prices (Pietinen et al. 2001). Blood pressure decreased as a result of better medical treatment, a lowered salt intake in the population and, possibly, through an increase in the intake of polyunsaturated fat from vegetable origin. Anti-smoking legislation was also enacted.

As a result, cardiovascular mortality, including from ischaemic heart disease and stroke, decreased faster in North Karelia than in the rest of Finland during the first five years of the intervention; after 1977 the trend was the same all over Finland (Pietinen et al. 2001) (Fig. 4.1). Today cardiovascular mortality is 80% lower than at its peak, which is a remarkable achievement. Most of this decrease has been explained by the fall in serum cholesterol brought about by dietary change (Puska 2009). Furthermore, life expectancy in Finland has increased during this period by almost ten years.

The developments in Finland provide an interesting example of how research on the links between blood lipids, diet, smoking and heart disease was translated into community action in 1972 and finally to health policy in 1978, when the Finnish National Nutrition Council made its proposal for Finland's first food and nutrition policy. In 1987, the Council published recommendations for improving health and diet, emphasizing the role of fat, salt and dietary fibre. Two years later, in 1989, a multisectoral action plan including the whole food sector was released. In 1995, the Finnish Nutrition Surveillance System was established and in 1997 there was a consensus meeting regarding a programme to reduce cardiovascular diseases. Today, health services, schools and voluntary organizations share responsibility for implementing nutrition and health education (Puska 2009). Even though the health trends in Finland have been paralleled by similar developments in other countries, nowhere else have health gains been as large as in Finland.

Denmark's ban on industrially produced trans-fatty acids

Milk and dairy products contain low amounts of TFAs (Micha and Mozaffarian 2008), but the major source in the diet today is industrially produced partially hydrogenated vegetable oils, which are used in bakery products, deep fried and frozen foods, packaged snacks and margarines. These contribute 2–4% of

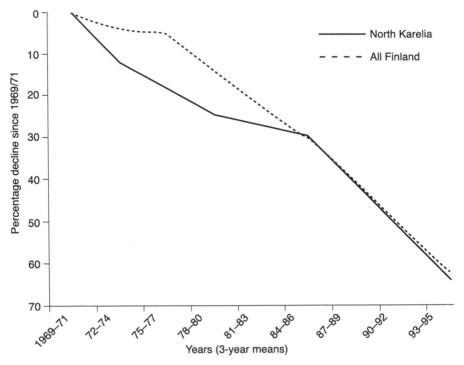

Figure 4.1 Percentage declines in mortality from ischaemic heart disease among men aged 35–64 years in North Karelia and the whole of Finland, 1969–1995

Source: Puska et al. 1998

energy intake in many countries. Some groups in the population may have even higher intakes, particularly those who consume large amounts of fast foods and snacks. The WHO recommends a maximum TFA intake corresponding to 1% of daily energy intake (Nishida and Uauy 2009). This can be accomplished by the elimination of partially hydrogenated vegetable oil in the human food supply.

Observational studies have linked a high intake of TFA to unfavourable effects on blood lipids, increased systemic inflammation, endothelial dysfunction and insulin resistance – all factors associated with an elevated risk of ischaemic heart disease (Mozaffarian et al. 2006). Calorie for calorie, TFAs have stronger relationships with ischaemic heart disease risk than seen for any other nutrient, including saturated fatty acids. A meta-analysis of four prospective cohort studies showed that each 2% increase in energy intake from TFA was associated with a 24–32% higher incidence of myocardial infarction and death from ischaemic heart disease (Mozaffarian et al. 2009).

In the 1970s, margarines and shortenings still contained large amounts of TFAs (up to 10%), but rising concerns about health risks in the 1990s prompted some food manufacturers to reformulate products to eliminate TFAs (Leth et al. 2006). A study from Denmark showed that in 1999 TFAs had been removed from margarines but were still found in shortenings and a number of common foods, such as frying fat, popcorn, cakes and biscuits (Hulshof et al. 1999). The Danish

Government, guided by experts, considered that labelling was insufficient to reach the appropriate level of protection and, therefore, eventually decided to pass legislation to ban TFAs in foods. Since January 2004, Denmark limits industrially produced TFAs in oils and fats for human consumption to 2% (Leth et al. 2006). The Danish experience showed that changes were economically feasible and did not affect the quality or cost of the foods involved (Tan 2009).

The events leading up to this legislation are a good example of how instrumental a policy coordination mechanism, such as the Danish Nutrition Council, is at country level. Key elements for success were the scientific integrity of the Council and sustained pressure on the food industry through media exposure and alliances with key policy-makers in the Ministry of Food and Agriculture (Astrup 2006). The Council installed a working group concerned with developing evidence for the potential harm of TFAs and issued three reports. The first, released in 1994, concluded that TFAs produce health problems such as thrombosis and atherosclerosis and are a threat to adults, unborn children and infants (Leth et al. 2006). It recommended that industrially produced TFAs should be removed from all foods within a few years. After that, TFAs started to be removed from margarines and were essentially gone by 1999. In a study covering the period 1998–2000, it was shown that median intake of industrially produced TFAs had declined to 0.4 g/day (Nielsen et al. 2011). However, consuming a 'high *trans* menu' composed of typical fast foods in 2001 could still result in an intake of far above the levels considered safe in Denmark (Stender et al. 2006).

The second report was issued in April 2001 and recommended legislation to reduce industrially produced TFAs to below 2% in all fats and oils for human consumption. After a battle involving EU legislation on unfair competition, Denmark was able to introduce its own legislation, which restricted the TFA content of all food products and ready meals to a maximum of 2% of the total fat content. The third report of the Council was issued in 2003 and went one step further by concluding that industrially produced TFAs could be eliminated from human diets without any adverse effect on taste, price or availability of foods. Denmark's TFA ban virtually eliminated artificial TFAs in the food supply by 2005 (Stender et al. 2006), even in products that are typically high in TFAs such as French fries, nuggets, biscuits/cakes/wafers and microwave popcorn. Food manufacturers gradually replaced TFAs with healthier options, with negligible negative impact on cost or revenue, and cost of foods to the population was not affected (Stender et al. 2006).

The effect of the removal of TFA on rates of cardiovascular diseases is difficult to estimate. Deaths from ischaemic heart disease decreased faster in Denmark after 1998, coinciding with the removal of TFAs from table margarines, than in most other countries in the region. However, as there are many other concurrent influences on ischaemic heart disease mortality, and as there may have been spill-over effects to other Scandinavian countries, the precise effect is difficult to estimate on the basis of trend analysis (L'Abbe et al. 2009).

The Danish ban on industrially produced TFAs has so far only been followed by Austria and Switzerland; other European countries such as the Netherlands have taken a voluntary approach initiated by the food industry (Appendix table 4.A1). In the Netherlands, this resulted in a major reduction in TFA content in retail foods in the 1990s, mainly through efforts of industry and with minimal government intervention. Further campaigns have also lowered the TFA content of frying fats. As a result, average TFA intake declined from 4% of energy intake in 1990 to slightly more than 1% in 2010. It has been estimated that this has reduced the annual number of deaths from ischaemic heart disease in the Netherlands by 1500, or 10% (Katan 2006). Some other countries have mentioned limitation of TFAs in their dietary goals, albeit without setting a target. Comparative data show that a ban is more effective than, for example, mandatory labelling or voluntary action in eliminating TFA from products that typically contain high amounts (Stender et al. 2006).

The United Kingdom's strategy to reduce salt intake

Throughout history, salt has been used by humans to preserve food. At the end of the 19th century, intake peaked and salt was the most taxed and traded commodity in the world (He and MacGregor 2009). The invention of the refrigerator and freezer gradually reduced the need for salt as a food-preserving agent, and intake started to decline. In Europe, salt intake has fallen from peak levels of 15–20 g/day to a current average intake of 9–12 g/day, which is still well above the recommended level of 5 g/day (2 g/day sodium, or 85 mmol/day) (Elmadfa 2009).

Salt intake above the recommended level has convincingly been linked to elevated blood pressure (Cutler et al. 1997). In populations with a salt intake <5 g/day, only a small rise in blood pressure is seen with advancing age (Elliott et al. 1996). A meta-analysis of prospective studies to assess the relation between the level of habitual salt intake and stroke or cardiovascular diseases showed that higher salt intake was associated with a significantly increased risk of stroke (23%) and of cardiovascular diseases (17%) (Strazzullo et al. 2009). Therefore, a reduction in salt intake from the current 9–12 g/day to the recommended level of 5–6 g/day is expected to have major effects on blood pressure and coronary heart disease and stroke, and may also have other beneficial effects on health (He and MacGregor 2009).

In 2003, the United Kingdom was one of the first European countries to start a national salt reduction strategy. This strategy had been preceded by 20 years of investigations into the health effects of salt. In 1994 an independent committee appointed by the United Kingdom Government (COMA) recommended that salt intake should be reduced to 6 g/day or less. However, this recommendation was opposed by the food industry (He and MacGregor 2009). As a response, in 1996, 22 scientific experts in the United Kingdom set up an advocacy group known as the Consensus Action on Salt and Health. Within a few years, this group succeeded in persuading a major supermarket and some food companies to start reducing salt in food products by 10–15%. The United Kingdom Department of Health finally endorsed new national recommendations on salt intake of less than 6 g/day in adults. The Food Standards Agency was assigned the role of bringing relevant stakeholders together to establish targets and parameters for review, to monitor progress, to provide technical expertise, to disseminate the results of relevant research, to report on progress and to develop further challenging recommendations. In 2001, salt intake in the population was 9.5 g/day, of which

80% was estimated to derive from processed foods (mainly cereals and baked goods) or caterer and restaurant meals. Therefore, a 40% reduction was required, in two to three steps that were small enough not to be sensed by consumers.

The United Kingdom strategy is based on three components: (1) collaboration with the food industry, (2) an advertising and social marketing campaign, and (3) introduction of traffic light labelling indicating whether foods are high or low in salt. This voluntary strategy has had some success so that salt levels in key processed foods were lowered by 25–45% by 2008 (Foods Standards Agency 2010). In addition, a public health campaign was launched in 2005 and this has raised awareness of the recommended salt intake from 3% to 34% of the population. From 2004, when the strategy was launched, until May 2008, the average salt intake had fallen by 10%, from 9.5 to 8.6 g/day. This is estimated to have saved some 6000 lives a year. It was hoped that the target of 6 g/day would be reached in 2012, but according to the National Institute for Health and Clinical Excellence, this is not likely to happen using the existing voluntary agreements (National Institute for Health and Clinical Excellence 2010). The National Institute is proposing that this goal should be reached in 2015 and has argued that legislation is now needed and that the United Kingdom should seek to convince other EU Member States to follow the United Kingdom in reducing salt intake.

In 2005, a global advocacy group World Action on Salt and Health (WASH) was established, with the United Kingdom Consensus Action on Salt and Health as its model and with the aim of reducing salt consumption worldwide. In 2011, WASH included participants from 80 countries (Webster et al. 2011). Pressure is exerted on multinational food companies to reduce the salt content of processed foods. In addition, WHO supports the development of national salt reduction strategies by establishing networks in partnership with regional organizations around the world (World Health Organization 2008). The European Union High Level Group on Diet, Physical Activity and Health has committed to implement the EU Salt Reduction Framework, which aims to reduce overall salt consumption by a minimum of 16% relative to levels in 2008 over four years (Tan 2009).

A recent report on salt reduction strategies around the world showed that, as of 2011, 32 national salt reduction initiatives are in progress, of which 19 are found in Europe (Webster et al. 2011). Most countries have set dietary intake targets for salt. Worldwide, only five countries have demonstrated some impact with their salt reduction initiatives, namely Finland, France, Ireland, Japan and the United Kingdom. Taken together, the lessons learned from the United Kingdom salt reduction strategy have been that it should be led by governments, be supported by convincing evidence on health effects and costs, involve reformulation of foods in collaboration with the food industry with realistic targets, include compulsory labelling of salt content, have intake targets and include media campaigns (Webster et al. 2011). Non-governmental organizations play an important role for advocacy and for placing and keeping the issue on the political agenda. The United Kingdom provides an example of how voluntary action can make some progress, particularly if overseen by a governmental body such as the Food Standards Agency, but also shows that legislation will often be necessary.

Trends in risk factors and health outcomes in Europe

After these three case studies, we will return to the picture in Europe as a whole and assess trends in nutrition-related risk factors and health outcomes. Over the past few decades, trends in the prevalence of nutrition-related risk factors for cardiovascular diseases in Europe have been mixed. To the extent that trends were favourable, they may have contributed to the decline in deaths from ischaemic heart disease. Yet, for most countries, it is unclear to what extent these changes reflect the implementation of food and nutrition policies or whether they are the result of other processes in society, such as a more liberal market approach, marketing and advertising, and globalization of trade. It is evident that changes in the food system, driven by economic and social factors, have an impact on food supply and demand, leading to both positive and negative changes in health outcomes.

For some nutrition-related risk factors, the situation has improved, but for others the situation has remained stable or even become worse. Time trend data on salt consumption in Europe are unavailable, but most European countries have now started to collect salt intake data systematically in the context of implementing the EU Salt Reduction Framework initiatives (European Commission 2009). Although most national policy initiatives to reduce salt intake are relatively recent, some of these declines in intake may reflect the impact of salt reduction policies, as in the case of Finland and the United Kingdom (see above). However, there is still a long way to go as most countries have only set dietary salt targets but have not yet implemented a comprehensive salt reduction strategy.

Total fat intake as a proportion of total energy intake has gone up in many parts of Europe, with the exception of north-western Europe where it has been stable. In Finland and other Nordic countries, the balance between dietary polyunsaturated and saturated fat has increased, resulting in a better fat quality of the diet. It is well documented that a higher dietary ratio of polyunsaturated to saturated fats is associated with a lower blood cholesterol and also has other heart protective effects (Hu and Willett 2002). Nutrition recommendations in most European countries include increasing the dietary polyunsaturated to saturated fats ratio; this has been proposed to have caused a decline in ischaemic heart disease mortality in Poland after 1991 (Zatonski and Willett 2005).

Another favourable trend is seen in fruit and vegetable consumption in many countries (Fig. 4.2). Fruit and vegetable consumption has gradually increased in western Europe, and even in central and eastern Europe, where consumption levels used to be low during the communist regimes, recent trends in many, but not all, countries have been favourable. To what extent this reflects shifts in consumer preferences based on health promotion efforts or broader economic and cultural changes is unclear.

However, trends in overweight and obesity are unfavourable, and the prevalence of diet-related non-communicable diseases such as diabetes type 2 is rising everywhere (Elmadfa 2009), partly as a result of an increasing overall supply of dietary energy (Food and Agriculture Organization 2012) and more sedentary lifestyles.

In summary, therefore, despite some favourable trends, the current situation is far from satisfactory, as shown in a recent report that described the nutrition

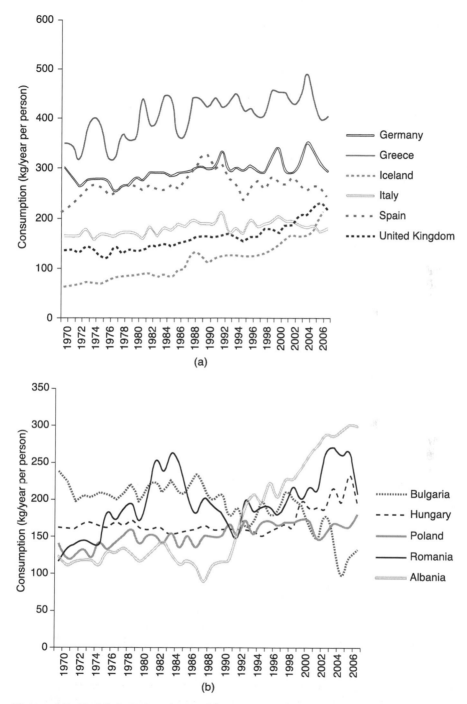

Figure 4.2 Trends in fruit and vegetable consumption in north-western (a) and central and eastern (b) Europe, 1970–2009

Source: WHO Regional Office for Europe 2012

situation in 21 EU Member States (Elmadfa 2009). Fat accounted for between 28.4 and 45.0% of total energy intake in men and between 29.9 and 47.2% in women. Therefore, in the majority of the participating countries, fat intake was above the maximum level recommended by WHO (30% of total energy intake). Furthermore, intake of saturated fatty acids was, in general, above the recommended level (<10% of total energy intake) and the proportion of polyunsaturated fatty acids in total energy intake was below the recommended intake range (6–11%) in most of the participating countries. Total energy intakes varied between 8.5 and 13.9 MJ in men and between 6.3 and 11.4 MJ in women, which is slightly below reference values and partly explained by under-reporting of food intake. In view of the high prevalence of overweight and obesity in adults, it can be assumed that most adults do not balance their energy intake with an appropriate amount of energy expenditure in the form of physical activity, as 41% of adults do not engage in any moderate physical activity in a typical week (European Commission 2006). In addition, there are large and persisting social inequalities in dietary intake, with lower socioeconomic groups consuming less-healthy diets, according to national and international recommendations, compared with groups with higher education and income (WHO Regional Office for Europe 2006b).

Even so, trends in mortality from ischaemic heart disease have been favourable over the last decades, at least in western Europe (Fig. 4.3). Some of this decline in mortality results from the favourable trends in nutrition-related health risks mentioned above. While many studies have tried to disentangle the causes of this decline for single countries, studies encompassing a broader range of European countries are scarce. The MONICA study included data from 16 European countries and showed that, on average, two-thirds of the decline in ischaemic heart disease mortality between the mid-1980s and mid-1990s in these countries was a result of declines in event rates, and one-third was from a decline in case fatality (Tunstall-Pedoe et al. 1999). The decline in event rates could partly be explained by changes in conventional risk factors, with the decline in smoking coming out as the most important contributor, particularly among men. Declines in blood pressure and cholesterol also made a contribution, while rising rates of over-weight and obesity would have a negative effect (Kuulasmaa et al. 2000).

Similar results were found in single-country studies, but these are available for a small number of countries only and show significant intercountry differences. In England and Wales, 60% of the decline in ischaemic heart disease mortality between 1981 and 2000 was explained by risk factor trends, mainly the decline in smoking but with additional contributions of declines in blood pressure (10%) and cholesterol (10%) (Unal et al. 2005). In Finland, risk factor trends explained a similar proportion of the reduction in ischaemic heart disease mortality, but here declines in cholesterol were the most important contributor (40%)(Laatikainen et al. 2005), perhaps reflecting the success of Finnish health policy over the last decades (see above).

A particularly detailed analysis has been undertaken of changes in ischaemic heart disease in Poland between 1991 and 2005 (Bandosz et al. 2012). This study found that about 37% of the decrease was attributable to better treatment and about 54% to changes in risk factors, mainly reductions in total cholesterol concentration (39%) and an increase in leisure time physical activity (10%).

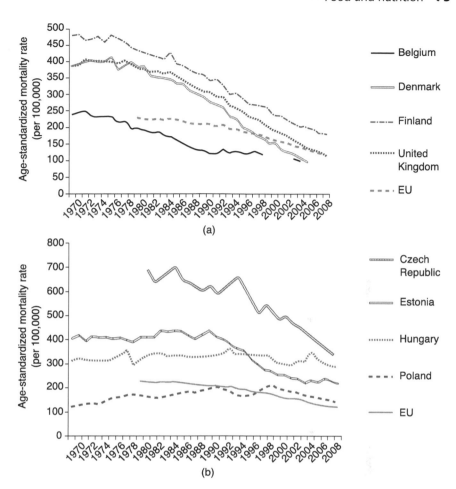

Figure 4.3   Male mortality from ischaemic heart disease in selected north-western (a) and central and eastern (b) European countries

Source: WHO Regional Office for Europe 2012

However, these were partially offset by increases in body mass index (~4%) and prevalence of diabetes (~2%). Changes in some of the risk factors have been ascribed to the abolition of government subsidies on animal products and the increased supply of fruits and vegetables following the opening up of the Polish food market after system changes occurring around 1990 (Zatonski et al. 2008).

Discussion and conclusions

Favourable changes in population diets have been reported in many countries in Europe since the 1970s. However, on the basis of the data presented here it is not possible to relate these changes directly to food and nutrition policies. Furthermore, some of the observed reduction in ischemic heart disease mortality was probably the result of changes in other risk factors such as smoking, in physical activity or in health promotion approaches in primary care delivery; there may also be effects of wider determinants of health such as changes in the economy, living conditions, gender roles, or environmental and ethical reasons. Another aspect that has to be taken into consideration in terms of evaluating the effectiveness of food and nutrition policies is their stage of development and degree of implementation, which we do not currently know much about. It is likely that the 2003 United Kingdom salt reduction strategy has yet to reach its full preventive potential in the population as complete implementation has not yet been achieved.

The examples presented here suggest that the following factors are of crucial importance for policy effectiveness.

1. Key decision-makers recognize that a nutritional problem exists and requires governmental attention.
2. The scientific evidence to support policy options and/or intervention is convincing.
3. All levels of government are involved in policy development and implementation (i.e. national, regional, local).
4. Actors from multiple sectors of society are engaged and work for common goals (e.g. public health, food industry, health care, media).
5. Long-term monitoring and surveillance is secured.

In the case studies from Finland, the United Kingdom and Denmark, these factors were fully or partially fulfilled. In contrast, the iodine story shows that key decision-makers, in spite of convincing evidence, have not yet taken forward the informed policy options, even though reports of negative effects of iodine deficiency on child development and behaviour keep coming from Europe (Costeira et al. 2011; Vanderpump et al. 2011).

After the eradication of hunger, oversupply of food, particularly in the form of fat and sugar, has led to new public health challenges; consequently, the need for evidence-based policy options is crucial. Commercial interests are much stronger than ever before and national governments have to take globalization of markets and rising food prices worldwide into consideration when developing their food and nutrition policies. Foods are crossing borders at an increasing rate, emphasizing the need for international agreements on food components such as salt and TFAs. A first step towards achieving a goal of better nutritional health would be to work for policy coherence, so that all policies should promote health goals or should at least be neutral in their effect on health and include a health impact assessment. Policies such as the EU Common Agricultural Policy (Elinder 2005; Lock and McKee 2005) still have a long way to go in supporting healthy eating habits.

Given the potential for a large part of the population in Europe to improve their diet and bring it closer to national and international recommendations, there is much scope for health gain in Europe. We hope that increased comparative studies, coupled with support from international agencies, will guide countries to the development and implementation of more effective food and nutrition policies. Monitoring progress on a continuous basis with feedback of results is an important element in this process as shown in policies concerning tobacco and alcohol.

Appendix

Table 4.A1 outlines food and nutrition policies in the EU Member States.

Table 4.A1 General and specific food or nutrition policies[a]

Country	Food/nutrition policy or action plan		Trans-fat strategy/policy	Salt strategy/policy	Iodinization of salt
	General	Fiscal measures			
Austria	*National Nutrition Action Plan 2011*[1]		*Trans Fat Regulation, 2009*[2]	Salt reduction plan included in the *National Nutrition Action Plan, 2011* Dietary salt target	Included in the *National Nutrition Action Plan, 2011* Auditing
Belgium	*Action Plan on Nutrition and Physical Activity 2009–2015*[3] Flemish Region *National Plan on Nutrition and Health 2005–2010*[4]			*Salt Strategy, Stop Salt:*[5] the food industry, distribution sector, restaurants and catering school sector adopted self-regulatory measures to be evaluated in 2012 by a taskforce led by the Federal Public Service of Health, Safety of the Food Chain and Environment Dietary salt target[6]	
Bulgaria	*National Food and Nutrition Action Plan 2005–2010*[7]			Included in the *National Food and Nutrition Action Plan 2005–2010* The 2007 *National Salt Initiative* set a target for consumption of 5 g/day. In 2009, an ordinance was established to reduce salt content of foods in school canteens. For 2011–2012, an updated ordinance includes healthy nutrition and salt reduction in kindergarten school canteens Dietary salt target	Included in the *National Food and Nutrition Action Plan 2005–2010*

(continued)

Table 4.A1 General and specific food or nutrition policies[a] (*continued*)

Country	Food/nutrition policy or action plan		Trans-fat strategy/ policy	Salt strategy/policy	Iodinization of salt
	General	*Fiscal measures*			
Cyprus	*National Nutrition Action Plan*[8]			Dietary salt target	
Czech Republic	*Food Safety and Nutrition Strategy for 2010–2013*[9]				
Denmark	*National Action Plan against Obesity: Recommendations and Perspectives*	Taxes on confectionary, soft drinks and saturated fat	*Trans-fat legislation*[12]	A strategy to reduce population salt intake was adopted for 2011–2012 by a partnership consisting of the Food Administration, DI Food, Agriculture & Food, Danish Chamber of Commerce, Heart Association, Consumer Council, Cancer Society, Association of Clinical Dieticians, Diabetes Association and Diet and Nutrition Association	
	Nordic Plan of Action on Better Health and Quality of Life through Diet and Physical Activity[10]			Dietary salt target	
	Agreement between the government and the Danish People's Party on a package of policies on growth, climate change and lower taxes[11]				

Country	Policy			
Estonia	*National Health Plan 2009–2020*[13] *The National Strategy for the Prevention of Cardiovascular Diseases 2005–2020*[14]		Included in the *National Strategy for the Prevention of Cardiovascular Diseases 2005–2020*	Included in the *National Health Plan 2009–2020* and in the *National Strategy for the Prevention of Cardiovascular Diseases 2005–2020*
Finland	*Nutrition in Finland*[15] *Nordic Plan of Action on Better Health and Quality of Life through Diet and Physical Activity*[10]	A tax of €0.95/kg on confectionery		*Nutrition in Finland*: guidelines on how to include nutritional criteria (such as salt) in food service procurements were implemented in late 2009 Dietary salt target
France	*Second National Nutrition and Health Programme 2006–2010: Actions and Measures*[16]	A tax on 'soft drinks containing sugar' through an increase of the *droit d'accise*: from €0.58/hl to €3.55/hl (this would represent approximately 1 cent on a 33 cl drink)		Included in *Second National Nutrition and Health Programme 2006–2010* Dietary salt target
Germany	*IN FORM: Germany's Initiative for a Healthy Nutrition and More Physical Activity*[17]			

(continued)

Table 4.A1 General and specific food or nutrition policies[a] (continued)

Country	Food/nutrition policy or action plan		Trans-fat strategy/ policy	Salt strategy/policy	Iodinization of salt
	General	Fiscal measures			
Greece	Action Plan for Implementation of the National Nutrition Policy National Action Plan for Nutrition and Eating Disorders 2008–2012[18]			Mentioned in the Action Plan for Implementation of the National Nutrition Policy	
Hungary	Hungarian National Nutrition Action Plan 2010–2013[19]	Act CIII of 2011 on the Public Health Product Tax		Included in the Hungarian National Nutrition Action Plan 2010–2013 Dietary salt target	Included in the 'Johan Bela' National Programme for the Decade of Health, 2003[20]
Ireland	Changing Cardiovascular Health, National Cardiovascular Health Policy 2010–2019[21]		Included in Changing Cardiovascular Health, National Cardiovascular Health Policy 2010–2019	Included in Changing Cardiovascular Health, National Cardiovascular Health Policy 2010–2019 Dietary salt target	
Italy	Gaining Health[22]		Included in Gaining Health	Mentioned in Gaining Health	

Country	Policy document	Increased taxes on food high in fat, salt and sugar nutrients (other than sodium)	Salt-specific programme	Dietary salt target	Trans fat initiative
Latvia	*Healthy Nutrition (2003–2013)*[23]		Salt-specific programme[6]	Dietary salt target	
Lithuania	The state strategy on the *Non-communicable Disease Prevention Programme for the years 2008–2010*				
	National Food and Nutrition Strategy and its Implementation Plan for 2003–2010[24]			Dietary salt target	
Luxembourg	*Action Plan for the Promotion of Healthy Nutrition and Physical Activity, 2007*[25]				
Malta	*A Strategy for the Prevention and Control of Noncommunicable Disease in Malta, 2010*[26]		Mentioned in *A Strategy for the Prevention and Control of Noncommunicable Disease in Malta*, 2010		
The Netherlands	*Health Close By: National Health Policy Note 2011–2015*[27]			Dietary salt target	*Trans* fat initiative
	Covenant Healthy Weight 2010–2014[28]				

Table 4.A1 General and specific food or nutrition policies[a] (continued)

Country	Food/nutrition policy or action plan		Trans-fat strategy/ policy	Salt strategy/policy	Iodinization of salt
	General	Fiscal measures			
Poland	National Prevention Programme of Overweight, Obesity and Non-communicable Diseases through Diet and Physical Activity Improvement 2007–2011[29]			Included in the National Prevention Programme of Overweight, Obesity and Non-communicable Diseases through Diet and Physical Activity Improvement 2007–2011 and the National Health Programme 2007–2015	
	National Health Programme 2007–2015[30]			Dietary salt target	
Portugal	National Platform against Obesity[31]			Included in National Platform against Obesity	
Romania	Ministerial Order 687 of 10.04.2008 for Establishing the National Committee for Food and Nutrition[32]			Dietary salt target	
Slovakia	National Obesity Prevention Programme[33]			Mentioned in the National Obesity Prevention Programme	

Slovenia	*National Programme of Food and Nutrition Policy 2005–2010*[34]		Included in the *National Programme of Food and Nutrition Policy 2005–2010*[6] Salt-specific programme[6] Dietary salt target
Spain	*Strategy for Nutrition, Physical Activity and Prevention of Obesity (NAOS)*[35]	Mentioned in the *Strategy for Nutrition, Physical Activity and Prevention of Obesity (NAOS)*	Included in the *Strategy for Nutrition, Physical Activity and Prevention of Obesity (NAOS)* Dietary salt target
Sweden	*Healthy Dietary Habits and Increased Physical Activity, the Basis for an Action Plan*[36] Sweden's national public health policy *Nordic Plan of Action on Better Health and Quality of Life through Diet and Physical Activity*[10]		Mentioned in *Healthy Dietary Habits and Increased Physical Activity, the Basis for an Action Plan* Dietary salt target
United Kingdom: England	*Healthy Lives, Healthy People: Our Strategy for Public Health in England*[37]		National salt reduction strategy 2003[6] National salt target

(continued)

Table 4.A1 General and specific food or nutrition policies[a] *(continued)*

Country	Food/nutrition policy or action plan		Trans-fat strategy/ policy	Salt strategy/policy	Iodinization of salt
	General	*Fiscal measures*			
United Kingdom: Scotland	*Preventing Overweight and Obesity in Scotland: A Route Map Towards Healthy Weight 2010–2030*[39]			National salt reduction strategy 2003[6] Included in *Preventing Overweight and Obesity in Scotland: A Route Map Towards Healthy Weight 2010–2030*	
United Kingdom: Northern Ireland	*Promoting Good Nutrition: Strategy for Good Nutritional Care for Adults in all Care Settings in Northern Ireland 2011–2016*[40]			National salt reduction strategy 2003[6]	
United Kingdom: Wales	*All Wales Obesity Pathway*[41]			National salt reduction strategy 2003[6]	

[a]Data included in the table are self-reported and included in the report *Monitoring Progress on Improving Nutrition and Physical Activity and Preventing Obesity in the European Union (EU)* (Bollars 2012); therefore, only EU countries are included.

Sources: [1]Austrian Federal Ministry of Health 2011; [2]Austrian Federal Ministry of Health 2009; [3]Flemish Institute for Health Promotion and Disease Prevention 2008; [4]Belgium Federal Public Service Health, Food Chain and Environment 2005; [5]Belgium Federal Public Service Health, Food Chain and Environment 2009; [6]Webster et al. 2011; [7]Bulgarian Council of Ministers 2005; [8]Cypriot Ministry of Health 2007; [9]Government of the Czech Republic 2010; [10]Nordic Council of Ministers 2006; [11]Danish Ministry of Finance 2009; [12]L'Abbe et al. 2009; [13]Estonian Ministry of Social Affairs 2008; [14]National Institute for Health Development 2003; [15]National Public Health Institute 2006; [16]French Ministry of Health and Solidarity 2006; [17]German Ministry of Food, Agriculture and Consumer Protection and Ministry of Health 2008; [18]Greek Ministry of Health and Social Welfare 2008; [19]Hungarian Ministry of Health, Social and Family Affairs 2010; [20]Hungarian Ministry of Health 2003; [21]Irish Department of Health and Children, Minister for Health and Children 2010; [22]Italian Ministry of Health 2007; [23]Latvian Cabinet of Ministers 2003; [24]Government of Lithuania 2003; [25]Luxembourg Ministry of Health 2007; [26]Maltese Ministry for Health, the Elderly and Community Care 2010; [27]Dutch Ministry of Health, Welfare and Sport 2011; [28]Dutch Ministry of Health, Welfare and Sport 2009; [29]Polish Ministry of Health 2006; [30]Portuguese Ministry of Health 2005; [32]Romania Ministry of Health 2008; [33]Slovakia Ministry of Health 2008; [34]Slovenian Ministry of Health 2005; [35]Spanish Ministry of Health and Consumer Affairs 2005; [36]Swedish National Institute of Public Health 2005; [37]Department of Health 2010; [38]Department of Health 2011; [39]Scottish Government, 2010; [40]Department of Health, Social Services and Public Safety 2010; [41]Welsh Assembly Government 2010.

References

Andersson, M., de Benoist, B., Darnton-Hill, I. and Delange, F. (2007) *Iodine deficiency in Europe: a continuing public health problem*. Geneva: World Health Organization.

Andersson, M., de Benoist, B. and Rogers, L. (2010) Epidemiology of iodine deficiency: salt iodisation and iodine status, *Best Practice and Research in Clinical and Endocrinology Metabolism*, 24(1):1–11.

Astrup, A. (2006) The *trans* fatty acid story in Denmark, *Atherosclerosis Supplement*, 7(2):43–6.

Austrian Federal Ministry of Health (2009) Verordnung des Bundesministers für Gesundheit über den Gehalt an trans-Fettsäuren in Lebensmitteln (Trans-Fettsäuren-Verordnung) [Regulation of the Ministry of Health on the Content of Trans Fatty Acids in Foods (Trans Fat Regulation)]. *Federal Law Journal of the Republic of Austria*, 20 August.

Austrian Federal Ministry of Health (2011) *Nationaler Aktionsplan Ernährung 2011 [National Nutrition Action Plan 2011]*. Vienna: Federal Ministry of Health, http://www.bmg.gv.at/home/Schwerpunkte/Ernaehrung (accessed 15 February 2012).

Bandosz, P., O'Flaherty, M., Drygas, W. et al. (2012) Decline in mortality from coronary heart disease in Poland after socioeconomic transformation: modelling study, *British Medical Journal*, 344:d8136.

Belgium Federal Public Service Health, Food Chain and Environment (2005) *Plan National Nutrition Santé 2005–2010 [National Plan on Nutrition and Health 2005–2010]*. Brussels: Belgium Federal Public Service Health, Food Chain and Environment, http://www.health.fgov.be/internet2Prd/groups/public/@public/@dg4/@consumerproducts/documents/ie2divers/19061891.pdf (accessed 16 February 2012).

Belgium Federal Public Service Health, Food Chain and Environment (2009) *Salt Strategy, Stop Salt*. Brussels: Belgium Federal Public Service Health, Food Chain and Environment, http://www.health.belgium.be/eportal/Myhealth/Healthylife/Food/FoodandHealth Plan2/SALT/Menu/index.htm (accessed 10 July 2012).

de Benoist, B., McLean, E., Andersson, M. and Rogers, L. (2008) Iodine deficiency in 2007: global progress since 2003, *Food and Nutrition Bulletin* 29(3):195–202.

Bollars, C. (2011) *Review of Food and Nutrition Policy Development and Legislation in the European Union (EU)*. Copenhagen: WHO Regional Office for Europe.

Brunner, E.J., Rees, K., Ward, K., Burke, M. and Thorogood, M. (2007) Dietary advice for reducing cardiovascular risk, *Cochrane Database of Systematic Reviews*, (4):CD002128.

Bulgarian Council of Ministers (2005) *National Food and Nutrition Action Plan 2005– 2010*. Sofia: Bulgarian Council of Ministers, http://www.seefsnp.org.rs/documents/bulgaria/Bul_FNAP.pdf (accessed 16 February 2012).

Costeira, M.J., Oliveira, P., Santos, N.C. et al. (2011) Psychomotor development of children from an iodine-deficient region, *Journal of Pediatrics*,159(3):447–53.

Cutler, J.A., Follmann, D. and Allender, P.S. (1997) Randomized trials of sodium reduction: an overview, *American Journal of Clinical Nutrition*, 65(2 Suppl):643S–51S.

Cypriot Ministry of Health (2007) *National Nutrition Action Plan*. Nicosia: Ministry of Health.

Danish Ministry of Finance (2009) *Aftale mellem regeringen og Dansk Folkeparti om forårspakke 2.0: vækst, klima, lavere skat [Agreement between the Government and the Danish People's Party about the Spring Package 2.0: Growth, Climate and Lower Taxes]*. Copenhagen: Ministry of Finance, http://www.fm.dk/Publikationer/2009/~/media/Files/Publikationer/2009/aftale%20forarspakke%202.0/aftale_forarspakke_2%200_web.ashx (accessed 15 February 2012).

Delange, F. (2002) Iodine deficiency in Europe and its consequences: an update, *European Journal of Nuclear Medical and Molecular Imaging* 29(suppl 2):S404–16.

Department of Health (2010) *Healthy Lives, Healthy People: Our Strategy for Public Health in England.* London: Department of Health, http://www.dh.gov.uk/prod_consum_dh/groups/dh_digitalassets/documents/digitalasset/dh_127424.pdf (accessed 19 February 2012).

Department of Health (2011) *Healthy Lives, Healthy People: A Call to Action on Obesity in England.* London: Department of Health, http://www.dh.gov.uk/prod_consum_dh/groups/dh_digitalassets/documents/digitalasset/dh_130487.pdf (accessed 19 February 2012).

Department of Health, Social Services and Public Safety (2010) *Promoting Good Nutrition: Strategy for Good Nutritional Care for Adults in all Care Settings in Northern Ireland 2011–2016.* Belfast: Department of Health, Social Services and Public Safety, http://www.dhsspsni.gov.uk/promoting_good_nutrition.pdf (accessed 19 February 2012).

Dutch Ministry of Health, Welfare and Sport (2009) *Convenant Gezond Gewicht 2010–2014 [Covenant Healthy Weight 2010–2014].* The Hague: Ministry of Health, Welfare and Sport, http://www.convenantgezondgewicht.nl/download/39/koepelconvenant_def_16112009.pdf (accessed 19 February 2012).

Dutch Ministry of Health, Welfare and Sport (2011) *Landelijke nota Gezondheidsbeleid: Gezondheid dichtbij 2011–2015 [Health Close By: National Health Policy Note 2011–2015].* The Hague: Ministry of Health, Welfare and Sport, http://www.rijksoverheid.nl/documenten-en-publicaties/notas/2011/05/25/landelijke-nota-gezondheidsbeleid.html (accessed 19 February 2012).

Elinder, L.S. (2005) Obesity, hunger, and agriculture: the damaging role of subsidies, *British Medical Journal*, 331(7528):1333–6.

Elliott, P., Stamler, J., Nichols, R. et al. (1996) Intersalt revisited: further analyses of 24 hour sodium excretion and blood pressure within and across populations. Intersalt Cooperative Research Group, *British Medical Journal*, 312(7041):1249–53.

Elmadfa, I. (2009) *European Nutrition and Health Report 2009.* Basel: Karger.

Estonian Ministry of Social Affairs (2008) *National Health Plan 2009–2020.* Tallinn: Ministry of Social Affairs, http://www.sm.ee/fileadmin/meedia/Dokumendid/Tervisevaldkond/Rahvatervis/RTA/National_Health_Plan_20092010.pdf (accessed 16 February 2012).

European Commission (2006) *Special Eurobarometer, Health and Food.* Brussels: European Commission.

European Commission (2009) *National Salt Initiatives: Implementing the EU Framework for Salt Reduction Initiatives.* Brussels: European Commission.

Flemish Institute for Health Promotion and Disease Prevention (2008) *Actie Plan Voeding en Beweging 2009–2015 [Action Plan on Nutrition and Physical Activity 2009–2015].* Brussels: Flemish Institute for Health Promotion and Disease Prevention, http://www.zorg-en-gezondheid.be/WorkArea/linkit.aspx?LinkIdentifier=id&ItemID=21484 (accessed 15 February 2012).

Food and Agriculture Organization (2012) *Food Balance Sheets.* Rome: Food and Agriculture Organization.

Foods Standards Agency (2010) Salt reduction targets. London, Foods Standards Agency, http://collections.europarchive.org/tna/20100927130941/http://food.gov.uk/healthier eating/salt/saltreduction (accessed 1 November 2012).

French Ministry of Health and Solidarity (2006) *Second National Nutrition and Health Programme 2006–2010: Actions and Measures.* Paris: Ministry of Health and Solidarity, http://www.sante.gouv.fr/IMG/pdf/pnns2.pdf (accessed 16 February 2012).

German Ministry of Food, Agriculture and Consumer Protection and Ministry of Health (2008) *IN FORM: Deutschlands Initiative für gesunde Ernährung und mehr Bewegung. Nationaler Aktionsplan zur Prävention von Fehlernährung, Bewegungsmangel, Übergewicht und damit zusammenhängenden Krankheiten [IN FORM: Germany's Initiative for a Healthy Nutrition and More Physical Activity]*. Berlin: Ministry of Food, Agriculture and Consumer Protection and Ministry of Health, http://www.bmelv.de/SharedDocs/Downloads/Broschueren/AktionsplanINFORM.pdf;jsessionid=AE8F3E87645E85 C363D60A621AA0FFA4.2_cid163?__blob=publicationFile (accessed 16 February 2012).

Government of Lithuania (2003) *Del Valstybines Maisto ir Mitybos Strategijos ir Jos Įgyvendinimo Priemonių 2003–2010 metų Plano Patvirtinimo [National Food and Nutrition Strategy and its Implementation Plan for 2003–2010]*. Vilnius: Government of Lithuania, http://www3.lrs.lt/pls/inter3/dokpaieska.showdoc_bin?p_id=219949 (accessed 17 February 2012).

Government of the Czech Republic (2010) *Food Safety and Nutrition Strategy for 2010– 2013*. Prague: Government of the Czech Republic.

Greek Ministry of Health and Social Welfare (2008) *National Action Plan for Nutrition and Eating Disorders 2008–2012*. Athens: Ministry of Health and Social Welfare.

He, F.J. and MacGregor, G.A. (2009) A comprehensive review on salt and health and current experience of worldwide salt reduction programmes, *Journal of Human Hypertension*, 23(6):363–84.

Hetzel, B. (2004) An overview of the elimination of brain damage due to iodine deficiency, In B. Hetzel (ed.) *Towards the Global Elimination of Brain Damage due To Iodine Deficiency*. New Delhi: Oxford University Press, pp. 24–37.

Hooper, L., Bartlett, C., Davey, S.G. and Ebrahim, S. (2004) Advice to reduce dietary salt for prevention of cardiovascular disease, *Cochrane Database of Systematic Reviews*, (1):CD003656.

Hooper, L., Summerbell, C.D., Thompson, R. et al. (2011) Reduced or modified dietary fat for preventing cardiovascular disease, *Cochrane Database of Systematic Reviews*, (7):CD002137.

Hu, F.B. and Willett, W.C. (2002) Optimal diets for prevention of coronary heart disease, *Journal of the American Medical Association*, 288(20):2569–78.

Hulshof, K.F., van Erp-Baart, M.A., Anttolainen, M. et al. (1999) Intake of fatty acids in western Europe with emphasis on *trans* fatty acids: the TRANSFAIR Study, *European Journal of Clinical Nutrition*, 53(2):143–57.

Hungarian Ministry of Health (2003) *'Johan Bela' National Programme for the Decade of Health 2003*. Budapest: Ministry of Health, http://www.eum.hu/English/public-health-programme/national-public-health (accessed 10 July 2012).

Hungarian Ministry of Health, Social and Family Affairs (2010) *Magyarország Nemzeti Táplálkozáspolitikájának 2010–2013 [Hungarian National Nutrition Action Plan 2010– 2013]*. Budapest: Ministry of Health, Social and Family Affairs, http://www.oeti.hu/download/mntpcst_terv_101115y.pdf (accessed 17 February 2012).

Irish Department of Health and Children, Minister for Health and Children (2010) *Changing Cardiovascular Health, National Cardiovascular Health Policy, 2010–2019*. Dublin: Department of Health and Children, Minister for Health and Children, http://www.dohc.ie/publications/pdf/changing_cardiovascular_health.pdf?direct=1 (accessed 17 February 2012).

Italian Ministry of Health (2007) *Guadagnare Salute [Gaining Health]*. Rome: Ministry of Health, 2007, http://www.salute.gov.it/imgs/C_17_pubblicazioni_605_allegato.pdf (accessed 17 February 2012).

James, W.P., Ralph, A. and Bellizzi, M. (1997) Nutrition policies in western Europe: national policies in Belgium, the Netherlands, France, Ireland, and the United Kingdom, *Nutrition Reviews*, 55(11):S4–20.

Johns Hopkins Bloomberg School of Public Health (2012) *Food and Nutrition Policy*. Baltimore, MD: Johns Hopkins Bloomberg School of Public Health, http://ocw.jhsph.edu/courses/FoodNutritionPolicy/index.cfm (accessed 25 June 2012).

Katan, M.B. (2006) Regulation of *trans* fats: the gap, the Polder, and McDonald's French fries, *Atherosclerosis Supplement*, 7(2):63–6.

Keys, A., Menotti, A., Karvonen, M.J. et al. (1986) The diet and 15-year death rate in the seven countries study, *American Journal of Epidemiology*, 124(6):903–15.

Kuszewski, K., Goryński, P., Wojtniak, B. and Halik, R. (eds) (2007) *Narodowy Program Zdrowia na lata 2007–2015 [National Health Programme 2007–2015]*. Warsaw: Council of Ministers, http://www.mz.gov.pl/wwwfiles/ma_struktura/docs/zal_urm_npz_90_15052007p.pdf (accessed 19 February 2012).

Kuulasmaa, K., Tunstall-Pedoe, H., Dobson, A. et al. (2000) Estimation of contribution of changes in classic risk factors to trends in coronary-event rates across the WHO MONICA Project populations, *Lancet*, 355(9205):675–87.

Laatikainen, T., Critchley, J., Vartiainen, E. et al. (2005) Explaining the decline in coronary heart disease mortality in Finland between 1982 and 1997, *American Journal of Epidemiology*, 162(8):764–73.

L'Abbe, M.R., Stender, S., Skeaff, M., Ghafoorunissa and Tavella, M. (2009) Approaches to removing *trans* fats from the food supply in industrialized and developing countries, *European Journal of Clinical Nutrition*, 63:S50–67.

Latvian Cabinet of Ministers (2003) *Pamatnostādnes 'Veselāgs uzturs (2003–2013)' [Healthy Nutrition (2003–2013)]*. Riga: Cabinet of Ministers, http://polsis.mk.gov.lv/view.do?id=846 (accessed 17 February 2012).

League of Nations (1938) *Survey of National Nutrition Policies, 1937/38*. Geneva: League of Nations.

Leth, T., Jensen, H.G., Mikkelsen, A.Æ. and Bysted, A. (2006) The effect of the regulation on *trans* fatty acid content in Danish food, *Atherosclerosis Supplements*, 7(2):53–6.

Lock, K. and McKee, M. (2005) Will Europe's agricultural policy damage progress on cardiovascular disease? *British Medical Journal*, 331(7510):188–9.

Luxembourg Ministry of Health (2007) *Plan d'action pour la promotion de l'alimentation saine et de l'activité physique [Action Plan for the Promotion of Healthy Nutrition and Physical Activity]*. Luxembourg: Ministry of Health, http://www.sante.public.lu/fr/catalogue-publications/rester-bonne-sante/alimentation/plan-national-alimentation-saine-activite-physique/index.html (accessed 17 February 2012).

Maltese Ministry for Health, the Elderly and Community Care (2010) *A Strategy for the Prevention and Control of Noncommunicable Disease in Malta*. Valletta: Ministry for Health, the Elderly and Community Care, https://ehealth.gov.mt/download.aspx?id=4793 (accessed 17 February 2012).

Mente, A., de Koning, L., Shannon, H.S. and Anand, S.S. (2009) A systematic review of the evidence supporting a causal link between dietary factors and coronary heart disease, *Archives of Internal Medicine*, 169(7):659–69.

Micha, R. and Mozaffarian, D. (2008) *Trans* fatty acids: effects on cardiometabolic health and implications for policy, *Prostaglandins, Leukotrienes and Essential Fatty Acids*, 79(3–5):147–52.

Mozaffarian, D., Katan, M.B., Ascherio, A., Stampfer, M.J. and Willett, W.C. (2006) *Trans* fatty acids and cardiovascular disease, *New England Journal of Medicine*, 354(15):1601–13.

Mozaffarian, D., Aro, A. and Willett, W.C. (2009) Health effects of *trans*-fatty acids: experimental and observational evidence, *European Journal of Clinical Nutrition*, 63(suppl 2):S5–21.

National Institute for Health and Clinical Excellence (2010) *Prevention of Cardiovascular Disease at Population Level*. London: National Institute for Health and Clinical Excellence.

National Institute for Health Development (2003) *National Strategy for the Prevention of Cardiovascular Diseases 2005–2020*. Tallinn: National Institute for Health

Development, http://www.who.int/fctc/reporting/Estonia_annex3_CVD_strategy.pdf (accessed 10 July 2012).

National Public Health Institute (2006) *Nutrition in Finland*. Helsinki: National Public Health Institute, http://www.ktl.fi/attachments/english/health_monitoring_and_promotion/nutrition_in_finland/nutrition_in_finland_pdf.pdf (accessed 16 February 2012).

Nielsen, B.M., Nielsen, M.M., Jakobsen, M.U. et al. (2011) A cross-sectional study on *trans*-fatty acids and risk markers of CHD among middle-aged men representing a broad range of BMI, *British Journal of Nutrition*, 106(8):1245–52.

Nishida, C. and Uauy, R. (2009) WHO scientific update on health consequences of *trans* fatty acids: introduction, *European Journal of Clinical Nutrition*, 63(suppl 2): S1–4.

Nordic Council of Ministers (2006) *A Better Life Through Diet and Physical Activity: Nordic Plan of Action on Better Health and Quality of Life through Diet and Physical Activity*. Copenhagen: Nordic Council of Ministers, http://www.norden.org/en/nordic-council-of-ministers/councils-of-ministers/council-of-ministers-for-fisheries-and-aquaculture-agriculture-food-and-forestry-mr-fjls/nordic-plan-of-action-on-better-health-and-quality-of-life-through-diet-and-physical-activity (accessed 16 February 2012).

Pietinen, P., Lahti-Koski, M., Vartiainen, E. and Puska, P. (2001) Nutrition and cardiovascular disease in Finland since the early 1970s: a success story, *Journal of Nutrition Health Aging*, 5(3):150–4.

Polish Ministry of Health (2006) *Narodowy Program Zapobiegania Nadwadze I Otyłości Oraz Przewlekłym Chorobom Niezakaźnym Poprzez PopraWę Żywienia I Aktywności Fizycznej Na Lata 2007–2011 [National Prevention Programme of Overweight, Obesity and Non-communicable Diseases through Diet and Physical Activity Improvement 2007–2011]*. Warsaw: Ministry of Health, http://www.mz.gov.pl/wwwmz/index?mr=b3&ms=0&ml=pl&mi=0&mx=0&mt=&my=246&ma=9064 (accessed 19 February 2012).

Portuguese Ministry of Health (2005) *Plataforma contra à Obesidade [National Platform against Obesity]*. Lisbon: Ministry of Health, http://www.plataformacontraaobesidade.dgs.pt/PresentationLayer/conteudo.aspx?menuid=115&exmenuid=113&SelMenuId=115 (accessed 19 February 2012).

Prattala, R. (2003) Dietary changes in Finland: success stories and future challenges, *Appetite*, 41(3):245–9.

Puska, P. (2009) Fat and heart disease: yes we can make a change – the case of North Karelia (Finland), *Annals in Nutrition Metabolism*, 54(suppl 1):33–8.

Puska, P., Vartiainen, E., Tuomilehto, J., Salomaa, V. and Nissinen, A. (1998) Changes in premature deaths in Finland: successful long-term prevention of cardiovascular diseases, *Bulletin of the World Health Organization*, 76(4):419–25.

Rokx, C. (2003) Prospects for improving nutrition in Eastern Europe and Central Asia. Washington, DC: World Bank.

Romania Ministry of Health (2008) *Ministerial Order 687 of 10.04.2008 for Establishing the National Committee for Food and Nutrition*. Bucharest: Ministry of Health.

Scottish Government (2010) *Preventing Overweight and Obesity in Scotland: A Route Map Towards Healthy Weight 2010–2030*. Edinburgh: Scottish Government, http://www.scotland.gov.uk/Resource/Doc/302783/0094795.pdf (accessed 19 February 2012).

Slovakia Ministry of Health (2008) *Národný Program Prevencie Obezity [National Obesity Prevention Programme]*. Bratislava: Ministry of Health, http://www.uvzsr.sk/docs/info/podpora/Narodny_program_prevencie_obezity.pdf (accessed 19 February 2012).

Slovenian Ministry of Health (2005) *Food and Nutrition Action Plan for Slovenia 2005–2010: Summary of the Resolution on the National Programme of Food and Nutrition Policy 2005–2010*. Ljubljana: Ministry of Health, http://www.mz.gov.si/fileadmin/mz.gov.

si/pageuploads/javno_zdravje_09/Nacionalni_program_prehranske_politike_ang.pdf (accessed 19 February 2012).

Spanish Ministry of Health and Consumer Affairs (2005) *Estrategia para la Nutrición, Actividad Física y Prevención de la Obesidad (NAOS) [Strategy for Nutrition, Physical Activity and Prevention of Obesity (NAOS)]*. Madrid: Ministry of Health and Consumer Affairs, http://www.coposa.es/docs/pdf/Estrategia_NAOS2.pdf (accessed 19 February 2012).

Stender, S., Dyerberg, J., Bysted, A., Leth, T. and Astrup, A. (2006) A *trans* world journey, *Atherosclerosis Supplement*, 7(2):47–52.

Strazzullo, P., D'Elia, L., Kandala, N.B. and Cappuccio, F.P. (2009) Salt intake, stroke, and cardiovascular disease: meta-analysis of prospective studies, *British Medical Journal*, 339:b4567.

Swedish National Institute of Public Health (2005) *Healthy Dietary Habits and Increased Physical Activity, the Basis for an Action Plan*. Stockholm: National Institute of Public Health, http://www.fhi.se/PageFiles/4175/healthydietaryhabits physicalactivitysummary0502.pdf (accessed 19 February 2012).

Tan, A.S. (2009) A case study of the New York City *trans*-fat story for international application, *Journal of Public Health Policy*, 30(1):3–16.

Tunstall-Pedoe, H., Kuulasmaa, K., Mahonen, M. et al. (1999) Contribution of trends in survival and coronary-event rates to changes in coronary heart disease mortality: 10-year results from 37 WHO MONICA project populations. Monitoring trends and determinants in cardiovascular disease, *Lancet*, 353(9164):1547–57.

Unal, B., Critchley, J.A. and Capewell, S. (2005) Modelling the decline in coronary heart disease deaths in England and Wales, 1981–2000: comparing contributions from primary prevention and secondary prevention, *British Medical Journal*, 331(7517):614.

Vanderpump, M.P.J., Lazarus, J.H., Smyth, P.P. et al. (2011) Iodine status of UK schoolgirls: a cross-sectional survey, *Lancet*, 377(9782):2007–12.

Vartiainen, E., Puska, P., Jousilahti, P. et al. (1994) Twenty-year trends in coronary risk factors in north Karelia and in other areas of Finland, *International Journal of Epidemiology*, 23(3):495–504.

Vitti, P., Delange, F., Pinchera, A., Zimmermann, M. and Dunn, J.T. (2003) Europe is iodine deficient, *Lancet*, 361(9364):1226.

Waters, E., de Silva-Sanigorski, A., Hall, B.J. et al. (2011) Interventions for preventing obesity in children, *Cochrane Database of Systematic Reviews*, (12):CD001871.

Webster, J.L., Dunford, E.K., Hawkes, C. and Neal, B.C. (2011) Salt reduction initiatives around the world, *Journal of Hypertension*, 29(6):1043–50.

Welsh Assembly Government (2010) *All Wales Obesity Pathway*. Cardiff: Welsh Assembly Government, http://wales.gov.uk/docs/phhs/publications/100824obesityen.doc (accessed 19 February 2012).

WHO Regional Office for Europe (2000) *The First Action Plan for Food and Nutrition Policy, WHO European Region, 2000–2005*. Copenhagen: WHO Regional Office for Europe.

WHO Regional Office for Europe (2006a) *Addressing the Socioeconomic Determinants of Healthy Eating and Physical Activity Levels Among Adolescents*. Copenhagen: WHO Regional Office for Europe.

WHO Regional Office for Europe (2006b) *European Charter on Counteracting Obesity*. Copenhagen: WHO Regional Office for Europe.

WHO Regional Office for Europe (2008) *WHO European Action Plan for Food and Nutrition Policy 2007–2012*. Copenhagen: WHO Regional Office for Europe.

WHO Regional Office for Europe (2012) *European Health for All Database (HFA-DB)*. Copenhagen: WHO Regional Office for Europe, http://data.euro.who.int/hfadb/ (accessed 4 June 2012).

World Health Organization (2004) *Global Strategy on Diet, Physical Activity and Health*. Geneva: World Health Organization.

World Health Organization (2007) *Iodine Deficiency in Europe. A Continuing Public Health Problem*. Geneva: World Health Organization.

World Health Organization (2008) *2008–2013 Action Plan for the Global Strategy for the Prevention and Control of Noncommunicable Diseases: Prevent and Control Cardiovascular Diseases, Cancers, Chronic Respiratory Diseases and Diabetes*. Geneva: World Health Organization.

World Health Organization (2009) *Global Health Risks: Mortality and Burden of Disease Attributable to Selected Major Risks*. Geneva: World Health Organization.

Zatonski, W., Campos, H. and Willett, W. (2008) Rapid declines in coronary heart disease mortality in Eastern Europe are associated with increased consumption of oils rich in alpha-linolenic acid, *European Journal of Epidemiology*, 23(1):3–10.

Zatonski, W.A. and Willett, W. (2005) Changes in dietary fat and declining coronary heart disease in Poland: population based study, *British Medical Journal*, 331(7510):187–8.

Zimmermann, M.B. and Andersson, M. (2011) Prevalence of iodine deficiency in Europe in 2010, *Annals in Endocrinology (Paris)*, 72(2):164–6.

chapter five

Fertility, pregnancy and childbirth

Jennifer Zeitlin, Béatrice Blondel and Babak Khoshnood

Introduction

In Europe, maternal and perinatal mortality and morbidity have declined markedly since the 1970s. Fertility, pregnancy and childbirth, however, remain important areas for public health policy. Although poor outcomes are increasingly rare, the population at risk is numerous. There are over 8,354,000 pregnant women and newborns each year in the 43 European countries covered by this book. For EU Member States, the annual number of births exceeds 5,300,000. Maternal and perinatal mortality and morbidity affect young people, and their consequences are long standing. For example, it is estimated that 8 out of 1000 children suffer from severe sensory or cognitive impairments (Cans et al. 2003) and that half of these impairments have their origin in complications of the perinatal period (Expertise Collective INSERM 2004). Perinatal health has also been linked to risks of chronic diseases, such as metabolic syndrome, in adulthood (Barker 1998). This burden of disease falls disproportionately on socially disadvantaged women and babies (Kramer et al. 2000) and contributes to lifelong health inequalities.

The declines in maternal and perinatal mortality and morbidity of the last decades have been partly the result of improvements in overall standards of living and partly from advances in the management of pregnancy and in care of high-risk infants, notably in neonatal intensive care. Advances in medical care were highly successful in improving survival among high-risk babies, and more improvement has occurred in the survival of high-risk babies (i.e. in birth weight or gestational age-specific mortality) than in the reduction of the incidence of high-risk births (Koupilova et al. 1998). In fact, in many countries, preterm birth rates and rates of low birth weight have increased (Goldenberg et al. 2008). Declines in stillbirths have also lagged behind those for neonatal and infant deaths; the reduction of stillbirths will require tackling population risk factors such as smoking and obesity (Flenady et al. 2011).

This chapter will explore advances in the prevention of problems in fertility, pregnancy and childbirth. For each domain a few areas have been selected for which there is an adequate evidence base linking policy initiatives with better health outcomes, and for which data are available that allow a comparison of successes and failures between European countries.

Fertility

Access to contraception and safe abortion

Providing women with the means to control their own fertility is an effective strategy for improving maternal and child health. Most directly, providing safe abortion services reduces maternal deaths. Unsafe abortion is a leading cause of maternal death in countries where abortions are not legal or where abortion services are inadequate. The Romanian experience is vivid testimony of this fact, as detailed in Box 5.1 and Fig. 5.1.

Most European countries allow terminations of pregnancy, with some exceptions (Table 5.1). Rates vary within Europe between the low rates (<8 per 1000 women aged 15–45 years) of Germany, Greece, Portugal, the Netherlands and Slovakia, and the high rates (>20 per 1000) of Bulgaria, Estonia and Romania. For women under 20 years of age, rates per 1000 women are high in Bulgaria (17.5), Estonia (24.1), Hungary (17.8), Romania (20.5), Sweden (24.4) and the United Kingdom (23.8). While abortion rates are lower in Europe than in North America and Oceania, there are countries in Europe where rates are substantially higher for all women and teens, suggesting an unmet need for contraceptive services. Countries with more restrictive access to early abortion services do not report lower rates than those with more liberal access (Gissler et al. 2012).

Most abortions in western, southern and northern Europe are safe, but unsafe abortions remain a public health concern in some countries of eastern Europe (Sedgh et al. 2012) (Table 5.2). Despite substantial declines in the abortion rate since the mid-1990s, 13% of abortions in eastern Europe are still unsafe. In an assessment as part of the International Federation of Gynaecology and Obstetrics initiative for the prevention of unsafe abortion, the following factors were identified as contributing to high rates of unsafe abortion: new legislative barriers to accessing pregnancy termination, unequal distribution of abortion services and the increased costs of abortion (Hodorogea and Comendant 2010).

Access to abortion is, of course, not enough; it is even more important to provide access to contraception. Provision of contraception makes it possible to reduce abortion rates. Induced abortions are associated with increased risks for adverse outcomes in subsequent pregnancies, particularly preterm birth (Lowit et al. 2010). Access to contraceptive services also reduces unwanted pregnancies and adolescent pregnancies. Having an unplanned or unintended pregnancy places women at greater risk for poor outcomes, such as preterm delivery or having a low-birth-weight infant (Shah et al. 2011).

Preterm birth, pre-eclampsia and perinatal death are also more common among adolescents, reflecting in part the prevalence of risk factors related to

Box 5.1   Maternal mortality: the Romanian experience

The extremely high levels of maternal mortality in the 1970s and 1980s in Romania (Fig. 5.1) resulted from a brutal pronatalist policy severely restricting abortion and banning modern contraceptives (Benson et al. 2011): 87% of the maternal deaths in 1989 were attributed to abortion complications (Benson et al. 2011). Following Ceausescu's fall in 1989, the restrictive abortion law was abolished and there was further liberalization in 1996. Furthermore, family planning and reproductive health policies increased access to safe abortion (financed in part by a grant from the World Bank in 1994). In 2001, the Romanian Government established the Romanian Family Health Initiative to increase access to family planning; other initiatives promoted family planning and reproductive health services at the primary health care level. As a result of these initiatives, modern contraceptive prevalence increased from 13.9% in 1993 to 38.2% in 2004 (Benson et al. 2011).

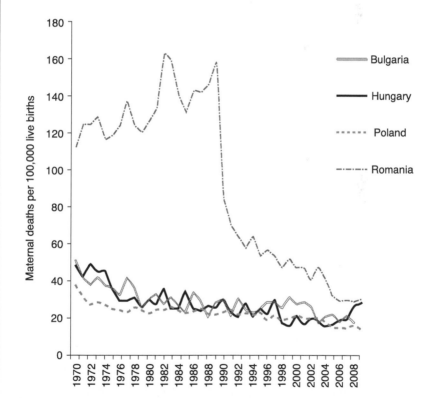

Figure 5.1   Maternal mortality rate in Romania and selected other countries in central and eastern Europe

Source: WHO Regional Office for Europe 2012

Table 5.1 Terminations of pregnancy in the European Union

Access criteria[a]	Number of abortions	Year	Per 1000 women aged 15–45 years
Prohibited (excluding to save woman's life)			
Ireland	0	2008	0
Malta	0	2008	0
Allowed for indications related to physical health			
Poland	506	2008	0.1
Allowed for indications related to physical and mental health			
Spain	115,812	2008	10.1
Allowed for indications related to physical and mental health and socioeconomic grounds			
Finland	10,427	2008	8.9
United Kingdom (excluding Northern Ireland)	209,191	2008	14.2
Allowed on request			
Belgium	18,595	2008	7.5
Bulgaria	36,593	2008	20
Czech Republic	25,760	2008	10.2
Denmark	16,394	2008	13.2
Estonia	8,420	2008	25.1
France	213,380	2007	14.3
Germany	114,484	2008	6
Greece	16,495	2005	6.1
Hungary	44,089	2008	18.4
Italy	121,301	2008	8.7
Latvia	10,425	2008	18
Lithuania	9,031	2008	10.3
The Netherlands	28,470	2008	7.3
Portugal	18,951	2009	7.3
Romania	127,909	2008	23.4
Slovakia	10,869	2008	7.7
Slovenia	4,946	2008	10.2
Sweden	38,053	2008	18.3

Source: Gissler et al. 2012
Note: [a]No data available for Austria, Cyprus and Luxembourg

Table 5.2 Total abortions and percentage of unsafe abortions in Europe by region

	2008		2003		1995	
	Abortions per 1000 women	*% unsafe*	*Abortions per 1000 women*	*% unsafe*	*Abortions per 1000 women*	*% unsafe*
Europe	27	9	28	11	48	12
Eastern Europe	43	13	44	12	90	13
Northern Europe	17	<0.5	17	<0.5	18	8
Southern Europe	18	<0.5	18	18	24	12
Western Europe	12	<0.5	12	<0.5	11	<0.5

Source: Sedgh et al. 2012

the lower social status of adolescent mothers. Detrimental consequences extend beyond those related to pregnancy outcome and include lower maternal educational attainment and higher unemployment. Adolescent pregnancies have become increasingly rare in many European countries: fewer than 3% of births are to mothers under 20 in many of the western European countries (EURO-PERISTAT 2008), and pregnancy rates are under 40 per 1000 in this group (Singh and Darroch 2000). But there are some countries with higher proportions of adolescent mothers, including Portugal and the United Kingdom (Table 5.3). Four countries were identified in one international review as having

Table 5.3 Percentage of live births to mothers under 20 years of age, 2008 or most recent year

<2%	2–3%	4–5%	6–7%	≥8% (%)
Switzerland	Cyprus	Croatia	Bosnia and	Latvia (8.1)
Netherlands	Luxembourg	Portugal	Herzegovina	Ukraine (9.5)
Slovenia	Finland	Albania	Hungary	Armenia (9.5)
Italy	France[a]	Poland	United Kingdom	Republic of
Denmark	Germany	Montenegro	Estonia	Moldova (10.5)
Sweden	Norway		Malta	Tajikistan (12.1)
Andorra	Israel		Kazakhstan	Romania (12.5)
	Belgium[b]		TFYR Macedonia	Bulgaria (13.0)
	Greece		Kyrgyzstan	Azerbaijan (13.6)
	Spain		Serbia	Georgia (13.7)
	Czech Republic		Belarus	
	Ireland		Lithuania	
	Uzbekistan		Slovakia	
	Iceland			
	Austria			

Source: WHO Regional Office for Europe 2012
Notes: TFYR Macedonia, the former Yugoslav Republic of Macedonia
[a]2010 (data from INSERM and French Ministry of Health 2012)
[b]2007

particularly high pregnancy rates among teens (Belarus, Bulgaria, Romania and the Russian Federation; Singh and Darroch 2000). The proportion of births to mothers under 20 is greater than 8% in nine countries. While the availability of contraceptive services is an important part of any strategy to prevent adolescent pregnancies, many other factors influence the proportion of births to teens, including the increased importance of education and changing life aspirations of women (Singh and Darroch 2000).

Prevention of multiple births in assisted reproduction

Another area where some successes have been achieved, with notable variations between countries, is the prevention of multiple births in assisted reproductive technology. The advent of these technologies has enabled many infertile couples to achieve parenthood. Since Louise Brown's birth in 1978, over 5 million babies have been born using assisted reproductive technology and Europe accounts for approximately 71% of all such cycles worldwide. In 2007, between 1 and 5% of all babies were conceived using in vitro fertilization (de Mouzon et al. 2010, European Society of Human Reproduction and Embryology 2012).

The spread of assisted reproductive technology has been accompanied by significant health risks, primarily because of the higher probability of multiple gestations in these pregnancies. The transfer of multiple embryos makes it possible to maximize pregnancy rates per cycle, but increases twin and higher-order births. About 60% of twins and 90% of triplets are preterm (before 37 weeks of gestation) and 10% and 30% are very preterm (before 32 weeks of gestation), in comparison to 6–7% and 1–2%, respectively, for singletons (Blondel 2002).

The diffusion of assisted reproductive technologies created an epidemic of twin and triplet births in many countries. Between the mid-1970s and 1998, the rate of twin pregnancies increased by 50–60% in England and Wales, France and the United States. The rate of triplet or higher-order multiple pregnancies increased by 310% in France, 430% in England and Wales and 696% in the United States (Blondel et al. 2002). In France, for example, twin births increased from 18.1 per 1000 births in 1972–1975 to 29.9 per 1000 in 2000–2003 (Khoshnood and Blondel 2007). Up to one-half of twins and over 75% of triplets can be born as a result of assisted reproductive technologies in countries with high rates of multiples (Blondel and Kaminski 2002).

In response to the alarming rises in multiple births, many countries enacted policies or established guidelines about the number of embryos transferred in a procedure. Alternative strategies were developed, including elective single embryo transfers, after it was found that, for women with two or more good quality embryos, transferring one embryo and freezing the other for future transfer could obtain similar overall pregnancy rates as double embryo transfers, without the risks associated with multiple birth. National policies for elective single embryo transfers have been adopted by several countries (Box 5.2) (Tiitinen and Gissler 2004; Cook et al. 2011). A powerful argument for these policies is that, although more cycles may be needed to achieve pregnancy, the additional costs are offset by the savings on neonatal intensive care needed for very preterm twins and triplets. Other European countries, however, have no

Box 5.2 Examples of policies in countries with high rates of single embryo transfer

---

Belgium (rate in 2006, 49%). In 2003, the Belgian Government agreed to reimburse laboratory expenses for six in vitro fertilization cycles for women up to the age of 42 years, in exchange for restriction of the number of embryos replaced. In the period after the introduction of the law, there were several evaluations of its impact. Overall, single embryo transfer increased from 14 to 49%. Pregnancy rates stayed the same and twin pregnancies decreased.

Sweden (rate in 2006, 70%). State policy is that only one embryo should be transferred, apart from exceptional circumstances. Only single embryo transfers are reimbursed, except with derogation.

Finland (rate in 2006, 55%). There is no official policy regarding elective single embryo transfer, but there is a large professional consensus about the importance of transferring only one embryo. This policy was initiated by professionals alarmed by adverse health outcomes associated with triplets and twins born after in vitro fertilization. Since 1993, data on the number of embryo transfers from each in vitro fertilization centre are published annually. While the data are anonymous, there are only 20 such centres in Finland. Compared with other countries, Finland has one of the most liberal insurance coverage systems for assisted reproduction, and this supports elective single embryo transfer practices (Ólafsdóttir 2012).

---

such policies. In Italy, the law requires transfer of all fertilized embryos in each cycle, although it limits the number of fertilized embryos to three (La Sala et al. 2012).

Both levels and trends of multiple birth rates differ greatly between countries (Fig. 5.2). Some countries have witnessed steep increases whereas others have experienced declines, especially in more recent periods, for example in the Netherlands. Countries where multiple births increased most steeply between 1996 and 2008 were those where rates of single embryo transfer were lowest (rates vary between under 10% and 70%) (de Mouzon et al. 2010).

Pregnancy

Protection of pregnant women and children

A range of policies aim to protect and to promote the health and well-being of pregnant women and their babies. These policies embody a collective recognition of the risks faced by women and infants during pregnancy and childbirth, in particular in vulnerable populations. The policies include measures to protect the health and safety of pregnant workers, workers who have recently given birth and women who are breastfeeding. There are EU Directives specifying minimum measures for protection of pregnant workers (European

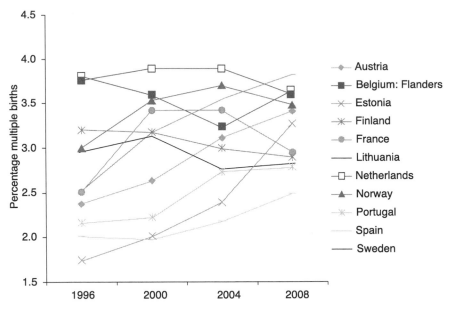

Figure 5.2 Rates and evolution of multiple births in Europe from 1996 to 2008

Source: Unpublished data from the EURO-PERISTAT Preterm Birth Group

Commission 1992). Paid leave is accorded to employed women during and after pregnancy and extends to fathers in many countries (European Foundation for the Improvement of Living and Working Conditions 2007). Income transfer policies for pregnant women have similar aims of protecting the woman and child during this key period. In many EU Member States, health insurance is extended to all women during pregnancy regardless of their employment, insurance or immigration status.

These policies are meant to improve a wide range of health outcomes, including stillbirth, preterm birth, low birth weight, infant mortality, breastfeeding and child health and development. The effectiveness of specific policies in achieving these goals has not been extensively documented, but research suggests that more comprehensive leave and social policies improve outcomes. One study on policies in 141 countries in 2007 reported that longer paid maternal leaves reduced infant mortality after adjustment for national income and expenditures on health (Heymann et al. 2011). A study from 1998 in nine European countries found that longer parental leave was associated with lower perinatal, infant and child mortality, with most marked effects for post-neonatal mortality (Ruhm 1998).

Analyses of the health effects of specific components of these social policies are complex, however. One example is the effect of work leave on employment-related risks of preterm birth. The associations between employment and poor pregnancy outcome are not straightforward, as employment, per se, is not a risk factor for poor outcome. Further, pregnant women who choose not to work may do so for health reasons, creating the well-documented healthy worker effect. Several recent meta-analyses have confirmed that employment is not a risk factor for preterm birth, but that physically strenuous work, shift work and exposures to specific products (gases, heavy metals, etc.) are associated with an increased risk of adverse perinatal and reproductive health outcomes (relative risks around 1.3) (Figa-Talamanca 2006; Savitz and Murnane 2010; Bonzini et al. 2011). One explanation for differences in employment-related risk may be the presence of work leave policies, as suggested by the results of a European case–control study of preterm birth (Saurel-Cubizolles et al. 2004). This study found that there was no significant impact of work conditions (long working hours and time in a standing position) on pregnancy outcomes in countries where it was easier for women to take work leave during pregnancy, yet these conditions had a negative impact in other countries. The proportion of employed pregnant women who were on leave in their third trimester of pregnancy in this study varied hugely: in France, Germany, Italy, Slovenia and the Czech Republic it was between 33 and 67%, whereas in Finland, Greece, Scotland, Spain, Sweden and the Netherlands it was only between 11 and 22% (INSERM and French Ministry of Health 2012).

Preventive care in the prenatal period

European countries usually provide women with a cost-free prenatal care package, and some include incentives for pregnant women to use these services. The aim of prenatal care is to screen for potential complications in the pregnancy and to prevent and to treat these complications. While many of these screening activities are likely to be effective, the evidence base is not always clear. Consequently, there is an enormous variability between European countries in what constitutes basic prenatal care during pregnancy.

One of the first European studies on perinatal health showed that, in the early 1980s, the legal number or recommended number of prenatal visits was 5 in Luxembourg; 7 in Belgium, France, and Italy; 10 in Denmark, and the Federal Republic of Germany; and over 12 in the United Kingdom, the Netherlands, Greece and Ireland (Blondel et al. 1985; Kaminski et al. 1986). This study also found differences in the type of medical personnel (obstetricians, midwives, general practitioners) responsible for prenatal care and in the place of care. Since this study, there have been several other descriptive studies of prenatal care in Europe, which continue to show great heterogeneity in prenatal care services (Kaminski et al. 1986; Hemminki and Blondel 2001). Figure 5.3 shows the results of a recent study looking at national guidelines for baseline clinical care of healthy women with uncomplicated singleton pregnancies (Bernloehr et al. 2005). This figure shows how many of the 20 of the 25 EU Member States with national guidelines recommended specific tests (data from 2006). For example, while all countries with national guidelines recommended taking blood pressure and rhesus factor determination, only 10 recommended tests for toxoplasmosis and only 11 for gestational diabetes.

A Cochrane review has shown that there is no difference in health outcomes between a larger and a smaller number of antenatal visits, although in low- and middle-income countries perinatal mortality was slightly higher in

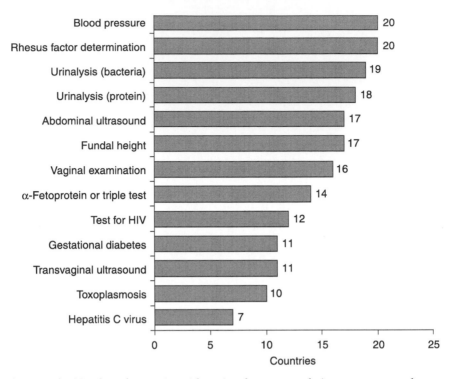

Figure 5.3 Number of countries with national recommendations on content of prenatal care

Source: Bernloehr et al. 2005

reduced schedule groups (Dowswell et al. 2010). Another Cochrane review found no benefit of repeated vaginal examinations (Alexander et al. 2010) and two other reviews concluded that there was not enough evidence to evaluate routine screening for gestational diabetes or fundal height measurement in pregnancy (Neilson 2000; Tieu et al. 2010). In many cases, there are simply not enough studies to enable conclusions to be drawn. In contrast, however, smoking cessation programmes reduce smoking and have an impact on low birth weight and preterm births (Lumley et al. 2009).

There are few studies linking prenatal care policies to actual outcomes in EU Member States. One analysis that related the number and the organization of prenatal visits to perinatal mortality found no association and concluded 'there is no single way to provide high-coverage services' (Hemminki and Blondel 2001). In some cases, data are not available on the policies in place as, for instance, the implementation of smoking cessation programmes. Smoking is an area where further investigation would be fruitful since smoking during pregnancy varies greatly in Europe (Fig. 5.4). The extent to which these differences are related to the effective integration of smoking cessation programmes into routine antenatal care is at present impossible to establish.

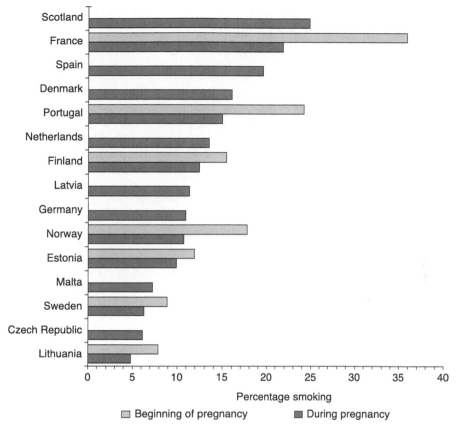

Figure 5.4 Smoking during pregnancy in European countries in 2004

Source: EURO-PERISTAT 2008

Screening for congenital anomalies

One area in which studies do show a link between policies and health outcomes is screening for congenital anomalies. Congenital anomalies constitute one of the principal causes of infant mortality, childhood morbidity and adverse neurodevelopmental outcomes (Hatton et al. 2000; Lee et al. 2001; Liu et al. 2002; Dolk et al. 2011). The aetiology of the majority of cases of congenital anomalies remains unknown. Hence, while primary prevention is important and should be a priority, prevention measures are currently limited to (1) the avoidance of known teratogens (notably certain medications and environmental risk factors), (2) optimal management of chronic maternal illnesses (in particular diabetes), and, most importantly, (3) use of folic acid to prevent neural tube defects.

Important progress has been made in prenatal diagnosis of congenital anomalies, particularly for Down syndrome (Taipale et al. 1997; Wald et al. 1999; Nicolaides et al. 2002), and in the postnatal clinical management and thereby outcomes of newborns with certain anomalies, in particular congenital heart defects and gastrointestinal anomalies (Bonnet et al. 1999; Lee et al. 2001;

Khoshnood et al. 2005; Blyth et al. 2008). The optimal medical and surgical management of many anomalies requires prenatal diagnosis of the anomaly in order to allow early transfer of the mother or the newborn to a specialized centre.

Most countries have included screening for congenital anomalies in routine antenatal care for pregnant women, including ultrasound scans and biochemical screening tests. There is now a consensus that the ultimate aim of prenatal screening should be to offer women and their families the opportunity to make informed choices regarding their pregnancy (Marteau 1995, 2002). Prenatal detection of an anomaly can give women the possibility of terminating a pregnancy with a severe ('incurable') anomaly and also allow better management of the anomaly at birth, thus allowing secondary prevention by improving the outcome for the newborn.

While national screening policies are associated with lower perinatal mortality, as discussed below, and also with a lower live birth prevalence of

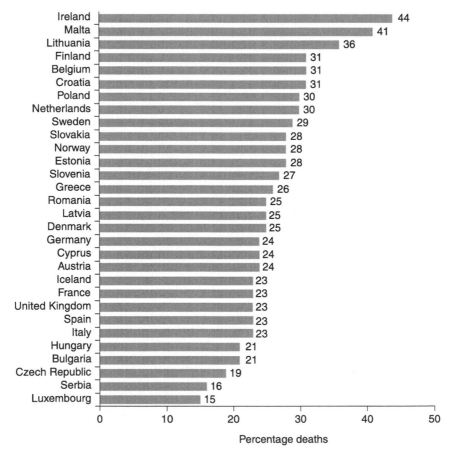

Figure 5.5   Percentage of neonatal deaths caused by congenital anomalies (average over years 2004 to 2008)

Source: WHO Regional Office for Europe 2012

certain lethal or incurable congenital anomalies, it is important to recognize that these policies do not prevent congenital anomalies (Dolk 2009). There is solid evidence that periconceptional supplementation with folic acid reduces the prevalence of neural tube defects. Evaluations of policies that simply recommend periconceptional folic acid did not find a major impact on the occurrence of neural tube defects (Busby et al. 2005), but recent data suggest there may be some effect (Khoshnood et al. 2011). However, prevalence of neural tube defects has decreased significantly in areas with mandatory folic acid fortification policies (Botto et al. 2006).

Figure 5.5 displays national data on the percentage of neonatal deaths for which the cause of death was coded as congenital anomaly over the period 2004–2008. While questions exist about the comparability of these data, they nonetheless illustrate the importance of congenital anomalies as a cause of neonatal death in Europe and reveal an important variability between countries (from 15 to 44%). Both Ireland and Malta, where terminations are not legal, have the highest proportion of neonatal deaths from congenital anomalies.

The proportion of infant mortality due to congenital anomalies is determined by many factors, including the frequency of other causes of mortality, the presence of screening programmes and postnatal clinical management of newborns with congenital anomalies. As infant mortality from other causes declines, the proportion of deaths linked to congenital anomalies tends to increase in countries without, or with limited, prenatal screening programmes. As an illustration, Fig. 5.6 shows data from Ireland where there are no policies to screen for congenital anomalies. As neonatal mortality rates decreased, the proportion of deaths from congenital anomalies grew to 46% in 2009. Time trends for France and Austria (selected because they have complete data over the period for these two indicators) do not show a similar increase in the proportion of congenital anomalies over time, although neonatal mortality has strongly declined as well. In both France and Austria, screening and termination for lethal anomalies is routinely carried out, although Austria does not have a national screening policy (Boyd et al. 2008).

EUROCAT, a European network of congenital anomaly registers established in 1979, has generated comparable data on screening and terminations for congenital anomalies in Europe. These studies reveal large differences in the existence and content of screening programmes and the regulations governing the termination of pregnancies. For example, there are national policies for Down syndrome screening in Belgium, Denmark, England and Wales, Finland, Germany, Italy, Poland, Portugal and Switzerland, but not in Austria, Croatia, Ireland, Malta, the Netherlands, Norway, Spain or Sweden (Boyd et al. 2008). Detection rates ranged from 32 to 95% in countries with some form of screening. While countries with national policies had high detection rates, some countries without national policies also had high detection rates. Perinatal mortality rates tend to be higher in EUROCAT registries where termination of pregnancy for fetal anomaly is illegal, such as Dublin and Malta (Khoshnood et al. 2011).

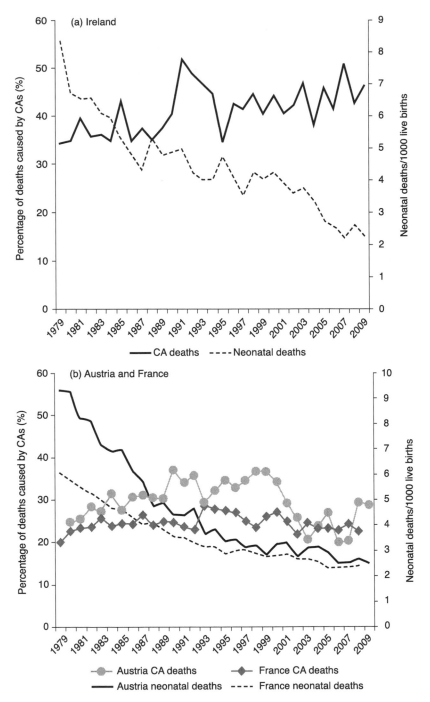

Figure 5.6 Trends in neonatal mortality and the percentage of neonatal deaths from congenital anomalies (CA) in Ireland (a), Austria and France (b)

Source: WHO Regional Office for Europe 2012

Delivery and postpartum care

Access to safe delivery care

The organization of delivery and postpartum services is an important domain for public policy. Pregnancy is not an illness and most pregnant women have normal pregnancies requiring little medical intervention. However, when risks arise, access to specialized care is essential for the survival of both mother and child. Organizing access to risk-appropriate health care for mothers and babies is, therefore, a central pillar of a successful perinatal health system, and one in which public policy and regulation play an important role.

Policies in this area have focused on two principal areas. The first is the regionalization of care, meaning the concentration of care for high-risk pregnancies in regional centres with specialized care. Regionalization programmes are targeted at pregnant women at risk of delivering a very preterm infant (before 32 weeks of gestation). These infants (about 1 to 1.5% of all births) account for one-third to one-half of all neonatal deaths and are at high risk of longer-term developmental and cognitive impairment (Bhutta et al. 2002; Ancel et al. 2006). Access to intensive care determines their survival and future quality of life. The delivery of these infants in maternity units with on-site neonatal intensive care (so-called level III units) is associated with lower mortality and higher survival without disability (Ozminkowski et al. 1988). This is the result of both the technical expertise and coordination between obstetric and neonatal teams in these facilities and the avoidance of potentially harmful neonatal transport after birth. Very preterm babies hospitalized in larger units have lower mortality after adjustment for case mix (Phibbs et al. 2007; Lasswell et al. 2010), but not everywhere (Field and Draper 1999). There is a wide variability in what constitutes a 'level III' unit for the care of preterm infants in Europe (Van Reempts et al. 2007; Blondel et al. 2009) and volume is only one of the attributes distinguishing these care settings. In some countries, minimum volume or activity levels have been integrated into the criteria for defining level III units (Van Reempts et al. 2007). Regionalization policies emphasize the transfer of pregnant women before delivery (also called in utero transfer) so that optimal care is available at birth. Neonatal transfer services are developed for situations where transfer is not possible.

The second area of policy focus is that of guaranteeing a minimal level of safety for low-risk pregnancies and for the unforeseen risks that can arise during childbirth and postpartum. These policies have entailed closing small maternity units, creating risk triage systems for delivery in non-medicalized settings or specifying minimum staffing and services for all maternity units, for example 24/24 presence of an obstetrician or anaesthetist and existence of operating theatres and blood transfusion capacity. Many countries have taken initiatives to close maternity units that have a low annual volume of deliveries (under 300 or under 500 per year). The move to close small maternity units has not been uniform across Europe, as shown by Fig. 5.7, which gives the percentage of births in maternity units with fewer than 500 births in 2004. Some studies have found that delivery in a small unit is associated with higher mortality, but the findings are not consistent (Bouvier-Colle et al. 1996; Moster et al. 1999).

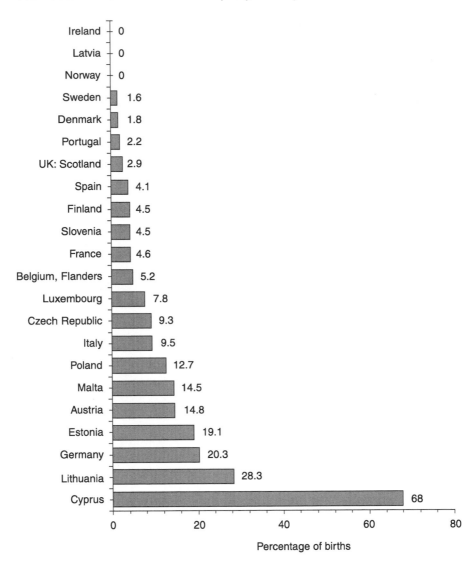

Figure 5.7   Percentage of births in maternity units with fewer than 500 births, 2004

Source: EURO-PERISTAT 2008

Randomized trials comparing delivery in traditional settings with alternative, less medicalized settings have not found that there are increased health risks in the latter, and they consistently show lower rates of obstetrical interventions (such as caesarean section or episiotomies) and higher maternal satisfaction (Hodnett et al. 2010). The question of whether delivery is safe in a less medicalized setting is high on the policy agenda in some countries. For example, in the Netherlands where home delivery is common (30% of deliveries take place at home), there is an active debate about whether this model entails excess risks and may be responsible for the higher than average perinatal mortality rate in the Netherlands. Recent studies of home versus hospital births have not been entirely reassuring and suggested elevated risks in specific subgroups (de Jonge et al. 2009; van der Kooy et al. 2011, Evers et al. 2010). The recent Birthplace in England study compared risks associated with deliveries at home, in freestanding midwifery units and in alongside midwifery units next to an obstetrical ward and obstetrical units. They found no differences in adverse outcomes between any of the non-obstetric settings and the obstetric units, although risks were slightly higher for nulliparous women selecting home birth (Birthplace in England Collaborative Group 2011). There were fewer interventions during pregnancy in all non-obstetric settings. However, providing care in non-obstetric settings requires an effective risk triage system for identifying eligible pregnant women as well as the organization of transfers between non-obstetric and obstetric settings. In the English study, between 20 and 26% of women in non-obstetric settings required transfer during or after delivery; these rates were 36 to 45% among first-time mothers. It is possible that, in the absence of the triage and the availability of transfer, delivery at home or in a smaller unit may be associated with higher risks; this may explain the results of studies that find worse outcomes in non-obstetric settings (Wax et al. 2010).

Promotion of breastfeeding

Breastfeeding gives babies crucial benefits, including important nutritional advantages and improved resistance to infections (Ip et al. 2007). Breastfeeding is an international public health priority; the World Health Assembly approved the Global Strategy on Infant and Young Child Feeding in 2003. This strategy includes developing national policies about breastfeeding, training health professionals and promoting best practices in hospitals, including controlling the use and endorsement of infant formula feeding through the baby friendly hospital initiative. Launched in 1991, the initiative awards maternity units 'baby friendly status'. Maternity facilities can be designated baby friendly when they do not accept free or low-cost breast-milk substitutes, feeding bottles or teats, and have implemented ten specific steps to support successful breastfeeding (World Health Organization 2002).

The EURODIET project described policies on breastfeeding in Europe and their conformity to international recommendations (Cattaneo et al. 2005, 2010). This project covered the EU Member States and assessed policies in 2002 and 2007. The project's overall conclusion was that although many countries had initiatives in place the implementation of the WHO global strategy was insufficient. Improvements were, however, noted between 2002 and 2007. In 2002, 48% of countries had national policies to help mothers to start breastfeeding as soon as possible after birth; this proportion was 63% in 2007.

Figure 5.8 juxtaposes the percentage of births in baby friendly hospitals in 2002 with data from 2004 on breastfeeding initiation. In general, countries with higher breastfeeding rates had more births in baby friendly hospitals, although there were some exceptions. This figure displays the wide difference in breast-feeding rates and the low breastfeeding rates in some countries. Throughout Europe, few women continue to breastfeed after the first few months. Data

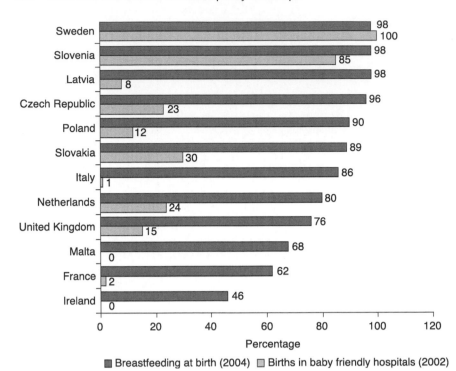

Figure 5.8   Percentage of births in baby friendly hospitals and percentage of babies breastfed at birth

Sources: EURO-PERISTAT 2008; Cattaneo et al. 2010

from around the year 2000 found ranges of between 10 and 80% for any breast-feeding and 1 and 35% for exclusive breastfeeding at six months (Cattaneo et al. 2005).

Discussion and conclusions

Policies in the area of fertility, pregnancy and childbirth have benefited from the long-standing existence of routine registration of births and deaths. International comparisons of data relating to pregnancy outcome and maternity care date back at least to the mid-19th century (Le Fort 1866; Semenow 1872; Report of the Special Committee on Infantile Mortality 1912). National and international expert groups have convened to define measures of maternal and child health care and outcomes for use in evaluating public health programmes, thereby facilitating benchmarking and mutual learning (Centers for Disease Control 1992; Graafmans et al. 2001). These efforts are continuing to the present day, as shown by the recent EURO-PERISTAT project, financed by the European Commission's Public Health Programme, which developed a set of indicators to form the basis for perinatal health surveillance in Europe and collected data for the year 2004 (EURO-PERISTAT 2008; Zeitlin et al. 2009). Some of these data have also been used in this chapter.

The scope for public policy in improving maternal and child health outcomes is broad and there have been effective actions in many domains, as shown in this chapter. Yet, many questions remain about the effectiveness of public action and its commonly used tools. Researchers attempting a cross-national comparison of the effectiveness of health policy in this area face three major difficulties. The first is the absence of comparative data on the regulatory and legislative contexts. Because of the heterogeneity in health system governance in Europe and the multiplicity and diversity of actors involved in maternal and child health policies, describing policy content is daunting (the language diversity further complicates access to government reports and so on). Further, while our focus has been on the country level, many policy initiatives in this area are taken on the subnational or local level. In general, our knowledge of policy is best for areas where there are long-standing networks of European researchers, such as EUROCAT (for congenital anomalies) or ESHRE (for assisted reproductive technologies). These collaborations create a common vocabulary among members and bring together experts who are able to analyse the policy environment and extract relevant laws, regulations and recommendations, despite institutional and political heterogeneity.

Second is the absence of a good evidence base for many preventive interventions. There is a long-standing tradition of clinical reviews in the fields of obstetrics and neonatology; indeed, the Cochrane Collaboration originally evolved from a British project for systematic reviews of perinatal trials in the mid-1970s (McGuire et al. 2010). While this tradition provides a good evidence base for medical interventions and procedures in obstetrics and neonatology, less evidence exists about preventive policies. Furthermore, data on implementation and effectiveness within the entire population are also needed. In the absence of clear evidence, there is a danger that these policies will be abandoned (particularly given current pressure on health budgets and the European debt crisis). At the same time, there are substantial differences in health outcomes between European countries; for example preterm birth rates in some countries have risen over the past decades whereas elsewhere rates have declined (Langhoff-Roos et al. 2006; Jakobsson et al. 2008; Norman et al. 2009; Schaaf et al. 2011). These and other findings suggest that there are population-level risk factors that are potentially amenable to intervention.

The third difficulty is that, while European countries embrace similar values about the responsibility of the state for the provision of health care for pregnant women and children, ways of achieving these aims differ. Recognition of the demographic, political and cultural diversity of Europe is a necessary backdrop to any discussion of the 'European' experience and complicates the evaluation of the successes or failures of national policies. Assessment of the appropriateness of care provided to women and children during pregnancy and childbirth must take into account historical and cultural components, as illustrated by national debates on what levels of medicalization are necessary, on what risks are acceptable and on what the ethical implications are of more screening for congenital anomalies or active resuscitation of sick babies. The answers to these questions differ within Europe, and these choices have a strong impact on care and health outcomes. A dialogue about society's priorities and values must, therefore, be integrated into the assessment of what constitutes success or failure of health policy.

References

Alexander, S., Boulvain, M., Ceysens, G., Haelterman, E. and Zhang, W.H. (2010) Repeat digital cervical assessment in pregnancy for identifying women at risk of preterm labour, *Cochrane Database of Systematic Reviews*, (6):CD005940.

Ancel, P.Y., Livinec, F., Papiernik, E., Saurel-Cubizolles, M.J. and Kaminski, M. (2006) Cerebral palsy among very preterm children in relation to gestational age and neonatal ultrasound abnormalities: the EPIPAGE cohort study, *Pediatrics*, 117(3):828–35.

Barker, D.J. (1998) In utero programming of chronic disease, *Clinical Science (Lond)*, 95(2):115–28.

Benson, J., Andersen, K. and Samandari, G. (2011) Reductions in abortion-related mortality following policy reform: evidence from Romania, South Africa and Bangladesh, *Reproductive Health*, 8(1):39.

Bernloehr, A., Smith, P. and Vydelingum, V. (2005) Antenatal care in the European Union: a survey on guidelines in all 25 member states of the Community, *European Journal of Obstetrics, Gynecology and Reproductive Biology*, 122(1):22–32.

Bhutta, A.T., Cleves, M.A., Casey, P.H., Cradock, M.M. and Anand, K.J. (2002) Cognitive and behavioral outcomes of school-aged children who were born preterm: a meta-analysis, *Journal of the American Medical Association*, 288(6):728–37.

Birthplace in England Collaborative Group (2011) Perinatal and maternal outcomes by planned place of birth for healthy women with low risk pregnancies: the Birthplace in England national prospective cohort study, *British Medical Journal*, 343:d7400.

Blondel, B. and Kaminski, M. (2002) Trends in the occurrence, determinants, and consequences of multiple births, *Seminars in Perinatology*, 26(4):239–49.

Blondel, B., Pusch, D. and Schmidt, E. (1985) Some characteristics of antenatal care in 13 European countries, *British Journal of Obstetrics and Gynecology*, 92(6):565–8.

Blondel, B., Kogan, M.D., Alexander, G.R. et al. (2002) The impact of the increasing number of multiple births on the rates of preterm birth and low birthweight: an international study, *American Journal of Public Health*, 92(8):1323–30.

Blondel, B., Papiernik, E., Delmas, D. et al. (2009) Organisation of obstetric services for very preterm births in Europe: results from the MOSAIC project, *BJOG: An International Journal of Obstetrics and Gynaecology*, 116(10):1364–72.

Blyth, M., Howe, D., Gnanapragasam, J. and Wellesley, D. (2008) The hidden mortality of transposition of the great arteries and survival advantage provided by prenatal diagnosis, *BJOG: An International Journal of Obstetrics and Gynaecology*, 115(9):1096–1100.

Bonnet, D., Coltri, A., Butera, G. et al. (1999) Detection of transposition of the great arteries in fetuses reduces neonatal morbidity and mortality, *Circulation*, 99(7):916–18.

Bonzini, M., Palmer, K.T., Coggon, D. et al. (2011) Shift work and pregnancy outcomes: a systematic review with meta-analysis of currently available epidemiological studies, *BJOG: An International Journal of Obstetrics and Gynaecology*, 118(12):1429–37.

Botto, L.D., Lisi, A., Bower, C. et al. (2006) Trends of selected malformations in relation to folic acid recommendations and fortification: an international assessment, *Birth Defects Research A: Clinical and Molecular Teratology*, 76(10):693–705.

Bouvier-Colle, M.H., Salanave, B., Ancel, P.Y. et al. (1996) Obstetric patients treated in intensive care units and maternal mortality. Regional Teams for the Survey, *European Journal of Obstetrics, Gynecology and Reproductive Biology*, 65(1):121–5.

Boyd, P.A., Devigan, C., Khoshnood, B., Loane, M., Garne, E. and Dolk, H. (2008) Survey of prenatal screening policies in Europe for structural malformations and chromosome anomalies, and their impact on detection and termination rates for neural tube defects and Down's syndrome, *BJOG: An International Journal of Obstetrics and Gynaecology*, 115(6):689–96.

Busby, A., Abramsky, L., Dolk, H. and Armstrong, B. (2005) Preventing neural tube defects in Europe: population based study, *British Medical Journal*, 330(7491):574–5.

Cans, C., Guillem, P., Fauconnier, J., Rambaud, P. and Jouk, P.S. (2003) Disabilities and trends over time in a French county, 1980–91, *Archives of Disease in Childhood*, 88(2):114–17.

Cattaneo, A., Yngve, A., Koletzko, B. and Guzman, L.R. (2005) Protection, promotion and support of breast-feeding in Europe: current situation, *Public Health Nutrition*, 8(1):39–46.

Cattaneo, A., Burmaz, T., Arendt, M. et al. (2010) Protection, promotion and support of breast-feeding in Europe: progress from 2002 to 2007, *Public Health Nutrition*, 13(6):751–9.

Centers for Disease Control (1992) *Proceedings of the International Collaborative Effort on Perinatal and Infant Mortality: Second International Symposium on Perinatal and Infant Mortality*. Bethesda, MD: US Centers for Disease Control, National Center for Health Statistics.

Cook, J.L., Collins, J., Buckett, W. et al. (2011) Assisted reproductive technology-related multiple births: Canada in an international context, *Journal of Obstetrics and Gynecology of Canada*, 33(2):159–67.

Dolk, H. (2009) What is the primary prevention of congenital anomalies? *Lancet*, 374(9687):378.

Dolk, H., Loane, M. and Garne, E. 2011 (2011) Congenital heart defects in Europe: prevalence and perinatal mortality, 2000 to 2005, *Circulation*, 123(8):841–9.

Dowswell, T., Carroli, G., Duley, L. et al. (2010) Alternative versus standard packages of antenatal care for low-risk pregnancy, *Cochrane Database of Systematic Reviews*, (10):CD000934.

European Commission (1992) *Council Directive 92/85/EEC of 19 October 1992 on the Introduction of Measures to Encourage Improvements in the Safety and Health at work of Pregnant Workers and Workers who have Recently Given Birth or are Breastfeeding.* [10th individual Directive within the meaning of Article 16 (1) of Directive 89/391/EEC.] Brussels: European Commission.

European Foundation for the Improvement of Living and Working Conditions (2007) *Parental Leave in European Companies*. Dublin: European Foundation for the Improvement of Living and Working Conditions, http://www.eurofound.europa.eu/pubdocs/2006/87/en/1/ef0687en.pdf (accessed 17 June 2012).

European Society of Human Reproduction and Embryology (2012). Information Resources. Beigem, ESHRE (www.eshre.eu/ESHRE/English/Press-Room/Information-resources/page.aspx/1719 (accessed 31 October 2012).

Evers A.C., Brouwers H.A., Hukkelhoven C.W. et al. (2010) Perinatal mortality and severe morbidilty in law and high risk term pregnancies in the Netherlands: prospective cohort study, *BMJ*, 2:341:c5639

EURO-PERISTAT (2008) *European Perinatal Health Report*. Paris: EURO-PERISTAT, http://www.europeristat.com/images/doc/EPHR/european-perinatal-health-report.pdf (accessed 4 June 2012).

Expertise Collective INSERM (2004) *Déficiences et handicaps d'origine périnatale. Dépistage et prise en charge*. Paris: INSERM.

Field, D. and Draper, E.S. (1999) Survival and place of delivery following preterm birth 1994–1996, *Archives of Disease in Childhood, Fetal and Neonatal Education*, 80:F111–15.

Figa-Talamanca, I. (2006) Occupational risk factors and reproductive health of women, *Occupational Medicine (Lond)*, 56(8):521–31.

Flenady, V., Middleton, P., Smith, G.C. et al. (2011) Stillbirths: the way forward in high-income countries, *Lancet*, 377(9778):1703–17.

Gissler, M., Fronteira, I., Jahn, A. et al. (2012) Terminations of pregnancy in the European Union, *BJOG: An International Journal of Obstetrics and Gynaecology*, 119(3):324–32.

Goldenberg, R.L., Culhane, J.F., Iams, J.D. and Romero, R. (2008) Epidemiology and causes of preterm birth, *Lancet*, 371(9606):75–84.

Graafmans, W.C., Richardus, J.H., Macfarlane, A. et al. (2001) Comparability of published perinatal mortality rates in Western Europe: the quantitative impact of differences in gestational age and birthweight criteria, *BJOG: An International Journal of Obstetrics and Gynaecology*, 108(12):1237–45.

Hatton, F., Bouvier-Colle, M.H., Blondel, B., Pequignot, F. and Letoullec, A. (2000) [Trends in infant mortality in France: frequency and causes from 1950 to 1997.] *Archives of Pediatrics*, 7(5):489–500.

Hemminki, E. and Blondel, B. (2001) Antenatal care in Europe: varying ways of providing high-coverage services, *European Journal of Obstetrics, Gynecology and Reproductive Biology*, 94(1):145–8.

Heymann, J., Raub, A. and Earle, A. (2011) Creating and using new data sources to analyze the relationship between social policy and global health: the case of maternal leave, *Public Health Report*, 126(suppl 3):127–34.

Hodnett, E.D., Downe, S., Walsh, D. and Weston, J. (2010) Alternative versus conventional institutional settings for birth, *Cochrane Database of Systematic Reviews*, (9): CD000012.

Hodorogea, S. and Comendant, R. (2010) Prevention of unsafe abortion in countries of Central Eastern Europe and Central Asia, *International Journal of Gynaecology and Obstetrics*, 110(suppl): S34–37.

INSERM and French Ministry of Health (2012) *Tables from the French National Perinatal Survey 2012*. Paris: INSERM, http://www.europeristat.com/bm.doc/french-national-perinatal-survey.pdf (accessed 15 June 2012).

Ip, S., Chung, M., Raman, G. et al. (2007) *Breastfeeding and Maternal and Infant Health Outcomes in Developed Countries*. [Evidence Reports and Technology Assessments 153.] Rockville, MD: Agency for Healthcare Research and Quality, US Department of Health and Human Services.

Jakobsson, M., Gissler, M., Paavonen, J. and Tapper, A.M. (2008) The incidence of preterm deliveries decreases in Finland, *BJOG: An International Journal of Obstetrics and Gynaecology*, 115(1):38–43.

de Jonge, A., van der Goes, B.Y., Ravelli, A.C. et al. (2009) Perinatal mortality and morbidity in a nationwide cohort of 529,688 low-risk planned home and hospital births, *BJOG: An International Journal of Obstetrics and Gynaecology*, 116(9):1177–84.

Kaminski, M., Bréart, G., Buekens, P. et al. (1986) *Perinatal Care Delivery Systems: Description and Evaluation in European Community countries*. Oxford: Oxford University Press.

Khoshnood, B. and Blondel, B. (2007) Regional variations in trends for multiple births: a population-based evaluation in France, 1972–2003, *Twin Research and Human Genetics*, 10(2):406–15.

Khoshnood, B., De Vigan, C., Vodovar, V. et al. (2005) Trends in prenatal diagnosis, pregnancy termination, and perinatal mortality of newborns with congenital heart disease in France, 1983–2000: a population-based evaluation, *Pediatric*, 115(1):95–101.

Khoshnood, B., Greenlees, R., Loane, M. and Dolk, H. (2011) Paper 2: EUROCAT public health indicators for congenital anomalies in Europe, *Birth Defects Research A: Clinical and Molecular Teratology*, 91(suppl 1):S16–22.

van der Kooy, J., Poeran, J., de Graaf, J.P. et al. (2011) Planned home compared with planned hospital births in the Netherlands: intrapartum and early neonatal death in low-risk pregnancies, *Obstetrics and Gynecology*, 118(5):1037–46.

Koupilova, I., McKee, M. and Holcik, J. (1998) Neonatal mortality in the Czech Republic during the transition, *Health Policy (New York)*, 46(1):43–52.

Kramer, M.S., Seguin, L., Lydon, J. and Goulet, L. (2000) Socio-economic disparities in pregnancy outcome: why do the poor fare so poorly? *Paediatric and Perinatal Epidemiology*, 14(3):194–210.

La Sala, G.B., Nicoli, A., Villani, M.T. et al. (2012) The 2004 Italian legislation on the application of assisted reproductive technology: epilogue, *European Journal of Obstetrics, Gynecology and Reproductive Biology*, 161(2):187–9.

Langhoff-Roos, J., Kesmodel, U., Jacobsson, B., Rasmussen, S. and Vogel, I. (2006) Spontaneous preterm delivery in primiparous women at low risk in Denmark: population based study, *British Medical Journal*, 332(7547):937–9.

Lasswell, S.M., Barfield, W.D., Rochat, R.W. and Blackmon, L. (2010) Perinatal regionalization for very low-birth-weight and very preterm infants: a meta-analysis, *Journal of the American Medical Association*, 304(9):992–1000.

Le Fort, L. (1866) *Des maternités de l'Europe*. Paris: Masson.

Lee, K., Khoshnood, B., Chen, L. et al. (2001) Infant mortality from congenital malformations in the United States, 1970–1997, *Obstetrics and Gynecology*, 98(4): 620–7.

Liu, S., Joseph, K.S., Kramer, M.S. et al. (2002) Relationship of prenatal diagnosis and pregnancy termination to overall infant mortality in Canada, *Journal of the American Medical Association*, 287(12):1561–7.

Lowit, A., Bhattacharya, S. and Bhattacharya, S. (2010) Obstetric performance following an induced abortion, *Best Practice Research, Clinical Obstetrics and Gynecology*, 24(5):667–82.

Lumley, J., Chamberlain, C., Dowswell, T. et al. (2009) Interventions for promoting smoking cessation during pregnancy, *Cochrane Database of Systematic Reviews*, (3):CD001055.

Marteau, T.M. (1995) Towards informed decisions about prenatal testing: a review, *Prenatal Diagnosis*, 15(13):1215–26.

Marteau, T.M. (2002) Prenatal testing: towards realistic expectations of patients, providers and policy makers, *Ultrasound in Obstetrics and Gynecology*, 19(1):5–6.

McGuire, W., Fowlie, P., and Soll, R. (2010) What has the Cochrane collaboration ever done for newborn infants? *Archives of Disease of Children, Fetal and Neonatal Education*, 95:F2–6.

Moster, D., Lie, R.T. and Markestad, T. (1999) Relation between size of delivery unit and neonatal death in low risk deliveries: population based study, *Archives of Disease in Childhood, Fetal and Neonatal Education*, 80(3):F221–225.

de Mouzon, J., Goossens, V., Bhattacharya, S. et al. (2010) Assisted reproductive technology in Europe, 2006: results generated from European registers by ESHRE, *Human Reproduction*, 25(8):1851–62.

Neilson, J.P. (2000) Symphysis–fundal height measurement in pregnancy, *Cochrane Database of Systematic Reviews*, (2):CD000944.

Nicolaides, K.H., Heath, V. and Cicero, S. (2002) Increased fetal nuchal translucency at 11–14 weeks, *Prenatal Diagnosis*, 22(4):308–15.

Norman, J.E., Morris, C. and Chalmers, J. (2009) The effect of changing patterns of obstetric care in Scotland (1980–2004) on rates of preterm birth and its neonatal consequences: perinatal database study, *PLoS Medicine*, 6(9):e1000153.

Ólafsdóttir, H.S. (2012) *Nordic and Infertile. A Study of Options and Decisions*. Gothenburg: Nordic School of Public Health.

Ozminkowski, R.J., Wortman, P.M. and Roloff, D.W. (1988) Inborn/outborn status and neonatal survival: a meta-analysis of non randomised studies, *Statistical Medicine*, 7:1207–21.

Phibbs, C.S., Baker, L.C., Caughey, A.B. (2007) Level and volume of neonatal intensive care and mortality in very-low-birth-weight infants, *New England Journal of Medicine*, 356(21):2165–75.

Van Reempts, P., Gortner, L., Milligan, D. et al. (2007) Characteristics of neonatal units that care for very preterm infants in Europe: results from the MOSAIC study, *Pediatrics*, 120(4):e815–825.

Report of the Special Committee on Infantile Mortality (1912) Infant mortality, *Journal of the Royal Statistical Society*, LXXVI: 27–87.

Ruhm, C. (1998) *Parental Leave and Child Health.* [NBER Working Paper 6554.] Cambridge, MA: National Bureau of Economic Research.

Saurel-Cubizolles, M.J., Zeitlin, J., Lelong, N. et al. (2004) Employment, working conditions, and preterm birth: results from the Europop case–control survey, *Journal of Epidemiology and Community Health*, 58(5):395–401.

Savitz, D.A. and Murnane, P. (2010) Behavioral influences on preterm birth: a review, *Epidemiology* 21(3):291–9.

Schaaf, J.M., Mol, B.W., Abu-Hanna, A. and Ravelli, A.C. (2011) Trends in preterm birth: singleton and multiple pregnancies in the Netherlands, 2000–2007, *BJOG: An International Journal of Obstetrics and Gynaecology*, 118(10):1196–1204.

Sedgh, G., Singh, S., Shah, I.H. et al. (2012) Induced abortion: incidence and trends worldwide from 1995 to 2008, *Lancet*, 379(9816):625–32.

Semenow, P. (1872) *Compte-rendu général des travaux du Congrès International de Statistique.* St Petersburg: Imprimerie de l'Academie Imperiale des Sciences.

Shah, P.S., Balkhair, T., Ohlsson. A. et al. (2011) Intention to become pregnant and low birth weight and preterm birth: a systematic review, *Maternal and Child Health Journal*, 15(2):205–16.

Singh, S. and Darroch, J.E. (2000) Adolescent pregnancy and childbearing: levels and trends in developed countries, *Family Planning Perspectives*, 32(1):14–23.

Taipale, P., Hiilesmaa, V., Salonen, R. and Ylostalo, P. (1997) Increased nuchal translucency as a marker for fetal chromosomal defects, *New England Journal of Medicine*, 337(23):1654–8.

Tieu, J., Middleton, P., Mcphee, A.J. and Crowther, C.A. (2010) Screening and subsequent management for gestational diabetes for improving maternal and infant health, *Cochrane Database of Systematic Reviews*, (7):CD007222.

Tiitinen, A. and Gissler, M. (2004) Effect of in vitro fertilization practices on multiple pregnancy rates in Finland, *Fertility and Sterility*, 82(6):1689–90.

Wald, N.J., Watt, H.C. and Hackshaw, A.K. (1999) Integrated screening for Down's syndrome on the basis of tests performed during the first and second trimesters, *New England Journal of Medicine*, 341(7):461–7.

Wax, J.R., Lucas, F.L., Lamont, M. et al. (2010) Maternal and newborn outcomes in planned home birth vs planned hospital births: a metaanalysis, *American Journal of Obstetrics and Gynecology*, 203(3):241–8.

WHO Regional Office for Europe (2012) *European Health for All Database (HFA-DB).* Copenhagen: WHO Regional Office for Europe, http://data.euro.who.int/hfadb/ (accessed 4 June 2012).

World Health Organization (2002) *Global Strategy on Infant and Young Child Feeding.* [55th World Health Assembly.] Geneva: World Health Organization.

Zeitlin, J., Mohangoo, A. et al. (2009) The European Perinatal Health Report: comparing the health and care of pregnant women and newborn babies in Europe, *Journal of Epidemiology and Community Health*, 63(9):681–2.

chapter six

Child health

Ingrid Wolfe

Introduction

The health of Europe's children has improved markedly over the decades from 1970 to 2010. But what has been the contribution of child health policies, and what were the determinants of their success? These are not easy questions to answer because relevant health policies and desired outcomes for an area as broad as child health are many compared with, for example, policies designed to tackle a specific risk factor such as tobacco consumption, where the immediate goal is to reduce smoking rates.

As in other areas covered in this book, the translation of evidence about child health needs and effective interventions into policy and practice is a complex non-linear and often non-rational process. Kingdon (1984) identified three essential conditions for successful policy-making: problem recognition, politics; and policies (this will be further elaborated in Chapter 15). The examples presented in this chapter will highlight important lessons about each of these aspects of children's health policy. Three groups of conditions will be discussed that together account for approximately two-thirds of deaths among children (Fig. 6.1): infectious diseases, external causes and ill-defined causes (the last being part of the 'other' group).

Infectious diseases

This section will examine two of the once common infectious diseases of childhood: first, from diphtheria, we learn about the need for systems resilience; second, through measles, we learn how – or how not – to respond to public uncertainty about vaccine safety.

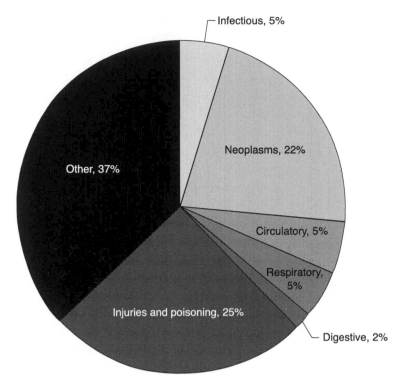

Figure 6.1   Causes of death among children aged 0–14 years in the EU-15, 2009–2010

Source: WHO Regional Office for Europe 2012

Diphtheria

Diphtheria vaccination

In the 1950s, before a diphtheria vaccination programme began, there were more than 750,000 cases of the disease in the USSR. A universal childhood vaccination programme, initiated in 1958 (Khazanov 1964), successfully controlled the disease for several decades (Vitek and Wharton 1998). By the 1970s, the incidence in the USSR was 0.08 per 100,000 population, comparable to western Europe figures. The Semashko model of a centralized health system with a strong public health service, known as 'San-Epid', was responsible for disease surveillance and prevention and made an important contribution to the successful control of vaccine-preventable diseases (Gotsadze et al. 2010).

A slow resurgence of diphtheria in the USSR started in the late 1970s until an epidemic began around 1990. Cases of the disease increased by 70% between 1989 and 1990, tripled by 1991, and by 1992 was almost 6000. Within a year the number affected had reached nearly 20,000 and an epidemic was firmly established.

The dissolution of the USSR that began in the late 1980s put pressures on the old San-Epid system of public health, which failed to adapt sufficiently to the changing relationships among states and institutions. The newly emerging states, to differing extents, allowed their public health systems to become weakened and fragmented, and organizational instability compromised the ability of their public health systems to perform optimally. The result was a catastrophic operational failure: the inability to manage the early stages of the diphtheria outbreak and prevent the epidemic that ensued.

Figure 6.2 shows precipitate declines in vaccine coverage in the Commonwealth of Independent States (CIS) in the early to mid-1990s. Concurrent with the dip in vaccination rates are large peaks in disease incidence. Between 1990 and 1996, there were approximately 125,000 cases and 4000 deaths in the former Soviet countries (Centers for Disease Control and Prevention 1996). Latvia and Sweden are shown as examples of neighbouring countries that had contrasting experiences with diphtheria. Sweden had a stable public health system and experienced no rise in diphtheria cases. Latvia underwent profound system upheaval, vaccine coverage rates fell and the largest epidemic in Europe occurred, which unusually was mostly among the adult population (Griskevica 2002). A mass vaccination campaign was supported by outside agencies and within a few years the Latvian vaccine coverage and disease incidence rates matched those of Sweden, where, from the mid-1970s onwards, vaccine coverage had continued to rise and diphtheria incidence to decline.

What happened in the CIS region that differed from the rest of Europe, and Sweden in particular? The epidemic occurred because of a complex and ultimately dangerous mix of influences. Vaccine-induced immunity wanes after some decades (Galazka and Robertson 1995) and, paradoxically, because of the success of the vaccination programme, the opportunity for naturally occurring immunity to emerge as a result of disease had diminished. There was no adult revaccination programme (Vitek and Wharton 1998), and increased susceptibility to diphtheria among adults was the result. Meanwhile, children had also become more vulnerable in the early 1990s because of a variety of changes in vaccination practice, such as lengthening the interval between booster

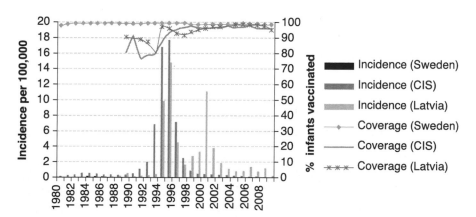

Figure 6.2   Diphtheria incidence and vaccine coverage in the Commonwealth of Independent States (CIS), Latvia and Sweden

Source: WHO Regional Office for Europe 2012.

doses, increasing numbers of children believed to have contraindications to vaccination and a growing popular belief that vaccination could be harmful (Vitek and Wharton 1998). The result was an increase in the number of cases in children, which became an important factor in spread of disease to the adult population. The vaccine itself was quickly excluded as a cause; case–control studies showed the vaccine itself was not faulty (Hardy 1993), and once vaccine coverage increased disease incidence fell quickly, confirming the vaccine's efficacy.

The crucial factors in the epidemic becoming established were the profound social and economic changes accompanying the break-up of the USSR in 1991. Overcrowded and impoverished urban housing conditions and reduced barriers to population movement between newly independent states also contributed. These events helped to create a perfect storm of conditions that allowed an epidemic to occur. Disrupted health systems made it impossible to recognize the early signals of concern rapidly; thus the first element of Kingdon's policy framework (problem recognition) failed. Once the problem became evident, unstable public health systems were unable to take effective early action to control the burgeoning epidemic (Hardy 1993). This represents a failure of the politics aspect of the policy framework. The visible participants were engaged in the destruction and rebuilding of nations.

Control of the diphtheria epidemic in the CIS was eventually achieved by international cooperation, with an Interagency Immunization Coordinating Committee. Effective policy development and implementation could only take place when external influences were brought in to overcome domestic weaknesses.

What general lessons can be learned from the diphtheria epidemic?

Diphtheria began to spread in the CIS because of particular conditions affecting the region. It developed into an epidemic that was beyond the abilities of local systems to contain. The operational failures of local public health systems were exacerbated by a series of policy failures, which provide important learning points. Disruption of public health systems and health services on the scale that accompanied the massive political changes in the former USSR are rare events, but health systems in all European countries are in transition of varying degrees and types, with consequences for the resilience of health protection systems (Castleden et al. 2011). This is particularly the case for preventive services such as vaccination and surveillance in straitened economic conditions.

Indeed, some recommendations made following the diphtheria epidemic have yet to be implemented in many European countries. For example vaccination programmes should be reviewed to ensure that population immunity continues to be adequate throughout the life course. This appears not to have led to changes in policy in the United Kingdom, for example, as there have been no changes to the schedule for diphtheria vaccination to ensure immunity persists into later adulthood, so susceptibility to resurgent disease may remain a problem (Health Protection Agency 2011).

Preventing epidemics of vaccine-preventable diseases requires stable and well-functioning public health systems that can anticipate and detect problems and with the resources to deal with problems when they arise. Those advocating policies that fragment public health functions, for whatever reason, should consider the possible unintended consequences that may accompany such change (McKee et al. 2011).

Measles

Measles vaccination

The combined vaccine against measles, mumps and rubella (MMR) was introduced in most European countries around 1980, taking the place of the single measles vaccines that had been used from the late 1960s. As will be discussed in Chapter 7, measles cases declined rapidly as vaccine coverage increased. However, in 1998, an early report about children with chronic colitis and regressive developmental disorders, which mentioned a possible association with the MMR vaccine, was published in the *Lancet* (Wakefield et al. 1998). A press conference accompanied the report, at which the lead author, Andrew Wakefield, recommended that parents should give their children a single measles vaccine instead of MMR, going far beyond the suggested hypothesis in the report. The MMR vaccine scare was born.

After the events surrounding Wakefield's unsubstantiated recommendations to parents, the United Kingdom's MMR coverage rate dropped from 99% in 2001 to 80% in 2003 (Parliamentary Office of Science and Technology 2004). There were 59 reported measles cases in 1998 just before the scare began, and 460 in 2003. Although the decline in cover rate is evident (Fig. 6.3) and a few hundred measles cases occurred, the incidence per 100,000 still remained very

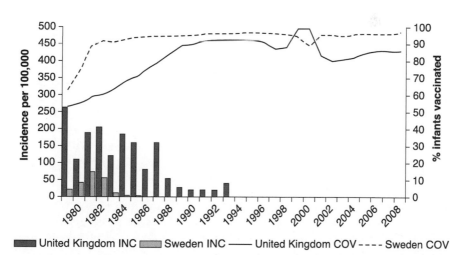

Figure 6.3   Measles incidence and vaccine coverage (MMR) in the United Kingdom and Sweden

Source: WHO Regional Office for Europe 2012
Notes: INC, incidence; COV, coverage

low. Since then, multiple inquiries and investigations have been conducted and the original case series was retracted. Wakefield was struck off the register of the General Medical Council after being found guilty of serious professional misconduct, and many subsequent studies have found no evidence of a link between MMR and autism (Institute of Medicine 2004; Honda et al. 2005). However, the repercussions of these events continue; vaccine coverage remains in parts of the United Kingdom suboptimal and sporadic measles outbreaks still occur.

Vaccine scares are not new, and the MMR scare is unlikely to be the last one. The United Kingdom was disproportionately affected by this scare, compared with Sweden for example, and vaccine coverage rates in the United Kingdom (86% in 2009) remain lower than the EU average (92% in 2009) (World Health Organization 2012). The only other European countries that experienced a notable decline in MMR coverage were Malta and Ireland, both countries with close cultural connections to the United Kingdom. The relatively constant level of circulating measles cases in France, which has never had uniformly high coverage rates, together with the events in the United Kingdom, contributed to a European resurgence of measles such that in the first eleven months of 2011 there were over 30000 cases of measles known in the EU; this is three to five times higher than in the same period in 2007–2009 (ECDC 2011).

The traditionally lower coverage rates for measles in France may be related to the fact that it has a private and decentralized public health system (World Health Organization 2011) which can make large-scale public health programmes difficult to implement (see Chapter 7). But regulated central-ized systems such as that in the United Kingdom can present disadvantages when there is a loss of public trust in government (Schmitt et al. 2003). The policy response by the United Kingdom Department of Health largely consisted of public information and education campaigns that reiterated the safety of MMR and 'catch-up campaigns' to improve coverage rates, together with pay-ments to general practitioners to encourage high vaccination coverage rates (Parliamentary Office of Science and Technology 2004).

Contemporaneous political and social events in the United Kingdom, for example the United Kingdom Government's response to the emergence of bovine spongiform encephalopathy (BSE) – laid the groundwork for a loss of public trust in official advice (McKee and Lang 1996). However, the specific policy responses to public concerns about the safety of MMR were also inadequate, mainly because the most important visible participants in vaccination, the parents, became alienated. This problem occurred for several reasons.

The first reason for concern was a lack of information. Mechanisms for detect-ing rare or less rare adverse effects resulting from vaccines in the United Kingdom were inadequate. Large-scale vaccine efficacy studies do not always detect rare effects, as was demonstrated by the eventual withdrawal of two of the three MMR vaccines that were available in 1992 (Immravax and Pluserix) because of rare asso-ciations with aseptic mumps meningitis, which were only noted once the vac-cines were in widespread use. A systematic review of studies examining adverse effects of MMR compared with single vaccines (Jefferson et al. 2003) found limited evidence on safety of MMR compared with single component vaccines, suggesting that the existing studies were inadequate or insufficient. The authors concluded that improvements were needed in vaccine safety studies. Indeed, the methods for collecting, disseminating and learning from reported adverse outcomes associated with MMR, pre- and postmarketing, were inadequate.

Second, there was no safe space to discuss uncertainty. The media furore following the Wakefield case series made it more difficult for researchers to raise hypotheses to be tested in further investigations lest this raised additional fears and thus unintended consequences for vaccination rates. Open debate and questioning of the causes of disease and the effects of vaccines became nearly impossible as personal attacks on the key actors increased and media scare stories multiplied. The scientific and public health community, together with the government, seemed reluctant to engage directly with parents who expressed doubts about MMR. Nor was there much public engagement on the uncertainties surrounding the cause of autism, a condition of still uncertain aetiology that affects 1% or more of the school-age population. Instead of engaging and rapidly rebutting Andrew Wakefield's recommendations, the Department of Health seemed fearful that to do so might legitimize his claims, given the climate of distrust in government. Their decision may have inadvertently enabled Wakefield to be perceived as a unique sympathetic figure ready to listen to parents whose children had developed autism, eager to help them to find an explanation. The failure by the academic community and the government to engage openly with the public gave the impression of a lack of compassion in the eyes of many anxious parents.

Third, social memory of measles and its potential dangers had faded, as it had for many infectious diseases that have been well controlled by successful vaccination programmes. Mothers said they were more influenced by the perceived risk of the MMR vaccine than those of measles (Parliamentary Office of Science and Technology 2004). The response to this shift in risk perception lacked a sufficiently convincing narrative. Presentations of statistics about likelihoods of disease complications, weighing them against vaccine reactions, may be technically correct but failed to engage and persuade parents. Guidelines on communication in science and health were subsequently issued (Social Issues Research Centre, the Royal Society and the Royal Institution of Great Britain 2001), but while the report noted the importance of credible sources, it focused on scientists and other figures of authority and were not about engaging with patients. There was little emphasis on the possible benefits of collaborating with other sources that could be more credible to the public. The Science Media Centre (www.sciencemediacentre.org) was founded as an independent organisation to facilitate communication between the scientific community and the media, however not directly with the public. The web sites of the United Kingdom Health Protection Agency and the NHS (Health Protection Agency 2012; NHS Choices 2012) have written information for parents, including a film of a parent's account of experience with measles, but they are strongly linked to the NHS name and logo (and therefore, to some parents, to a less-credible source of advice on vaccines). They have also yet to engage fully with modern information technology (Macario et al. 2011). In Canada, the British Columbian Centre for Disease Control tackled these problems head-on, instituting a parent-led forum for telling stories about what had happened to their children, for sharing experiences and discussing fears (Macario et al. 2011).

Fourth, there was an inconsistency in the approach to policy that further undermined the public's trust. The United Kingdom Government had seen 'choice' as an important element of its market-focused policy of the NHS for some years. However, when it came to MMR, this principle did not apply. The Department of Health argued that the safety record of MMR was well established while that of single measles vaccines was not; that a single-vaccine regimen would leave children unvaccinated for longer periods of time; and that failure to complete the course, therefore, increased the risk of disease compared with the standard vaccine schedule. A poll of parents showed that 64% thought that both MMR and single measles vaccinations should be available. Some professionals agreed (Parliamentary Office of Science and Technology 2004). The problems caused by the perceived policy of 'choice – but only on my terms' – was compounded when the Prime Minister refused to confirm that his young son had received MMR. In addition, concerns about conflict of interest influenced many people when it emerged that general practitioners received incentive payments for meeting their vaccination targets.

Finally, there was a lack of sufficient planning and coordination about how the hypothesis presented in the paper would be presented to the public. Andrew Wakefield wrote to the Department of Health and the Chief Medical Officer to discuss his plans for recommending single vaccines. The Department of Health, therefore, had advance notice of the events of the press conference at which Wakefield went beyond the published paper, but it took no action. Meanwhile the *Lancet*, which published the original paper, had not been involved in the authors' discussions with the Department of Health and was caught unaware when the recommendations to split the vaccine were made at the press conference. The lesson here is that all the actors involved in an important paper with relevance for public health, even an early report raising hypotheses for further investigation, should be involved in planning and preparing for publication to ensure that there are no surprises and that the message is crafted as carefully as possible.

What general lessons can be learned from the MMR scare?

Vaccination, perhaps uniquely among public health interventions, can inspire fear. It involves administering an intervention to a healthy child to prevent an illness that may not happen. There are tensions between the interests of the child and the parents' autonomy over their child, and between consideration of the individual and the population (Finn and Savulescu 2011). The success of vaccination programmes depends on confidence, social good will and a bond of trust between the scientific and medical communities, government and the public. These essential invisible threads were strained to breaking point in the United Kingdom.

What can be done? There seems still to be an unwillingness to engage openly in discussion when there is public doubt, or to acknowledge the loss of public trust in institutions. This is fuelled by a reluctance of official authorities to hear the other side of a story. Parents and other members of the public have legitimate concerns and questions that deserve to be addressed openly and honestly. Uncertainty can and should be acknowledged. More compassion for the plight of parents and patients is needed. Furthermore, to address the uncertainty, a thorough, systematic and reliable means of collecting data on vaccines before and after marketing is needed. Importantly, there needs to be a means for raising hypotheses about effects and unintended consequences of medical interventions, and a safe space for public and professional discourse about uncertainty. Careful coordination between key actors involved in potentially important scientific publications and policy-relevant findings is needed to ensure that there are no surprises and that the message is crafted as carefully as possible.

Injuries

Injuries, which remain a leading cause of preventable death in childhood and which vary markedly across Europe (Armour-Marshall et al. 2012). Drowning is a common cause of injury-related death, and clearly demonstrates the scope for success in reducing incidence through public policy. RTIs are discussed in Chapter 10.

Prevention of drowning

Unintentional injuries are the commonest cause of deaths among children aged 0–14 years in Europe (World Health Organization 2012 (data updated March 2011)) and highly amenable to prevention. If Europe could reduce the childhood injury death rate to 3.5 per 100,000 (the best country-rate), approximately 15,000 childhood deaths could be prevented each year (Sethi et al. 2008). Drowning is the second most common cause of injury-related deaths.

Causing more than 5000 deaths among children every year in Europe, accounting for 14% of all deaths among those aged 0–19 years (Mathers et al. 2008; Sethi et al. 2008). Boys are at greater risk than girls, and risk is strongly related to poverty (Mathers et al. 2008). The highest overall risk is for children under five years of age, but the specific causes vary with age. Infants are most at risk of bathtub drowning while toddlers are at greatest risk from swimming pools, garden ponds, wells and agricultural irrigation ditches. Deaths from drowning are, however, an incomplete measure of the damage from water-related injury. For each death there are approximately 4 hospital admissions, 14 emergency department attendances and 10 'near misses' (Spyker 1985; Wintemute 1990).

Childhood deaths from drowning have declined in all countries, but stark geographic inequalities remain. Countries in the Baltic and Central European region have markedly higher rates than countries in the western part of Europe (Fig. 6.5). What policies in the western areas might be useful for countries in the east? And how might western European countries prevent more children from drowning?

The European Child Safety Alliance has developed a performance score to assess countries according to the presence, implementation and enforcement of evidence-based policies for drowning prevention and water safety (Fig. 6.6). Although these safety scores should be interpreted with caution, the three

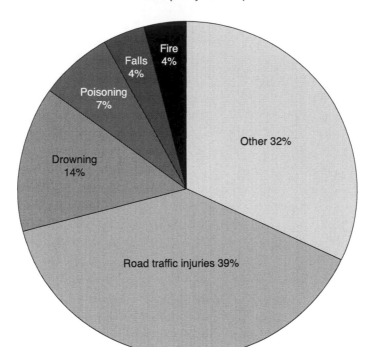

Figure 6.4 Proportion of unintentional injury deaths in children aged 0–19 years

Source: Mathers et al. 2008

Baltic countries Latvia, Lithuania and Estonia have markedly higher death rates from drowning and score poorly on the composite measure, with an average score lower than the countries with drowning mortality rates clustered at the lower end of the scale.

Differences between countries in individual drowning-prevention policies that are not reflected in the composite scores shown in the figure may offer useful insights to the national differences in outcomes. Pool fencing significantly reduces the risk of drowning (Thompson and Rivara 1998). France has led the way in Europe by passing a law in 2003 requiring private pool owners to fit a safety device – fence, shutter, alarm or shelter (Box 6.1). In addition there is an annual education campaign about adequate supervision for children around water (Sethi et al. 2008). Austria, Sweden, Italy and the Czech Republic have laws mandating fencing for public pools (European Child Safety Alliance 2009) but overall, fewer than 50% of European countries have implemented and enforced laws on pool fencing (WHO Regional Office for Europe 2007). The United Kingdom has no laws requiring private or public pool fencing, but exposure is low and deaths from drowning in garden ponds (especially by toddlers) and in pools abroad are more common causes (Sibert et al. 2002). The latter point highlights the importance of Europe-wide action.

Providing trained lifeguards at pools and beaches is an effective means of preventing deaths from drowning (Branche and Stewart 2001). Many European

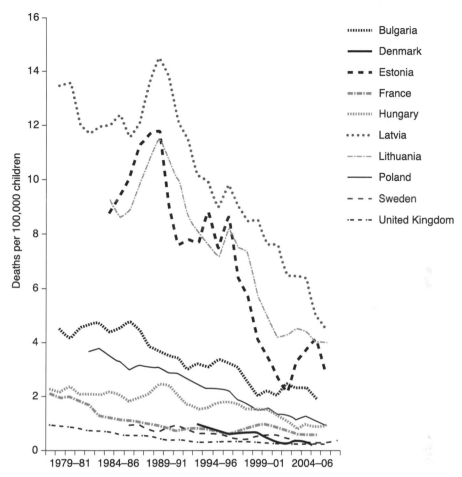

Figure 6.5 Childhood death rates from drowning

Source: World Health Organization 2012

countries, such as Italy, Greece, Spain and France, that have high levels of leisure-related water exposure legislate for a minimum number of lifeguards and for their certification and recertification standards. Between 50 and 69% of European countries have mandatory water safety education, including swimming lessons, as part of their national curricula, which seems a sensible precaution although there is no strong evidence supporting its effectiveness as a drowning-prevention policy for children (WHO Regional Office for Europe 2007), possibly because of the difficulties of evaluating such a policy.

The highest risk of drowning is in the toddler years, but the frequency of specific causes varies among countries and includes drowning in pools, garden ponds, agricultural irrigation ditches and baths. Consequently, legislation to prevent drowning deaths in the youngest age group should comprise a mix of universal policies and those targeted according to likely exposures. For example, children in the CIS and Baltic countries are more likely to encounter open water, such

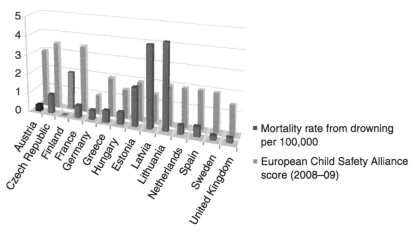

Figure 6.6 Childhood death rates from drowning and European drowning prevention and water safety scores

Sources: European Child Safety Alliance 2009; World Health Organization 2012

as irrigation ditches for agriculture. Policies directed towards promoting adult supervision, together with barriers around ditches, would be appropriate in such settings. Effective coordinated policy-making across different government ministries would be required for such an approach. However until injury prevention becomes a priority for governments (Armour-Marshall et al. 2012), backed up with sufficient funding, it is unlikely that legislation will be enacted or enforced.

Box 6.1 Drowning prevention policy in France

France had the highest rate of swimming pool drowning deaths among children under five years of age in swimming pools in the world. It also has more private swimming pools than any other European country (MacKay et al. 2006). Acknowledging these problems, France has led the world in legislating to improve pool safety and save lives. All private pools now must have safety systems consisting of fences or other specific barriers. Failure to comply with the law carries a substantial penalty, including criminal sanctions. Early evaluation of the impact of the French swimming pool safety law suggests a reduction in the numbers of deaths from drowning. Since the law in France was implemented in 2006, the drowning death rate in France has remained stable despite a 50% increase in the number of private pools (Sethi et al. 2008).

The swimming pool industry was initially against the legislation, arguing that it would negatively impact on business. In fact the opposite occurred, and numbers of swimming pools have continued to increase.

Legislation was facilitated by the strong participation of a non-governmental organization, *Sauve qui Veut*, and the support of a vocal legislator (MacKay et al. 2006).

What general lessons can be learned from drowning prevention?

Drowning and other external causes of injury and death represent an enormous, but largely preventable, child health problem. Poor children, and those living in eastern Europe, are particularly vulnerable to injury and death from external causes. Effective policies for preventing child injury are known. Few governments have, however, been willing to place accident prevention high on their list of policy priorities (McKee et al. 2000). Until they do, preventable injuries and deaths among children will continue.

Sudden infant death syndrome

The rise and fall of cot death

Sudden unexpected deaths in infancy have been described for centuries. In the 17th century, Florentine nuns invented a device called an *arcutio* to protect infants by preventing 'overlying', which was thought to be the cause of death in babies found dead in their shared beds (Savitt 1979). It was not until 1834 that it was realized that something else was happening; a letter in the *Lancet* described babies who had clearly not been suffocated or overlain and yet were found dead in their beds (Fearn 1834).

Sudden infant death syndrome (SIDS) was recognized and given an *International Classification of Disease* code in 1965 (World Health Organization 1965), although disagreement persisted into the 1980s about whether it existed, partly because of the difficulties of a diagnosis by exclusion, and the lack of a clear pathophysiological explanation. SIDS is now defined as the sudden unexpected death of an infant younger than 1 year of age without sufficient explanation, despite a postmortem examination performed to agreed standards, a review of clinical history and scrutiny of the circumstances of the death. Prone sleeping position was noted as a risk factor in 1944 (Abramson 1944) and by the 1970s there was reliable evidence of an increased risk of SIDS from prone sleeping compared with supine sleep position, but this did not become accepted widely until the 1980s (Gilbert et al. 2005). Systematic efforts to prevent SIDS did not begin until the early 1990s, and then only in some countries. A precipitate decline in SIDS occurred from that point onwards (Fig. 6.7).

As can be seen in Fig. 6.7, before the decline started there had been a rise in deaths from SIDS in western Europe. This coincided with a fashion for promoting prone sleeping by child care experts that began in the 1940s, possibly as a means of preventing choking if the infant vomited while lying prone (Gilbert et al. 2005). This advice was indirectly supported by misinterpretation of a paper presented at a conference in the 1980s that involved extrapolating from a small series of premature infants (McKee et al. 1996). Traditional supine sleeping practices persisted in central and eastern Europe, which had been isolated from these erroneous ideas that had been taken up in western countries, and as a consequence SIDS rates did not rise (Fig. 6.8).

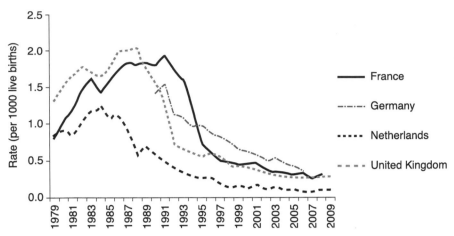

Figure 6.7 Sudden infant death syndrome in four European countries

Source: WHO Regional Office for Europe 2012

Prone sleeping position was still being recommended in child care manuals until the late 1980s (Gilbert et al. 2005). Public health campaigns to prevent SIDS by advising that infants be placed to sleep on their back only began in the early 1990s, and this was followed by a rapid fall in the rates of SIDS. Policy responses in the four countries portrayed in Fig. 6.7 illustrate how differences in response can have an immediate impact on population health outcomes. The chief difference between these four countries was that the Netherlands and the United Kingdom had nationwide campaigns, while France and Germany had regional ones, and only in some areas. As a result, declines started earlier in the Netherlands and United Kingdom than in France and Germany, where it also took longer to reach comparable lower rates.

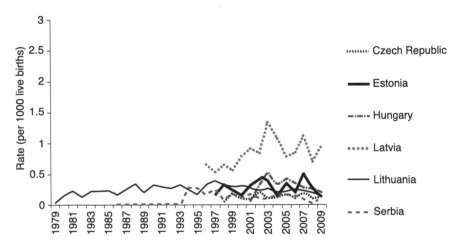

Figure 6.8 Sudden infant death syndrome in central and eastern Europe

Source: WHO Regional Office for Europe 2012

The Netherlands was the first country to recommend a change in infant sleeping position, following the presentation of research demonstrating an association between sleeping position and SIDS in a public lecture in 1987. Media interest in the findings, rather than a public health campaign or policy change, led to significant changes in parenting practices: 46% of babies born before the lecture slept face down while among those born afterwards only 19% slept face down (McKee et al. 1996). Sudden infant deaths fell from 1.04 to 0.44 per 1000 live births in the subsequent five years (de Jonge et al. 1993).

In the United Kingdom, a small study demonstrated a convincing rise in risk of SIDS associated with prone sleeping (Fleming et al. 1990). This led to a local public health campaign followed by a nationwide campaign led by a charity, the Foundation for the Study of Infant Deaths (FSID), which distributed information and public health advice to health professionals throughout the country (Box 6.2). National media interest was fuelled when the baby of a television presenter died of SIDS and she allowed her family's experience to strengthen the campaign initiated by FSID. The efforts of local public health campaigners, the FSID charity and the media prompted the United Kingdom Government to issue a policy statement. Although the statement was circulated to health professionals, the policy was not widely implemented until late 1991, when a national campaign using multimedia advertising and information leaflets was launched, involving the combined efforts of FSID and the government. The existence of an effective national public health infrastructure, with effective means of disseminating information, as in the United Kingdom, helped to implement the public information campaign.

Box 6.2   The Foundation for the Study of Infant Deaths: non-governmental organizations as vital participants in policy

FSID was instrumental when the Reduce the Risk campaign was launched in the early 1990s in the United Kingdom and then rolled out across the country. The numbers of babies who died from SIDS dropped by half within a year (Foundation for the Study of Infant Deaths 2009a). Their success highlights the value of strong partnerships among government, charities and non-governmental organizations.

FSID has continued to grow and diversify; it funds research, provides support for parents and families and information for public and professionals. It is also involved in improving the investigation of sudden unexpected infant deaths. It has been so successful that it now provides advice for others to launch campaigns on reducing risks of SIDS. Much of its information on campaign preparation, forming collaborations with health professionals, communication strategies and working with the media is useful for other types of public health campaign.

FSID continues to work closely with the Department of Health and has an ongoing campaign to reduce the risk of cot death (Foundation for the Study of Infant Deaths 2009b).

In France, a national campaign had been planned but was abandoned when elections intervened. In Germany, efforts were initially confined to two of the *länder*. Both countries had weak public health structures at the time.

What general lessons can be learned from the prevention of SIDS?

The ways in which evidence informs policy and in which implementation is supported in different countries can provide useful lessons about the policy process. In SIDS, the problem was difficult to elucidate and there were doubts about generalizability of evidence obtained from other countries; this delayed action. It took many years to generate sufficient agreement about the diagnosis and risk factors before policy could be devised or implemented. Visible participants outside of government played important roles in the success of official public health campaigns in both the United Kingdom and the Netherlands, illustrating that strong partnerships between governmental and non-governmental actors can play a key role in driving effective public health action. However, there was surprisingly little exchange of thinking among European countries, or even among regions in the same country, Germany. The need for knowledge brokers is apparent.

Discussion and conclusions

The examples presented in this chapter illustrate that European countries differ importantly in their child health policies, and that these differences sometimes have dramatic impacts on child health outcomes. The examples also highlight some of the critical factors that can contribute to success in child health policy. Systems and processes that enable policy-makers to recognize problems are essential. Evidence can be difficult to acquire, as demonstrated in the examples of diphtheria and SIDS. Recognition of the importance of a problem can be lacking, as is the case in eastern European countries for childhood drowning. The politics of the problem also have to be right. Visible participants such as parents can be hugely influential in the success or failure of a policy, as in the case of MMR. Policies can be developed if the problem and politics align, but success relies on cooperation of the visible participants and on mechanisms for implementation.

References

Abramson, H. (1944) Accidental mechanical suffocation in infants, *Pediatrics*, 25:404–13.
Armour-Marshall, J., Wolfe, I., Richardson, E., Karanikolos, M. and McKee, M. (2012) Trends in childhood external causes of mortality; inequalities within Europe and a shifting burden of disease, *European Journal of Public Health*, 22(1):61–5.
Branche, C. and Stewart, S. (2001) *Lifeguard Effectiveness: A Report of the Working Group*. Atlanta, GA: US Centers for Disease Control and Prevention.

Castleden, M., McKee, M., Murray, V. and Leonardi, G. (2011) Resilience thinking in health protection, *Journal of Public Health*, 33(3):369–77.

Centers for Disease Control and Prevention (1996) Update: diphtheria epidemic: new independent states of the former Soviet Union, January 1995–March 1996. *MMWR Morbidity and Mortality Weekly Report*, 45(32):693–7.

European Child Safety Alliance (2009) *Child Safety Report Card 2009. Europe Summary for 24 Countries.* Amsterdam: European Child Safety Alliance.

Fearn, S. (1834) Sudden and unexplained death of children, *Lancet*, 1:246.

Finn, A. and Savulescu, J. (2011) Is immunisation child protection? *Lancet*, 378(9790): 465–8.

Fleming, P., Gilbert, R., Azaz, Y. et al. (1990) Interaction between bedding and sleeping position in the sudden infant death syndrome: case–control study, *British Medical Journal*, 301:85–9.

Foundation for the Study of Infant Deaths (2009a) *Research Background to the Reduce the Risk of Cot Death Advice by the Foundation for the Study of Infant Deaths.* [Factfile 2.] London: Foundation for the Study of Infant Deaths, http://fsid.org.uk/document. doc?id=42 (accessed 10 June 2012).

Foundation for the Study of Infant Deaths (2009b) *Reducing the Risk of Cot Death.* London: The Stationery Office for Department of Health and the Foundation for the Study of Infant Deaths, http://www.dh.gov.uk/prod_consum_dh/groups/dh_digitalassets/ documents/digitalasset/dh_096299.pdf (accessed 10 June 2012).

Galazka, A.M. and Robertson, S.E. (1995) Diphtheria: changing patterns in the developing world, *European Journal of Epidemiology*, 11:107–17.

Gilbert, R., Salanti, G., Harden, M. and See, S. (2005) Infant sleeping position and the sudden infant death syndrome: systematic review of observational studies and historical review of recommendations from 1940 to 2002, *International Journal of Epidemiology*, 34:874–87.

Gotsadze, G., Chikovani, I., Goguadze, K., Balabanova, D. and McKee, M. (2010) Reforming sanitary-epidemiological service in Central and Eastern Europe and the former Soviet Union: an exploratory study, *BMC Public Health*, 10:440.

Griskevica, A. (2002) Epidemic of diphtheria in Latvia. *Seventh International Meeting of the European Laboratory Working Group on Diphtheria.* Vienna, Austria: A3.3.

Hardy, I. (1993) Effectiveness of diphtheria vaccine: results of studies in Russia and Ukraine. Paper presented to the Meeting on Diphtheria Epidemic in Europe. St Petersburg: Foundation Marcel Merieux and WHO.

Health Protection Agency (2011) *Vaccination Schedule for United Kingdom*, http://www. hpa.org.uk/Topics/InfectiousDiseases/InfectionsAZ/VaccineCoverageAndCOVER/ VaccinationSchedule/COVERVaccinepolicydevelopments/ (accessed 15 June 2012).

Health Protection Agency (2012) *Infectious Diseases*, http://www.hpa.org.uk/infections (accessed 15 June 2012).

Honda, H., Shimizu, Y. and Rutter, M. (2005) No effect of MMR withdrawal on the incidence of autism, *Journal of Child Psychology and Psychiatry*, 46:24–6.

Institute of Medicine (2004) *Immunization Safety Review: Vaccines and Autism.* Washington DC: Institute of Medicine.

Jefferson, T., Price, D., Demicheli, V. et al. (2003) Unintended events following immunization with MMR: a systematic review, *Vaccine*, 21:3954–60.

de Jonge, G., Burgmeijer, R., Engleberts, A. et al. (1993) Sleeping position for infants and cot deaths in the Netherlands 1985–91. *Archives of Disease in Childhood*, 69: 660–3.

Khazanov, M.I. (1964) [On the problem of eradication of diphtheria morbidity]. *Vestnik Akademii Meditsinskikh Nauk SSSR*, 19:13–20.

Kingdon, J. (1984) *Agendas, Alternatives and Public Policies.* Boston, MA: Little Brown.

Macario, E., Ednacot, E., Ullberg, L. and Reichel, J. (2011) The changing face and rapid pace of public health communication, *Journal of Communication in Healthcare*, 4(2):145–50.

MacKay, M., Vincenten, J., Brussoni, M. and Towner, L. (2006) *Child Safety Good Practice Guide: Good Investments in Unintentional Child Injury Prevention and Safety Promotion*. Amsterdam; European Child Safety Alliance, Eurosafe.

Mathers, C., Boerma, T. and Fat, D.M. (2008) *The Global Burden of Disease 2004 Update*. Geneva: World Health Organization.

McKee, M. and Lang, T. (1996) Secret government: the Scott report, *British Medical Journal*, 312(7029):455–6.

McKee, M., Fulop, N., Bouvier, P. et al. (1996) Preventing sudden infant deaths: the slow diffusion of an idea, *Health Policy*, 37:117–35.

McKee, M., Zwi, A., Koupilova, I., Sethi, D. and Leon, D. (2000) Health policy-making in central and eastern Europe: lessons from the inaction on injuries? *Health Policy Planning*, 15(3):263–9.

McKee, M., Hurst, L., Aldridge, R.W. et al. (2011) Public health in England: an option for the way forward? *Lancet*, 378(9790):536–9.

NHS Choices (2012) [website]., http://www.nhs.uk/Planners/vaccinations/Pages/Landing. aspx (accessed 15 June 2012).

Parliamentary Office of Science and Technology (2004) *Vaccines and Public Health*. [Postnote 219.] London: Parliamentary Office of Science and Technology.

Savitt, T. (1979) The social and medical history of crib death, *Journal of the Florida Medical Association*, 66:853–9.

Schmitt, H.-J., Booy, R., Weil-Olivier, C. et al. (2003) Child vaccination policies in Europe: a report from the Summits of Independent European Vaccination Experts, *Lancet Infectious Diseases*, 3:103–8.

Sethi, D., Towner, E., Vincenten, J., Segui-Gomez, M. and Racioppi, F. (2008) *European Report on Child Injury Prevention*. Copenhagen: WHO Regional Office for Europe.

Sibert, J., Lyons, R., Smith, B. et al. (2002) Preventing deaths by drowning in children in the United Kingdom: have we made progress in 10 years? Population based incidence study, *British Medical Journal*, 324:1070–1.

Spyker, D.A. (1985) Submersion injury: epidemiology, prevention and management, *Pediatrics Clinics of North America*, 32:113–25.

Social Issues Research Centre, the Royal Society and the Royal Institution of Great Britain (2001) *Guidelines on Science and Health Communication*. Oxford, Social Issues Research Centre, http://www.sirc.org/publik/revised_guidelines.shtml (accessed 10 June 2012).

Thompson, D. and Rivara, F. (1998) Pool fencing for preventing drowning of children, *Cochrane Database of Systematic Reviews*, (1):CD001047.

Vitek, C.R. and Wharton, M. (1998) Diphtheria in the former Soviet Union: reemergence of a pandemic disease, *Emerging Infectious Diseases*, 4(4):539–50.

Wakefield, A., Murch, S., Anthony, A. et al. (1998) Ileal-lymphoid-nodular hyperplasia, non-specific colitis, and pervasive developmental disorder in children, *Lancet*, 351:637–41.

Wintemute, G.J. (1990) Childhood drowning and near-drowning in the United States, *American Journal of Disease in Childhood*, 144(6):663–9.

WHO Regional Office for Europe (2007) *Policies to Reduce Unintentional Injuries from Falls, Drowning, Poisoning, Fires and Choking in Children and Adolescents*. Copenhagen: WHO Regional Office for Europe.

WHO Regional Office for Europe (2012) *European Health for All Database (HFA-DB)*. Copenhagen: WHO Regional Office for Europe, http://data.euro.who.int/hfadb/ (accessed 4 June 2012).

World Health Organization (1965) *International Classification of Diseases*, revision 8. Geneva: World Health Organization.

World Health Organization (2011) Fourth meeting of the Global Polio Eradication Initiative's Independent Monitoring Board. Increased transmission and outbreaks of measles, European Region, 2011. *Weekly Epidemiological Record*, 86(49): 557–64.

World Health Organization (2012) *Mortality Database*. Geneva: World Health Organization, http://www.who.int/healthinfo/morttables/en/ (accessed 4 June 2012).

chapter seven

Infectious disease

Ralf Reintjes and Martin McKee

Introduction

An area of great historical successes

Historically, the first successes of health policy were in the area of infectious disease. The year 1848 is remembered in Europe for two things, revolutions and epidemics. When Marx wrote of a spectre stalking Europe at the time, he could as easily have substituted cholera for communism. No-one was safe, with notable victims including Tchaikovsky and the Prussian military theorist Carl von Clausewitz. The demonstration by John Snow that cholera was transmitted by contaminated water has gone down in history as one of the greatest public health successes. Other successes, such as Pasteur's confirmation of the germ theory, showing that it was microorganisms that caused many then common diseases, and Koch's development of his postulates, which made it possible to link specific microorganisms to particular diseases, laid the foundation for a wide range of measures, from clean water to safe food production, that have allowed Europe's citizens to be safeguarded from many of the dangers that once surrounded them. Cholera has been eliminated from Europe and the few cases of typhoid are largely contracted elsewhere. Perhaps less obviously, the practice of paediatrics has been transformed, as the hospital wards that were, as recently as the 1970s, filled with children with gastroenteritis, jaundice and chest infections are now long closed.

As recently as the 1950s, an estimated 50 million cases of smallpox occurred each year worldwide. Although immunization had eliminated the disease from most industrialized countries by then, Europe remained at risk and as recently as 1972, a pilgrim from Kosovo brought the disease back from the Middle East, infecting 175 people and causing 35 deaths. Yet, by 1975, the disease had been confined to a small war-torn area in the horn of Africa where, on 26 October 1979, Ali Maow Maalin, a Somali cook, was the last person in the world to be diagnosed with naturally occurring smallpox. Exactly two years later, a commission of leading scientists declared that smallpox had been eradicated, a decision upheld by the World Health Assembly on 8 May 1980 (Pennington 2003).

So far, smallpox is the only infectious disease that had been affecting humans for long periods of time to have been eradicated. However, a number of other diseases are targeted for global or regional eradication, with varying degrees of success. One of those is polio. It was the development of vaccines against polio in the 1950s that provided an opportunity to target it for eradication. In 1960, one European country, Czechoslovakia, became the first to eliminate it, and other industrialized countries soon followed. In 1988, WHO, Rotary International, UNICEF and the United States Centers for Disease Control launched the Global Polio Eradication Initiative. In 1994, the Americas became the first of the WHO's regions to be declared polio free, followed in 2002 by the WHO European Region. However, the experience with polio serves as a warning. In 2010, polio returned to the central Asian part of the WHO European Region, with a major outbreak in Tajikistan. Genetic sequencing indicated that the virus had originated in northern India. As this example and several of the others in this chapter show, the price of success against infectious disease is constant vigilance.

This chapter will examine some of the major successes, and failures, in the struggle against infectious disease in Europe in recent decades. First, however, it is useful to review briefly the burden of disease attributable to infectious disease in Europe in comparison with the rest of the world.

The burden of disease attributable to infections in Europe

In the past century, Europe has undergone a profound epidemiological transition (Omran 1971). Access to clean water, safe food production and distribution, immunization and antibiotics, among other things, have brought about a steady decline in what were once very common, and often fatal, infectious diseases. In Stockholm, for example, when piped water was introduced in 1861, 25% of babies still died within their first year and only 50% survived until the age of 15, with the vast majority of deaths caused by infection (Burstrom and Bernhardt 2001). By 2010, the infant mortality rate in Sweden had fallen to 2.5 per 1000 live births, partly as a result of improved sanitation and other public health interventions. Consequently, the contribution that infectious diseases make to the total burden of disease in Europe is now very low, compared with that in the world as a whole (Fig. 7.1), although it is greater in the low- and middle-income countries of the region.

Table 7.1 shows a more detailed breakdown. Of the specific diseases identified, sexually transmitted diseases contribute most in the high-income countries, followed by human immunodeficiency virus (HIV) infection and the acquired immunodeficiency syndrome (AIDS). In the low- and middle-income countries, respiratory infections and tuberculosis are the largest single contributors, at levels much higher than in the high-income countries of Europe.

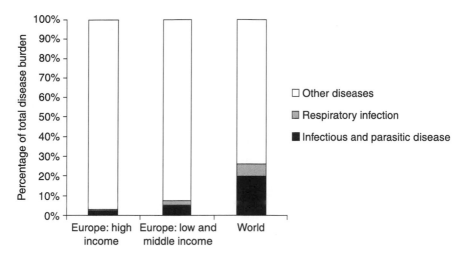

Figure 7.1 Contribution of infectious and parasitic diseases and respiratory infections to the total burden of disease

Source: Mathers et al. 2008
Note: High-income countries in Europe are Andorra, Austria, Belgium, Cyprus, Denmark, Finland, France, Germany, Greece, Iceland, Ireland, Israel, Italy, Liechtenstein, Luxembourg, Malta, Monaco, the Netherlands, Norway, Portugal, San Marino, Slovenia, Spain, Sweden, Switzerland, the United Kingdom

Two categories of successes and failures

The successes and failures that we will deal with in this chapter fall into two broad categories. The first involves putting in place systems that protect the public from new or persisting threats. Public health can do this in several ways. One, which also numbers among the greatest historical successes in public health, is to immunize people against disease. This will confer protection on the individual but, as importantly, if enough people are immunized it will also confer protection on the few that are not by breaking the chain of transmission – a process known as herd immunity. Another is to identify behaviours that place people at risk and take action to reduce that risk. Many of the best known examples relate to sexually transmitted diseases and, collectively, involve the dissemination of messages about 'safe sex'.

The second category involves securing previous gains. After systems have been put in place that protect the public from a particular threat, these need to be carefully maintained and updated when needed. This is less obvious than it seems: the history of infectious disease control is full of examples where systems have failed to be maintained or updated, and we will discuss a few examples in this chapter. A particular challenge in this category is that microorganisms are able to exploit new opportunities and to avoid barriers placed in their way. This leads to a continued struggle between those microorganisms and the public health community, which must strive to stay one step ahead. There are many examples that affect Europe, particularly as a consequence of the massive

Table 7.1 Burden of disease from specific infectious causes in disability-adjusted life-years and its percentage of the total disease burden, 2004

	Europe: high income			Europe: low and middle income			World		
	Total DALYS	DALYS per 1000 population	Percentage of total disease burden	Total DALYS	DALYS per 1000 population	Percentage of total disease burden	Total DALYS	DALYS per 1000 population	Percentage of total disease burden
Infectious and parasitic disease	**838**	**2.1**	**1.7**	**5203**	**10.9**	**5.1**	**302,144**	**46.9**	**19.8**
Tuberculosis	40	0.1	0.1	1695	3.6	1.7	34,217	5.3	2.2
Sexually transmitted diseases (excluding HIV)	77	0.2	0.2	290	0.6	0.3	10,425	1.6	0.7
HIV	196	0.5	0.4	983	2.1	1.0	58,513	9.1	3.8
Diarrhoeal disease	114	0.3	0.2	1279	2.7	1.3	72,777	11.3	4.8
Childhood cluster illness[a]	20	0.0	0.0	47	0.1	0.0	30,226	4.7	2.0
Meningitis	50	0.1	0.1	284	0.6	0.3	11,426	1.8	0.8
Hepatitis B	32	0.1	0.1	104	0.2	0.1	2,068	0.3	0.1
Hepatitis C	34	0.1	0.1	37	0.1	0.0	955	0.1	0.1
Respiratory infections	**488**	**1.2**	**1.0**	**2419**	**5.1**	**2.4**	**97,786**	**15.2**	**6.4**

Source: Mathers et al. 2008

Notes: DALY, disability-adjusted life-years; HIV, human immunodeficiency virus

[a]Childhood cluster includes pertussis, polio, diphtheria, measles and tetanus

increase, in volume and pace, of global movement of people and goods. The proximity of humans and domestic poultry provided the perfect conditions for genetic mixing of generic material from humans and birds, leading to avian influenza. A similar situation, although this time involving industrial production of pigs in Mexico, has allowed human influenza to mix with the swine version. The speed with which influenza spreads from person to person means that the emergence of a new strain of influenza can rapidly develop into a pandemic. Another threat arises from the overuse of antibiotics. Frequently, within a colony of infecting microorganisms, there will be a few that have a mutation that confers resistance to a particular antibiotic. Especially where treatment is inadequate to allow the body's natural defences to eliminate the infection, these mutated organisms may thrive, eventually replacing all the microorganisms that were sensitive to the antibiotic.

Protecting the health of the public from new or persisting threats

Measles

According to the OECD (2011), 'childhood vaccination continues to be one of the most cost-effective health policy interventions. . . . Coverage of these programmes can be considered as a quality-of-care indicator.' This is particularly the case for measles, a disease that, although often mild and self-limiting, can on occasions be fatal or leave severe neurological sequelae. Because of its proven effectiveness, with an efficacy of over 99% (van Boven et al. 2010), measles vaccination has been recommended for general administration since the 1990s, but there is still considerable variation in uptake. About half of the countries in the European Economic Area fail to achieve the 95% coverage considered necessary to achieve herd immunity (Fig. 7.2) (van Boven et al. 2010). Many of those failing to do so are among the wealthiest countries in Europe, with the highest levels of health resources. Moreover, even these figures may be considerable overestimates as those countries without centralized systems, such as Germany, are unable to track accurately their coverage levels. Consequently, it has been argued that 'immunization is not rated equally high on political agendas across countries in the EU' (Schmitt et al. 2003). The result is that major outbreaks continue to occur regularly in some European countries (Table 7.2), while others have essentially eliminated the disease except for imported cases. Yet, despite these very mixed results, the countries of the WHO have committed to eliminating measles from its European Region by 2015 (Martin et al. 2011).

The association between measles immunization rates and measles incidence is apparent from a study of data from the 30 countries of the European Economic Area in the years 2008 to 2011. Only nine of these countries maintained immunization rates at 95% or above (group 1) while 16 countries had rates of less than 95% (group 2) and five did not report coverage data to the European Centre for Disease Prevention and Control or WHO (group 3). The mean measles incidence in the four year period was 0.09 per 100,000 in

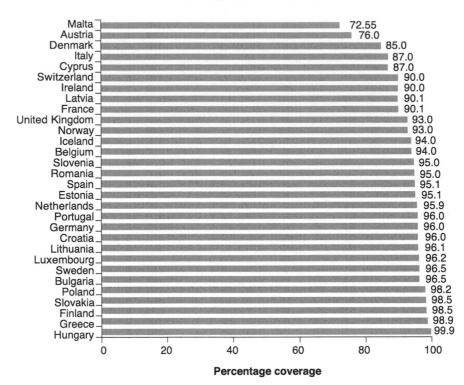

Figure 7.2   Coverage by measles immunization in the European Economic Area and Switzerland, 2010 or most recent available year

Source: WHO Regional Office for Europe 2012
Note: See warning about the quality of data in the text

Table 7.2   Burden of measles in countries with the highest incidence in first half of 2011

	Cases	*Incidence density[a]*
Europe	21,326	N.A
France	12,699	14.45
Romania	1,619	5.00
Switzerland	589	4.25
Spain	2,261	2.78
Italy	1,500	1.65
Belgium	382	1.37

Source: European Centre for Disease Prevention and Control 2011a
Note: [a]Incidence per 10 million per day in the surveillance period

group 1, 6.72 per 100,000 in group 2 and 3.57 per 100,000 in group 3 (Riemann-Lorenz 2012).

Why do the coverage levels achieved in these countries differ so much? National immunization systems differ widely. In broad terms they can be classified as centralized or decentralized. Typical examples of centralized systems are those in Finland and the Netherlands. In Finland, vaccines are purchased centrally by the National Public Health Institute. Parents receive invitations to bring their children to be immunized when they reach the appropriate age. Vaccines are administered, free of charge, in child care centres by public health nurses, who register the coverage rates and report them to a central office on a regular basis. A government-funded compensation scheme exists for the very rare occasion when a complication arises (Schmitt et al. 2003).

Germany and France are examples of countries with private or decentralized systems. Here the systems run with minimal input from the governments. In Germany, an advisory committee, the Ständige Impfkommission, develops national immunization plans, listing vaccines against diseases considered of public health importance and recommending the timing of immunization (Wiese-Posselt et al. 2011). The 16 federal German states (*Länder*) are advised to adopt and recommend this plan publicly. Such a public recommendation is the legal basis for compensation following a potential vaccine-induced event. Immunization is generally undertaken by private paediatricians or general practitioners. Those vaccines recommended by the Ständige Impfkommission are generally paid for by health insurance companies (Schmitt et al. 2003). Yet, at least until recently, there is evidence that many health workers and members of the public are unaware of these recommendations (Lauberau et al. 2001). Unlike the situation in Finland, parents must take the initiative to bring their children to be immunized. There is no mechanism to invite them systematically and no centralized registration that would allow monitoring of coverage, and thus institute intervention where it is low. This also means that the available data on coverage are largely taken from surveys or from data collected at school entry, although the use of social health insurance data is also being explored (Kalies et al. 2008).

There are many factors involved in the success or otherwise of an immunization programme. Consequently, there is no simple relationship between the degree of centralization and the coverage rate. For example, coverage rates in the United Kingdom, a country with a centralized system, fell markedly as a consequence of a concern about the safety of the combined MMR vaccine (discussed in Chapter 6). Nonetheless, many of the countries in Europe with low coverage rates have decentralized systems and many of those with high rates have centralized systems. Schmitt and colleagues (2003) have argued that centralized systems have certain obvious advantages over decentralized systems. Centralized systems can often procure vaccine at lower cost through bulk purchasing. They can optimize distribution systems to minimize wastage. Proactive invitations to parents, follow-up of non-attenders and the ability to undertake investigations to identify barriers facing marginalized groups (Cohuet et al. 2009) are all likely to increase coverage. In contrast, in decentralized systems plans, targets and deadlines are less well defined.

Influenza

Influenza affects hundreds of thousands of European citizens each year. It is often complicated by pneumonia, and it is a frequent cause of hospital admissions and sometimes death, particularly among children, the elderly and those with chronic diseases. In May 2003, the 56th World Health Assembly recommended influenza vaccination for all people at high risk defined as the elderly and persons with underlying diseases (World Health Organization 2003). All EU Member States committed to the goal of attaining vaccination coverage of the elderly population of at least 50% by 2006 and 75% by 2010. Many national guidelines also recommend yearly vaccination against influenza for all elderly people.

These recommendations are based on studies of vaccine effectiveness, which have been summarized in regularly updated *Cochrane Systematic Reviews*. A review published in 2006 concluded that vaccination prevented pneumonia, hospital admissions and deaths among elderly people residing in long-term care facilities, and also had modest effectiveness against complications of influenza among elderly living in the community (Rivetti et al. 2006). A recent update of this review was more sceptical of the evidence. It found only one randomized controlled trial (showing effectiveness of vaccination against influenza symptoms) against 74 observational studies, which were judged to be of insufficient quality to be used in assessing the effectiveness of influenza vaccination (Jefferson et al. 2010).

European countries have been very diverse in their uptake of these vaccination policies, and among countries that have national influenza vaccination policies there is large variation in the universality of the programmes (Mereckiene et al. 2008a, 2010). Some countries have been very successful in increasing vaccination uptake, others much less so. As a result, vaccination uptake among the elderly also differs strongly between countries. Not all countries have a system in place to monitor uptake, but among those who do, vaccination coverage in 2008 among those aged 65 and older ranged from 2% in Lithuania to 82% in the Netherlands (Mereckiene et al. 2008b). While vaccination uptake has gone up over time, achieving the target of 75% coverage remains a challenge (Mereckiene et al. 2010). Countries that require a co-payment from elderly people appear to have lower coverage rates than countries that do not (Kroneman et al. 2003). Figure 7.3 illustrates these variations.

While variations in uptake rates between countries should provide good opportunities to study the population health impact of influenza vaccination, the data needs to be analysed carefully because influenza is a relatively unreliable cause of death, and many influenza deaths may be hidden in other cause-of-death categories such as pneumonia and ischaemic heart disease. Some studies have indeed found that increased vaccination coverage is associated with lower mortality at the population level (Kwong et al. 2008; Fireman et al. 2009), but others have not (Rizzo et al. 2006; Simonsen et al. 2007). In any case, the effect is likely to be small and difficult to detect. As excess mortality attributable to influenza has been between 5% and 10%, on average, during the influenza seasons in the past several decades (Simonsen et al. 2007), and the protection of vaccination against excess death is likely to be lower than 50%, one would

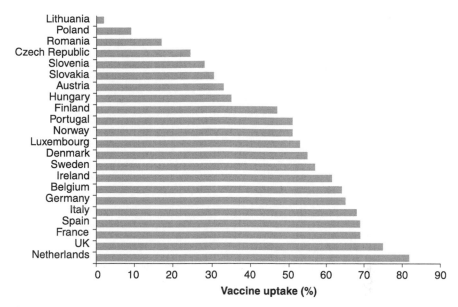

Figure 7.3   Uptake of influenza immunization by individuals older than 65 years of age vaccinated in 2008 or nearest year

Source: Mereckiene et al. 2008b

expect a coverage rate of say 60% to be associated with a few percentage points reduction of total mortality at most (Fireman et al. 2009).

We conclude that some countries have been highly successful in achieving a high uptake of influenza vaccination among the elderly, and while this has probably reduced complications, the population health impact remains somewhat elusive.

HIV infection and AIDS

The first cases of AIDS in Europe, the disease caused by HIV infection, were reported in 1982 (Francioli et al. 1982; Rozenbaum et al. 1982; Vilaseca et al. 1982). By the end of 2010, an estimated 2.3 million people in the European region were living with an HIV infection and many millions had died of AIDS and its complications in the preceding three decades.

The story of AIDS in Europe is one of some successes, many failures, and many missed opportunities (Atun et al. 2008). The epidemic took very different forms in different countries. To some extent, these reflected intrinsic differences in the countries involved, such as the very limited scale of movement of people into the USSR in the 1980s; consequently, the epidemic in countries such as the Russian Federation and Ukraine came much later than in western countries. However, to a considerable extent the differing forms of the epidemic also reflected differences in the policies that were adopted by the authorities in each country.

Prevention of the transmission of HIV requires a multifaceted strategy combining measures of proven effectiveness in reducing the transmission of HIV in general and those specific to different modes of transmission. The former include voluntary counselling and testing to enable those infected to become aware of their status (Voluntary HIV-1 Counseling and Testing Efficacy Study Group 2000) and treatment with antiretroviral drugs, as those with a very low viral load are unlikely to transmit the infection (Donnell et al. 2010). Mass media campaigns increase uptake of testing for HIV in the short term but evidence of long-term effects is lacking (Vidanapathirana et al. 2005). Reduction of risks of sexual transmission can be achieved by programmes using active learning methods to address sexual risk-taking behaviour (Peersman and Levy 1998) – but not abstinence-only programmes, which have not been found to be effective (Underhill et al. 2007) – and use of condoms (Weller and Davis 2002). Measures effective in reducing blood-borne spread include establishing safe blood supply systems (World Health Organization 2010) and needle exchange programmes for intravenous drug users (Wodak and Cooney 2004). The risk of mother-to-child transmission can be reduced by the use of antiretroviral drugs at the time of delivery (Siegfried et al. 2011). Figure 7.4 shows the trends in incidence of AIDS in some European countries.

In some countries, the public health authorities responded rapidly, with mass media campaigns to educate the public about the disease and the factors that increased the risk of getting infected. These included the Netherlands and the United Kingdom. The campaigns sought to promote both tolerance of what was recognized as a potentially highly stigmatizing disease and harm reduction measures among those whose lifestyles placed them at risk (de Vroome et al. 1990; Stimson 1995). In Switzerland, the success of pioneering initiatives

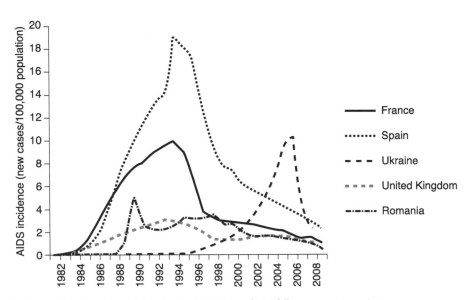

Figure 7.4 Trends in incidence of AIDS in selected European countries

Source: WHO Regional Office for Europe 2012

in Zurich convinced the federal government to adopt what were then courageous, and technically illegal, needle exchange programmes to reduce the risks associated with intravenous drug use (Csete and Grob 2012). In countries such as Spain and France, the response was considerably delayed (Barrio et al. 2011).

In other countries, however, such as Ireland and Poland, it was difficult to mount an effective response because of prevailing cultural attitudes to the major risk factors (Danziger 1996; Smyth 1998). Some countries, despite having strong public health systems, have also struggled to put in place effective systems. For example, harm reduction activities, such as needle exchange, are estimated to reach only about 5% of intravenous drug users in Sweden (Harm Reduction International 2008). Romania requires special mention. A deeply misguided policy of giving malnourished infants micro-transfusions of blood created a cohort of HIV-infected children (Dolea et al. 2002). However, the Ceausescu regime was in denial, viewing AIDS as a 'capitalist' disease that was absent from Romania, and it was not until after the revolution that any serious response was mounted. Delay similarly characterized many of the other countries of the former USSR and Central Europe, although some, such as Czechoslovakia, moved rapidly with public education and harm reduction programmes once the new governments were in place. The situation was even worse in the countries that emerged from the break-up of the USSR. Responses in Ukraine and the Russian Federation were fragmented and unfocused (Atun et al. 2005).

Many of those most affected by HIV, such as men who have sex with men, sex workers and intravenous drug users, had historically few links with public health authorities. The more progressive authorities recognized this and reached out to support and work with civil society organizations. In many cases, these organizations, such as the Terence Higgins Trust in the United Kingdom and the Dutch AIDS Foundation East West, which is active in the former USSR, have been very effective in promoting health promotion messages, running needle exchange programmes, and distributing condoms. However, their ability to act as advocates for people living with HIV, which has been very effective in many western countries, has been highly constrained in many countries of the former USSR (Spicer et al. 2011).

Since the early 1980s, there has been a vast increase in understanding of the factors that increase the risk of contracting infection with HIV. This has enabled many governments in western and central Europe to mount effective responses to at least some of the risk factors. For example, in 2010 there were only 250 cases of mother-to-child transmission reported in western and central Europe, a rate that is far lower than in most other parts of the world (European Centre for Disease Prevention and Control 2011b). The risk of contracting HIV infection from blood transfusions is now virtually eliminated (Likatavicius et al. 2007). However, in other areas, such as prevention of infection among intravenous drug users, the record is less consistent, with some countries integrating provision of needle exchange programmes and opioid substitution into their mainstream health services while in other such services cling on to the margins, provided by often poorly funded non-governmental organizations (Harm Reduction International 2010). There are also worrying signs of reversals in some countries, such as the rapid increase in new cases in men who have sex with men in countries such as Finland, Germany, Norway and the United

Kingdom (Likatavicius et al. 2008), which is thought to reflect an increasingly widespread complacency about HIV infections and AIDS given the availability of treatment (Marcus et al. 2006). There are also a growing number of infections among people from some countries, such as the United Kingdom, who are travelling abroad as 'sex tourists' (Rice et al. 2012).

While the picture is decidedly mixed in western and central Europe, it is consistently worse in eastern Europe. Since 2001, the prevalence of HIV infections has increased by 250%, making it the region with the fastest expanding epidemic in the world. Within this region, 90% of the new cases of HIV infections are in two countries, the Russian Federation and Ukraine. Intravenous drug users, sex workers and prisoners are at greatest risk, although the scale of the epidemic in men who have sex with men may be under-recorded because of the associated stigma and discrimination. In the Ukraine, for example, an estimated 40–50% of intravenous drug users are infected (Harm Reduction International 2010). Yet availability of harm reduction programmes is extremely limited, reaching an estimated 7% of intravenous drug users in the Russian Federation (Mathers et al. 2010). Opioid substitution therapy remains illegal in the Russian Federation, reflecting the persistence of an authoritarian approach to substance misuse that developed in isolation from developments in the west (Rechel et al. 2011), although such therapy has been introduced in Ukraine.

While it is necessary to take account of differences in the contribution to the overall incidence rates of migrants who contracted their infections abroad, the diversity of policies in place is a significant factor in the wide variation in incidence of HIV in Europe today (Fig. 7.5).

Bovine spongiform encephalopathy

Perhaps one of the best studied examples of a failure to protect the public from new health hazards in Europe in recent decades has been the emergence of variant Creutzfeldt–Jakob disease in humans following ingestion of beef from cows infected with BSE. This was a public health failure in one country, the United Kingdom, but with lessons for everyone. Since the first case was detected in 1987, there have been another 200,000 cases in cattle in Europe, the overwhelming majority in England (Fig. 7.6), with estimates of 1–3 million infected but slaughtered before developing the disease (Smith and Bradley 2003). As of 2011, over 200 humans were reported to have developed the disease (175 in the United Kingdom, 25 in France, 5 in Spain, 4 in Ireland, 3 in the Netherlands, 2 in Italy and 2 in Portugal (World Health Organization 2012). The measures that were eventually put in place included a worldwide ban on the export of British beef and cost the United Kingdom economy an estimated €4.8 billion.

The origins of BSE are believed to lie in changes in the process of manufacturing meat and bone meal, a foodstuff for cattle derived from animal waste such as animals dying on farms and animal parts unsuitable for human consumption. This took place in the 1970s in the United Kingdom, earlier than in other countries, and involved lowering the temperature used to separate protein from fat. The main justification was commercial, in that it was cheaper. Although

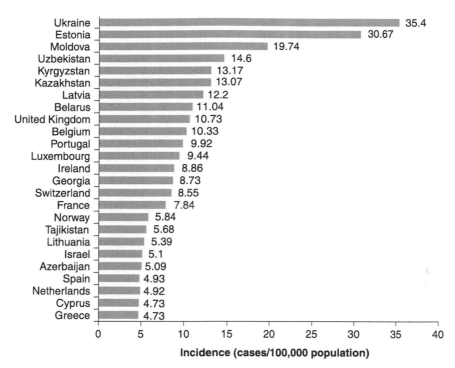

Figure 7.5 Incidence of HIV infections in Europe, 2010 or nearest year (25 highest countries)

Source: WHO Regional Office for Europe 2012

the subsequent inquiry commissioned by the United Kingdom Government appears to exonerate the public health authorities, a more detailed examination of the evidence it collected paints a much less positive picture (Abbasi 2000). There were three main public health failures (McKee et al. 1996). The first was a presumption in favour of deregulation by then Conservative Government, which saw regulations as an unnecessary restriction on business. Although concerns about the new meat and bone meal processing method had been raised in 1979, these were ignored. The government consistently adopted an optimistic interpretation of the evidence, eschewing the precautionary principle. This climate of deregulation would subsequently have many other serious consequences, particularly as a consequence of its application to the financial services industry.

The second failure was the process used by the government to obtain specialist information. Because of its public insistence that BSE was an animal disease that posed no significant threat to humans, it was very reluctant to involve public health specialists until the link between BSE and variant Creutzfeldt–Jakob disease could no longer be denied. The specialist committee took a very narrow approach, confining its deliberations to what had already happened. There was no attempt to think outside the box and to ask 'what if' or to model the consequences of different scenarios. There was no serious attempt to question

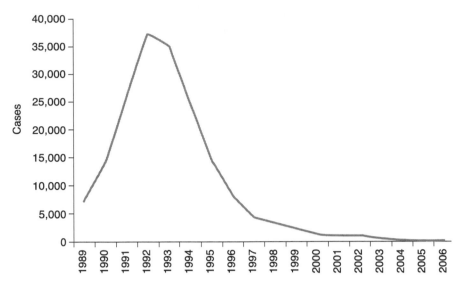

Figure 7.6 Annual incidence of bovine spongiform encephalopathy in cattle in the United Kingdom

Source: Ducrot et al. 2008
Note: In no year were there more than 350 cases in any other European country

the assumption that the species barrier was insurmountable. The committee also took on trust what it was told by government officials. This led it, erroneously, to conclude that the measures that had already been adopted to require that abattoirs remove those tissues most at risk were actually being implemented. Yet the government was well aware that in 30–40% their inspections revealed that they were not.

The third failure was the priority given by the government to the interests of industry above public health. The then Ministry of Agriculture, Fisheries and Food was widely viewed as having been captured by the industries over which it had regulatory oversight.

Severe acute respiratory syndrome

In contrast to the situation with variant Creutzfeldt–Jakob disease, where the public health authorities were slow in their response, when an outbreak caused by another new infectious agent, severe acute respiratory syndrome (SARS), occurred in November 2002 in Guangdong Province, China, they soon moved ahead to tackle the problem. Within days, the Canadian Global Public Health Intelligence Network, part of the WHO's Global Outbreak and Alert Response Network, identified an upsurge of reports on the Internet, in Chinese, of a 'flu outbreak' in China.

At the time the Chinese authorities had not informed WHO and, for several months, they continued to downplay its significance and deny access to WHO investigators. Quiet, but largely ineffective, diplomacy continued in the background, but this changed in February 2003 when an American businessman travelling from Guangdong to Singapore changed planes in Hanoi. He was severely ill and taken to a Vietnamese hospital where he died. Soon afterwards, several hospital staff developed the same previously unknown illness and one, an Italian doctor, also died. On 12 March 2003, WHO issued a global alert. However, by that time, two clusters had occurred in Hong Kong, one in a hotel in which a number of international visitors were staying. Within a short while, it had spread to Europe and single cases had been diagnosed in Ireland, Romania, the Russian Federation, Switzerland and Spain.

It could, however, have been much worse. Although over 8000 cases were reported from 29 countries, its transmission was interrupted successfully within less than four months of the first spread outside China. This was a consequence of 21st century methods of electronic communication (Ahmad et al. 2009) combined with 19th century public health tools, including case detection, contact tracing, quarantine and isolation, and infection control. This was only possible through the coordinated efforts of governments, international organizations and health care institutions. Countries were willing to forego their exclusive sovereign rights to solve a global threat (World Health Organization 2003a,b; Heymann 2005). Although WHO led the effort to contain spread given its global nature, the EU also played a role.

The European Commission established a multidisciplinary SARS expert group to provide advice on SARS-related issues. In June 2003, the Commission reported on the *Measures Undertaken by Member States and Accession Countries to Control the Outbreak of SARS* in Europe, and noted that 'on the whole, European countries have adopted rapid and consistent measures on early detection of cases, implementation of isolation measures and guidance to health professionals and the public on the identification of possible SARS cases' (European Commission 2003).

Yet the experience with SARS exposed major weaknesses in the health infrastructure in EU Member States and identified areas that needed strengthened European collaboration. It reinforced the need for a European centre that would provide an operational platform to bring together the expertise in EU Member States, delivering a systematic EU-wide approach to control communicable disease and strengthening cooperation with international partners. This culminated in the establishment of the European Centre for Disease Prevention and Control in 2005 as well as the initiation of research projects to advise policy-makers on how best to prepare for potential new epidemics (Ahmad et al. 2009).

Securing what has been achieved

System breakdown during economic crises

After systems have been put in place that protect the public from a particular threat, these need to be carefully maintained and updated when needed. This requires continued investment in the measures that have been taken in the past and constant vigilance based on effective systems of surveillance. Unfortunately, in the climate of austerity that has afflicted many European countries since 2008, there is a real danger that both of these could be compromised. Indications of what might happen can be gleaned from a recent systematic review of the effects of economic and political crises on infectious disease (Suhrcke et al. 2011). This review was based on a conceptual model of the factors that might change in times of difficulty.

The first potential factor is changes in the population at risk, for example as a consequence of reduced immunization coverage. The second is changes in the infection rate, by greater opportunities for person-to-person spread through either common vehicles or vectors. The third is changes in access to treatment to prevent progression of the illness and its onward spread.

All three factors can be identified in Europe in recent decades. The USSR had achieved a high level of vaccine coverage and, by the 1960s, it was believed that it might be possible to eliminate diphtheria. However, the systems that had been put in place did not survive the massive disruption that accompanied the dissolution of the USSR in 1989. Immunization rates fell precipitously and, exacerbated by declining socioeconomic conditions, a major epidemic occurred. The number of cases increased dramatically, from 839 in 1989 to almost 20,000 in 1993 (Vitek and Wharton 1998). The reasons for this outbreak and what was done to control it are discussed in detail in Chapter 6.

The second factor is a change in the infection rate. Economic downturns are often associated with increases in crime (Police Federation of England and Wales 2009) and incarceration of those convicted. However, prisons, particularly in poorer countries where conditions are poor, can act as incubators for disease, particularly tuberculosis (Basu et al. 2011), with subsequent spread into the general population when infected prisoners are released without adequate follow-up. Consequently, there is a close association between rates of incarceration in countries of eastern Europe and the growth of tuberculosis in the general population during the 1990s (Stuckler et al. 2008a). Increased infection rates may also be associated with increases in other high-risk behaviours, such as intravenous drug use, which has been implicated in the recent marked increase in infections with HIV in Greece (Kentikelenis et al. 2011). Disease may also arise through infectious agents transmitted by common vehicles, such as water supplies. This is what happened in Uzbekistan, when a lack of investment in infrastructure led to leaking pipes and low pressure, with cross-contamination of drinking-water and sewerage (Semenza et al. 1998). It may also arise as a result of changes in populations of vectors, or of changes in human behaviour that increase exposure to vectors. Examples include the recent reappearance of malaria in Greece (Health Protection Agency 2011), a substantial increase in cases of tick-borne encephalitis in the Baltic states in the 1990s (associated with a growth in foraging for food in forests; Randolph 2008) and an outbreak of Chikungunya fever in Italy (Angelini et al. 2007). Such events are likely to become more frequent in future as a consequence of climate change. However, the dangers are not only from insect vectors; an outbreak of tularaemia in Kosovo in 1999 was linked to an increase in rodents following the abandonment of food storage facilities (Reintjes et al. 2002).

The third factor is reduced access to care, leading to both progression of disease, in some cases with fatal consequences, and to continued spread of infection. Countries receiving loans from the International Monetary Fund are subject to strict conditions, in particular for reductions in public spending. This has been linked to increases in incidence and mortality from tuberculosis (Stuckler et al. 2008b).

Individually, each of these examples is a public health failure. Collectively, they illustrate what happens if governments fail to maintain the infrastructure that has safeguarded the people of Europe from many once common causes of disease.

Methicillin-resistant Staphylococcus aureus

Soon after penicillin became widely available, *Staphylococcus aureus*, a common cause of infections of skin, soft tissue, bone and the lining of the heart, demonstrated its ability to develop resistance (National Nosocomial Infections Surveillance 2003). Each time a new antibiotic was introduced, staphylococcal resistance was not far behind, and by 1961, strains were emerging that were resistant to methicillin, the only antibiotic that had until then been effective. Methicillin-resistant *Staphylococcus aureus* (MRSA) is now widespread in health care facilities in many countries and is a major concern because of its potential to spread, its high mortality rate in patients whose condition is already weakened and the stringent hygienic requirements needed to manage patients who are harbouring it (Cosgrove et al. 2003; Muto et al. 2003; Mellmann et al. 2006). It has been estimated that approximately 150,000 patients each year are infected with MRSA, with substantial additional costs for health care providers (Kock et al. 2010). Especially worrying is the emergence of strains that are also resistant to the few remaining effective antibiotics, such as vancomycin (Chang et al. 2003). Interestingly, the prevalence of MRSA varies extensively among countries (Fig. 7.7), with resistance found in 53.4% of *S. aureus* isolates in Portugal but only 0.5% in Sweden (European Centre for Disease Prevention and Control 2012). However, effective countermeasures do exist and, while it is difficult to differentiate the effects of the individual elements, a wide-ranging programme launched in 2004 in the United Kingdom, which then had one of the highest rates in Europe, was associated with a fall of 57% by 2008 (Edgeworth 2011). Factors believed to be responsible for this reduction included universal hand hygiene, contact precautions and admission screening, as well as decolonization using agents such as chlorhexidine and mupirocin.

These variations are likely to reflect differences in health policy. A comparison of national guidelines to prevent and control MRSA and the corresponding frequency of MRSA in isolates was undertaken in 2008 in 13 European countries (Kalenic et al. 2010). This revealed wide variation in when national (or regional in federal countries) guidelines were first issued – from 1970 in Sweden to 2008 in Spain and Croatia – and whether they were voluntary or compulsory. There were also considerable variations in surveillance systems, including what information was collected, with some, such as the Czech Republic and United Kingdom, collecting data on bacteraemia with others, such as Croatia, collecting data on isolates at any site. The content of guidelines also varied. Kalenic et al. (2010) drew four broad conclusions from their data. First, the

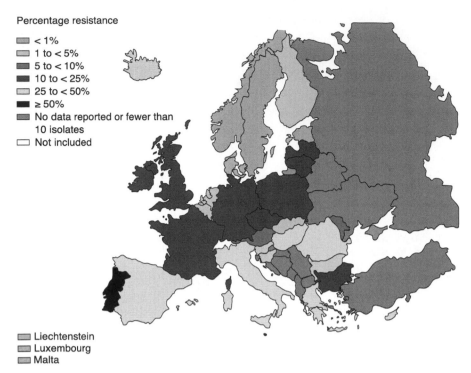

Percentage resistance

- ▨ < 1%
- ▨ 1 to < 5%
- ▨ 5 to < 10%
- ■ 10 to < 25%
- ▨ 25 to < 50%
- ■ ≥ 50%
- ▨ No data reported or fewer than 10 isolates
- ▢ Not included

▨ Liechtenstein
▨ Luxembourg
▢ Malta

Figure 7.7 *Staphylococcus aureus*: invasive isolates resistant to methicillin (MRSA), 2010

Source: European Centre for Disease Prevention and Control 2012

countries with the lowest rates of MRSA (Norway, Sweden, Denmark and the Netherlands) had first produced guidelines before 2000 while five of the nine with higher rates had produced them later. These low-prevalence countries also had guidelines for nursing homes, general practice and home care, which were lacking in many of the other countries. Second, all four low-prevalence countries prescribed single rooms for those infected while other countries also permitted cohorting, in which patients with the same infection are treated together. The authors speculated that this may reflect lower numbers of single rooms in the latter countries. It may also reflect broader issues of capacity, given evidence linking the growth of MRSA to understaffing and overcrowding in health facilities in some countries that operate close to capacity (Clements et al. 2008). The authors draw on other research, in particular the Europe-wide ARPAC study (Antibiotic Resistance, Prevention and Control), which found that hospitals in countries with low prevalence are more likely to have drug and therapeutic or antibiotic committees (Bruce et al. 2009) and that there was a significant association between low rates and the use of both isolation rooms and alcohol hand washes, while the inability to provide isolation facilities was associated with higher rates (Bruce et al. 2009).

The emerging evidence on factors associated with MRSA infection led to the introduction of a policy termed 'search and destroy', initially in the

Netherlands (Wertheim et al. 2004). It involves active surveillance by culture of samples from persons at risk, pre-emptive isolation of patients at risk, strict isolation of known MRSA carriers and the eradication of carriage. Although not subjected to formal evaluation, a modelling study of the cumulative impact of its component parts concluded that it was effective, but also that the addition of rapid diagnostic testing would significantly increase its feasibility (Bootsma et al. 2006). In addition, a number of economic evaluations have reported cost savings compared with estimates of traditional methods (Vriens et al. 2002; Simoens et al. 2009). This model is now being implemented in other European countries (Bocher et al. 2010; Higgins et al. 2010).

Discussion and conclusions

This chapter catalogues a series of successes and failures in public health, and both offer lessons for those engaged in protecting and promoting the health of the population. It began by celebrating some remarkable historical successes, creating safe environments so that it is no longer necessary for one in four babies to die in their first year, as was the case in Sweden only 140 years ago. But it is also evident how precarious these successes can be.

Although immunization is cheap and easy to perform, some of Europe's richest countries seem unable to achieve coverage levels adequate to interrupt transmission. One reason, it seems, is differences in how countries have chosen to organize their immunization programmes. Not unexpectedly, it seems easier to achieve high coverage in countries that have actively managed their immunization programmes than in those that leave matters to individual parents and health professionals. To some extent, this reflects the underlying health system. Countries funded by social insurance are more likely to leave it to the parents and their independent physicians to make things happen. This, however, is not inevitable, as can be seen in the Netherlands, a country with a social health insurance system where the government has intervened to centrally manage the immunization programme.

The story of HIV/AIDS provides a mixed picture. Despite the opportunities available to scientists and policy-makers in the 1980s, including large international conferences, many countries pursued policies in seeming isolation from each other. As a consequence, many people contracted the infection who might have been spared if they had, by some chance, lived elsewhere. Of course, it was not always easy to implement an evidence-based response, particularly where it had been a taboo to discuss some of the major risk factors. Many politicians had to undergo a crash course in some of the less common sexual practices (or at least pretend that they were learning about them for the first time). They faced powerful vested interests who saw harm reduction measures, such as distribution of condoms, as a mortal sin. But their varying ability to respond effectively has left a legacy to this day in the very different rates of new infections across Europe.

This chapter has also illustrated how important it is to maintain and update our protection systems after they have been put in place. At times of political or economic turmoil, or when we become complacent and fail to maintain the investments that have safeguarded us, microorganisms are waiting to exploit our weakness.

Many of the challenges of infectious disease control relate to the unpredictability of the constant evolutionary struggle between humans and microorganisms. Several lessons emerge from the examples considered here. The first is the importance of anticipating situations in which the epidemiology of an infectious disease might be expected to change, whether through a new means of food processing, as with BSE, or through the indiscriminate use of antibiotics, as with MRSA. The second is the importance of effective surveillance, such as that provided by the Global Public Health Intelligence Network, which searches the Internet for clues about emerging problems, or as an element of the search and destroy policies pioneered in hospitals in the Netherlands. The third is the importance of responding rapidly. This did not happen with BSE in the United Kingdom, but the lessons learned from this failure may have enabled the world to be better prepared for the later emergence of SARS. It is this need to learn from mistakes that underpins the case for writing this book.

References

Abbasi, K. (2000) BSE inquiry plays down errors, *British Medical Journal*, 321(7269): 1097.

Ahmad, A., Krumkamp, R., Richardus, J.H. and Reintjes, R. (2009) [Prevention and control of infectious diseases with pandemic potential: the EU-project SARSControl] *Gesundheitswesen*, 71:351–7.

Angelini, R., Finarelli, A.C., Angelini, P. et al. (2007) An outbreak of chikungunya fever in the province of Ravenna, Italy, *Eurosurveillance*, 12(9):281–2.

Atun, R.A., McKee, M., Drobniewski, F. and Coker, R. (2005) Analysis of how the health systems context shapes responses to the control of human immunodeficiency virus: case-studies from the Russian Federation, *Bulletin of the World Health Organization*, 83(10):730–8.

Atun, R.A., McKee, M., Coker, R. and Gurol-Urganci, I. (2008) Health systems' responses to 25 years of HIV in Europe: inequities persist and challenges remain, *Health Policy*, 86(2–3):181–94.

Barrio, G., Bravo, M.J., Brugal, M.T. et al. (2011) Harm reduction interventions for drug injectors or heroin users in Spain: expanding coverage as the storm abates, *Addiction*, 480(7375):123–7.

Basu, S., Stuckler, D. and McKee, M. (2011) Addressing institutional amplifiers in the dynamics and control of tuberculosis epidemics, *American Journal of Tropical Medicine and Hygiene*, 84(1):30–7.

Bocher, S., Skov, R.L., Knudsen, M.A. et al. (2010) The search and destroy strategy prevents spread and long-term carriage of methicillin-resistant *Staphylococcus aureus*: results from the follow-up screening of a large ST22 (E-MRSA 15) outbreak in Denmark, *Clinical Microbiology and Infection*, 16(9):1427–34.

Bootsma, M.C., Diekmann, O. and Bonten, M.J. (2006) Controlling methicillin-resistant *Staphylococcus aureus*: quantifying the effects of interventions and rapid diagnostic testing, *Proceedings of the National Academy of Sciences, USA*, 103(14):5620–5.

van Boven, M., Kretzschmar, M., Wallinga, J. et al. (2010) Estimation of measles vaccine efficacy and critical vaccination coverage in a highly vaccinated population, *Journal of Royal Society: Interface*, 7(52):1537–44.

Bruce, J., MacKenzie, F.M., Cookson, B. et al. (2009) Antibiotic stewardship and consumption: findings from a pan-European hospital study, *Journal of Antimicrobial Chemotherapy*, 64(4):853–60.

Burstrom, B. and Bernhardt, E. (2001) Social differentials in the decline of child mortality in nineteenth century Stockholm, *European Journal of Public Health*, 11(1):29–34.

Chang, S., Sievert, D.M., Hageman, J.C. et al. (2003) Infection with vancomycin-resistant *Staphylococcus aureus* containing the *vanA* resistance gene, *New England Journal of Medicine*, 348(14):1342–7.

Clements, A., Halton, K., Graves, N. et al. (2008) Overcrowding and understaffing in modern health-care systems: key determinants in meticillin-resistant *Staphylococcus aureus* transmission, *Lancet, Infectious Disease*, 8(7):427–34.

Cohuet, S., Bukasa, A., Heathcock, R. et al. (2009) A measles outbreak in the Irish traveller ethnic group after attending a funeral in England, March–June 2007, *Epidemiology and Infection*, 137(12):1759–65.

Cosgrove, S.E., Sakoulas, G., Perencevich, E.N. et al. (2003) Comparison of mortality associated with methicillin-resistant and methicillin-susceptible *Staphylococcus aureus* bacteremia: a meta-analysis, *Clinical Infectious Diseases*, 36(1):53–9.

Csete, J. and Grob, P.J. (2012) Switzerland, HIV and the power of pragmatism: lessons for drug policy development, *International Journal of Drug Policy*, 23(1):82–6.

Danziger, R. (1996) An overview of HIV prevention in central and eastern Europe, *AIDS Care*, 8(6):701–7.

Dolea, C., Nolte, E. and McKee, M. (2002) Changing life expectancy in Romania after the transition, *Journal of Epidemiology and Community Health*, 56(6):444–9.

Donnell, D., Baeten, J.M., Kiarie, J. et al. (2010) Heterosexual HIV-1 transmission after initiation of antiretroviral therapy: a prospective cohort analysis, *Lancet*, 375(9731):2092–8.

Ducrot, C., Arnold, M., de Koeijer, A., Heim, D. and Calavas, D. (2008) Review on the epidemiology and dynamics of BSE epidemics, *Vetinary Research*, 39(4):15.

Edgeworth, J.D. (2011) Has decolonization played a central role in the decline in UK methicillin-resistant *Staphylococcus aureus* transmission? A focus on evidence from intensive care, *Journal of Antimicrobial Chemotherapy*, 66(suppl 2:ii41–47.

European Centre for Disease Prevention and Control (2011a) *Surveillance Report: European Monthly Measles Monitoring*. Stockholm: European Centre for Disease Prevention and Control.

European Centre for Disease Prevention and Control (2011b) *HIV/AIDS Surveillance in Europe 2010*. Stockholm: European Centre for Disease Prevention and Control.

European Centre for Disease Prevention and Control (2012) *Susceptibility of Staphylococcus aureus isolates to Methicillin in Participating Countries in 2010*. Stockholm: European Centre for Disease Prevention and Control, http://ecdc.europa.eu/en/activities/surveillance/EARS-Net/database/Pages/table_reports.aspx (accessed 24 June 2012).

European Commission (2003) *Measures Undertaken by Member States and Accession Countries to Control the Outbreak of SARS*. Brussels: European Commission.

Fireman, B., Lee, J., Lewis, N. et al. (2009) Influenza vaccination and mortality: differentiating vaccine effects from bias, *American Journal of Epidemiology*, 170(5):650–6.

Francioli, P., Vogt, M., Schadelin, J. et al. (1982) [Acquired immunologic deficiency syndrome, opportunistic infections and homosexuality. Presentation of 3 cases studied in Switzerland]. *Schweizerische medizinische Wochenschrift*, 112(47):1682–7.

Harm Reduction International (2008) *The Global State of Harm Reduction 2008*. London: Harm Reduction International.

Harm Reduction International (2010) *The Global State of Harm Reduction 2010*. London: Harm Reduction International.

Health Protection Agency (2011) *Malaria Cases in Greece*, http://www.hpa.org.uk/ NewsCentre/NationalPressReleases/2011PressReleases/110823malariaingreece/ (accessed 24 June 2012).

Heymann, D. (2005) SARS: a global perspective, in M. Peiris, L.J. Anderson, A. Osterhaus, K. Stöhr and K. Y. Yuen (eds) *Severe Acute Respiratory Syndrome*. Malden, MA: Blackwell, pp.13–20.

Higgins, A., Lynch, M. and Gethin, G. (2010) Can 'search and destroy' reduce nosocomial methicillin-resistant *Staphylococcus aureus* in an Irish hospital? *Journal of Hospital Infection*, 75(2):120–3.

Jefferson, T., Di Pietrantonj, C., Rivetti, A. et al. (2010) Vaccines for preventing influenza in the elderly, *Cochrane Database of Systematic Reviews*, (2):CD004876.

Kalenic, S., Cookson, B., Gallagher, R. et al. (2010) Comparison of recommendations in national/regional guidelines for prevention and control of MRSA in thirteen European countries, *Internationa Journal of Infection Control* 6:i2.

Kalies, H., Redel, R., Varga, R., Tauscher, M. and von Kries, R. (2008) Vaccination coverage in children can be estimated from health insurance data, *BMC Public Health*, 8:82.

Kentikelenis, A., Karanikolos, M., Papanicolas, I. et al. (2011) Health effects of financial crisis: omens of a Greek tragedy, *Lancet*, 378(9801):1457–8.

Kock, R., Becker, K., Cookson, B. et al. (2010) Methicillin-resistant *Staphylococcus aureus* (MRSA): burden of disease and control challenges in Europe, *Eurosurveillance*, 15(41):12–20.

Kroneman, M., Paget, W.J. and van Essen, G.A. (2003) Influenza vaccination in Europe: an inventory of strategies to reach target populations and optimise vaccination uptake, *Eurosurveillance*, 8(6):130–8.

Kwong, J.C., Stukel, T.A., Lim, J. et al. (2008) The effect of universal influenza immunization on mortality and health care use, *PLoS Medicine*, 5(10):e211.

Lauberau, B., Hermann, M., Weil, J., Schmitt, H. and von Kries, R. (2001) Durchimpfungsraten bei Kindern in Deutschland 1999, *Monatsschrift Kinderheilkunde*, 149:367–72.

Likatavicius, G., Hamers, F.F., Downs, A.M., Alix, J. and Nardone, A. (2007) Trends in HIV prevalence in blood donations in Europe, 1990–2004, *AIDS*, 21(8):1011–18.

Likatavicius, G., Klavs, I., Devaux, I., Alix, J. and Nardone, A. (2008) An increase in newly diagnosed HIV cases reported among men who have sex with men in Europe, 2000–6: implications for a European public health strategy, *Sexually Transmitted Infections*, 84(6):499–505.

Marcus, U., Voss, L., Kollan, C. and Hamouda, O. (2006) HIV incidence increasing in MSM in Germany: factors influencing infection dynamics, *Eurosurveillance*, 11(9):157–60.

Martin, R., Jankovic, D., Goel, A. et al. (2011) Increased transmission and outbreaks of measles: European Region, 2011, *Morbidity and Mortality Weekly Report*, 60(47):1605–10.

Mathers, C., Boerma, T. and Fat, D.M. (2008) *The Global Burden of Disease 2004 Update*. Geneva: World Health Organization.

Mathers, B.M., Degenhardt, L., Ali, H. et al. (2010) HIV prevention, treatment, and care services for people who inject drugs: a systematic review of global, regional, and national coverage, *Lancet*, 375(9719):1014–28.

McKee, M., Lang, T. and Roberts, J.A. (1996) Deregulating health: policy lessons from the BSE affair, *Journal of the Royal Society of Medicine*, 89(8):424–6.

Mellmann, A., Friedrich, A.W., Rosenkotter, N. et al. (2006) Automated DNA sequence-based early warning system for the detection of methicillin-resistant *Staphylococcus aureus* outbreaks, PLoS *Medicine*, 3(3):e33.

Mereckiene, J., Cotter, S., Nicol, A. et al. (2008a) National seasonal influenza vaccination survey in Europe, 2008, *Eurosurveillance*, 13(43):4–10.

Mereckiene, J., Cotter, S., Weber, J.T. et al. (2008b) Low coverage of seasonal influenza vaccination in the elderly in many European countries, *Eurosurveillance*, 13(41):2–4.

Mereckiene, J., Cotter, S., D'Anconi, F. et al. (2010) Differences in national influenza vaccination policies across the European Union, Norway and Iceland 2008–2009, *Eurosurveillance*, 15(44):11–20.

Muto, C.A., Jernigan, J.A., Ostrowsky, B.E. et al. (2003) SHEA guideline for preventing nosocomial transmission of multidrug-resistant strains of *Staphylococcus aureus* and enterococcus, *Infection Control and Hospital Epidemiology*, 24(5):362–86.

National Nosocomial Infections Surveillance (2003) National Nosocomial Infections Surveillance (NNIS) System Report, data summary from January 1992 through June 2003, issued August 2003, *American Journal of Infection Control*, 31(8): 481–98.

OECD (2011) *Health at a Glance 2011: OECD Indicators*. Paris: Organisation for Economic Co-operation and Development.

Omran, A.R. (1971) The epidemiologic transition. A theory of the epidemiology of population change, *Milbank Quarterly*, 49(4):509–38.

Peersman, G.V. and Levy, J.A. (1998) Focus and effectiveness of HIV-prevention efforts for young people. *AIDS* 12(suppl A): S191–6.

Pennington, H. (2003) Smallpox and bioterrorism, *Bulletin of the World Health Organization*, 81(10):762–7.

Police Federation of England and Wales (2009) *Crime and the Economy*. London: Police Federation of England and Wales.

Randolph, S. (2008) Tick-borne encephalitis incidence in central and eastern Europe: consequences of political transition, *Microbes and Infection*, 10(3):209–16.

Rechel, B., Kennedy, C. and McKee, M. (2011) The Soviet legacy in diagnosis and treatment: Implications for population health, *Journal of Public Health Policy*, 32(3):293–304.

Reintjes, R., Dedushaj, I., Gjini, A. and Jorgensen, T.R. (2002) Tularemia outbreak investigation in Kosovo: case control and environmental studies, *Emerging Infectious Diseases*, 8:69–73.

Rice, B., Gilbart, V.L., Lawrence, J. et al. (2012) Safe travels? HIV transmission among Britons travelling abroad, *HIV Medicine*, 13(5):315–17.

Riemann-Lorenz, K. (2012) *Comparison of Measles Incidence between 2008 and 2011 in Selected European Countries in Relation to Vaccination Coverage*. [MPH assignment]. Hamburg: Hamburg University of Applied Sciences.

Rivetti, D., Jefferson, T., Thomas, R. et al. (2006) Vaccines for preventing influenza in the elderly, *Cochrane Database of Systematic Reviews*, (3):CD004876.

Rizzo, C., Viboud, C., Montomoli, E., Simonsen, L. and Miller, M.A. (2006) Influenza-related mortality in the Italian elderly: no decline associated with increasing vaccination coverage, *Vaccine*, 24(42–43):6468–75.

Rozenbaum, W., Coulaud, J.P., Saimot, A.G. et al. (1982) Multiple opportunistic infection in a male homosexual in France, *Lancet*, 1(8271):572–3.

Schmitt, H.-J., Booy, R., Weil-Olivier, C., Van Damme, P., Cohen, R. and Peltola, H. (2003) Child vaccination policies in Europe: a report from the Summits of Independent European Vaccination Experts, *Lancet Infectious Diseases*, 3:103–8.

Semenza, J., Roberts, L., Henderson, A., Bogan, J., Rubin, C.H. (1998) Water distribution system and diarrheal disease transmission: a case study in Uzbekistan, *American Journal of Tropical Medicine & Hygiene*, 59(6):941–6.

Siegfried, N., van der Merwe, L., Brocklehurst, P. and Sint, T.T. (2011) Antiretrovirals for reducing the risk of mother-to-child transmission of HIV infection, *Cochrane Database of Systematic Reviews*, (7):CD003510.

Simoens, S., Ophals, E. and Schuermans, A. (2009) Search and destroy policy for methicillin-resistant *Staphylococcus aureus*: cost–benefit analysis, *Journal of Advances in Nursing*, 65(9):1853–9.

Simonsen, L., Taylor, R.J., Viboud, C., Miller, M.A. and Jackson, L.A. (2007) Mortality benefits of influenza vaccination in elderly people: an ongoing controversy, *Lancet Infectious Diseases*, 7(10):658–66.

Smith, P.G. and Bradley, R. (2003) Bovine spongiform encephalopathy (BSE) and its epidemiology, *British Medical Bulletin*, 66:185–98.

Smyth, F. (1998) Cultural constraints on the delivery of HIV/AIDS prevention in Ireland, *Social Science and Medicine*, 46(6):661–72.

Spicer, N., Harmer, A., Aleshkina, J. et al. (2011) Circus monkeys or change agents? Civil society advocacy for HIV/AIDS in adverse policy environments, *Social Science and Medicine*, 73(12):1748–55.

Stimson, G.V. (1995) AIDS and injecting drug use in the United Kingdom, 1987–1993: the policy response and the prevention of the epidemic, *Social Science and Medicine*, 41(5):699–716.

Stuckler, D., Basu, S., McKee, M. and King, L. (2008a) Mass incarceration can explain population increases in TB and multi-drug resistant TB in European and central Asian countries, *Proceedings of the National Academy of Sciences USA*, 105(36): 13280–5.

Stuckler, D., Basu, S. and King, L. (2008b) International Monetary Fund programs and tuberculosis outcomes in post-communist countries, *Public Library of Science Medicine*, 5(7):e143.

Suhrcke, M., Stuckler, D., Suk, J.E. et al. (2011) The impact of economic crises on communicable disease transmission and control: a systematic review of the evidence, *PLoS One*, 6(6):e20724.

Underhill, K., Operario, D. et al. (2007) Abstinence-only programs for HIV infection prevention in high-income countries, *Cochrane Database of Systematic Reviews*, (4):CD005421.

Vidanapathirana, J., Abramson, M.J., Forbes, A. and Fairley, C. (2005) Mass media interventions for promoting HIV testing, *Cochrane Database of Systematic Reviews*, (3):CD004775.

Vilaseca, J., Arnau, J.M., Bacardi, R. et al. (1982) Kaposi's sarcoma and *Toxoplasma gondii* brain abscess in a Spanish homosexual, *Lancet*, 1(8271):572.

Vitek, C.R. and Wharton, M. (1998) Diphtheria in the former Soviet Union: reemergence of a pandemic disease, *Emerging Infectious Diseases*, 4(4):539–50.

Voluntary HIV-1 Counseling and Testing Efficacy Study Group (2000) Efficacy of voluntary HIV-1 counselling and testing in individuals and couples in Kenya, Tanzania, and Trinidad: a randomised trial. The Voluntary HIV-1 Counseling and Testing Efficacy Study Group, *Lancet*, 356(9224):103–12.

Vriens, M., Blok, H., Fluit, A. et al. (2002) Costs associated with a strict policy to eradicate methicillin-resistant *Staphylococcus aureus* in a Dutch University Medical Center: a 10-year survey, *European Journal of Clinical Microbiology and Infectious Diseases*, 21(11):782–6.

de Vroome, E.M., Paalman, M.E., Sandfort, T.G. et al. (1990) AIDS in the Netherlands: the effects of several years of campaigning, *International Journal of STD & AIDS*, 1(4):268–75.

Weller, S. and Davis, K. (2002) Condom effectiveness in reducing heterosexual HIV transmission, *Cochrane Database of Systematic Reviews*, (1):CD003255.

Wertheim, H.F., Vos, M.C., Boelens, H.A. et al. (2004) Low prevalence of methicillin-resistant *Staphylococcus aureus* (MRSA) at hospital admission in the Netherlands: the value of search and destroy and restrictive antibiotic use, *Journal of Hospital Infections*, 56(4):321–5.

Wiese-Posselt, M., Tertilt, C. and Zepp, F. (2011) Vaccination recommendations for Germany, *Deutsches Ärzteblatt International*, 108(45):771–9; quiz 780.

Wodak, A. and Cooney, A. (2004) *Effectiveness of Sterile Needle and Syringe Programming in Reducing HIV/AIDS among Injecting Drug Users*. Geneva: World Health Organization.

WHO Regional Office for Europe (2012) *European Health for All Database (HFA-DB)*. Copenhagen: WHO Regional Office for Europe, http://data.euro.who.int/hfadb/ (accessed 4 June 2012).

World Health Organization (2003a) *Consensus Document on the Epidemiology of Severe Acute Respiratory Syndrome (SARS)*. Geneva: World Health Organization.

World Health Organization (2003b) *Summary of Probable SARS Cases with Onset of Illness from 1 November 2002 to 31 July 2003 (based on data as of the 31 December 2003)*. Geneva: World Health Organization.

World Health Organization (2010) *Screening Donated Blood for Transfusion–Transmissible Infections: Recommendations*. Geneva: World Health Organization.

World Health Organization (2012) *Variant Creutzfeldt–Jakob Disease*. [Fact Sheet 180.] Geneva: World Health Organization.

World Health Organization (2003) *Influenza: Report by the WHO Secretariat to the 56th World Health Assembly*. [Report A56/23.] Geneva: World Health Organization.

chapter eight

Hypertension

Martin McKee and Johan Mackenbach

Introduction

Globally, high blood pressure is the number one leading risk factor for mortality, and the fifth leading risk factor for loss of DALYs (Rodgers et al. 2004). In middle- and high-income countries, such as those in Europe, high blood pressure accounts for around 17% of all deaths, and 5–6% of all DALYs lost (World Health Organization 2009).

Hypertension is a silent killer, because it is usually symptomless and can only be discovered if it is measured. Current clinical practice guidelines define hypertension as a systolic blood pressure >140 mmHg and/or a diastolic blood pressure >90 mmHg (Joint National Committee on Prevention, Detection, Evaluation and Treatment of High Blood Pressure 2004). Hypertension is an important risk factor for cardiovascular diseases, both ischaemic heart disease and cerebrovascular disease (or stroke). There are two main subtypes of stroke, ischaemic stroke and haemorrhagic stroke. The risk of both is elevated among those with hypertension, but the contribution of hypertension to ischaemic stroke is lower because it is more strongly affected by other risk factors.

Hypertension is very common. Estimates of the prevalence of hypertension in European countries typically range between 30 and 60% of the adult population (Wolf-Maier et al. 2003; Kearney et al. 2005). Within Europe, average blood pressure levels vary significantly between countries, as shown by Figs 8.1 and 8.2. Average blood pressure levels tend to be higher in central and eastern Europe than in western Europe (Danaei et al. 2011).

Important risk factors for hypertension include high salt consumption, lack of physical exercise, obesity, smoking, excessive alcohol consumption, low intake of fruit and vegetables and psychosocial factors (Hajjar et al. 2006). The prevalence of hypertension usually rises with age, but this age-related increase is not seen in populations with low salt consumption (INTERSALT 1988). Clearly, therefore, hypertension is amenable to primary prevention. This has partly been dealt with in Chapter 4. This chapter will focus on another

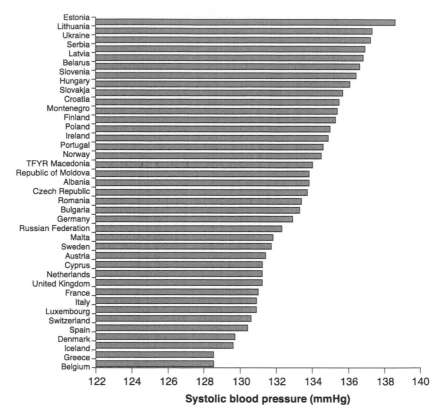

Figure 8.1 Average systolic blood pressure in men, 2008

Source: Data compiled for the *Global Burden of Disease* study (Mathers et al. 2008), from national and regional surveys with measured blood pressure, and adjusted using complex algorithms (Danaei et al. 2011; web appendix, web table 4)
Note: TFYR Macedonia, the former Yugoslav Republic of Macedonia

hypertension control strategy: secondary prevention by timely detection of individuals with elevated blood pressure and subsequent treatment with lifestyle advice and drugs.

Effectiveness of hypertension detection and control

Before the 1950s, hypertension was untreatable with medication. Many pages in medical textbooks were given over to its complications, including kidney and heart disease and stroke. It was not unusual, in advanced industrialized countries, to see patients with what was termed 'malignant hypertension', a life-threatening condition characterized by very high blood pressure and signs and symptoms of raised intracranial pressure. The situation changed markedly in the 1960s when the first modern drugs for the treatment of hypertension, thiazide diuretics, were introduced. These were later followed by beta-blockers,

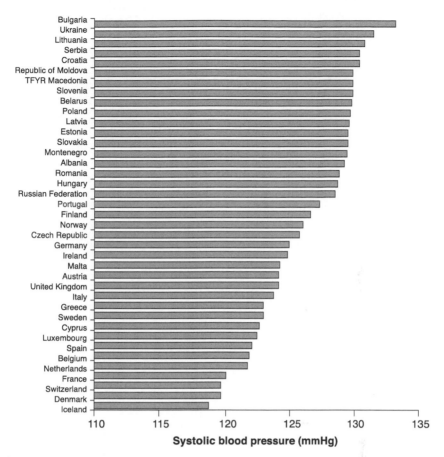

Figure 8.2 Average systolic blood pressure in women, 2008

Source: Data compiled for the *Global Burden of Disease* study (Mathers et al. 2008), from national and regional surveys with measured blood pressure, and adjusted using complex algorithms (Danaei et al. 2011; web appendix, web table 4)
Note: TFYR Macedonia, the former Yugoslav Republic of Macedonia

introduced in the 1970s, and angiotensin-converting enzyme inhibitors, angiotensin-receptor blockers and calcium antagonists, introduced in the 1980s. Early studies demonstrated dramatic results in reducing the complications of hypertension (Hamilton et al. 1964) and this has been confirmed in many subsequent studies. Systematic reviews show that adequate control of hypertension by drugs reduces risks of cardiovascular diseases considerably (Blood Pressure Lowering Treatment Trialists' Collaboration 2003; Wright and Musini 2009), also among elderly people, the main group at risk (Musini et al. 2009). For those drug treatments that have been tested against placebo, the average effect is in the order of a 30% reduction in stroke incidence, a 20% reduction in ischaemic heart disease incidence, a 20% reduction in cardiovascular death, and a 10% reduction in mortality from all causes (Blood Pressure Lowering Treatment Trialists' Collaboration 2003).

Targets for treatment have gradually been lowered, as evidence emerged that tighter control of hypertension gives better results (Medical Research Council 1985; Blood Pressure Lowering Treatment Trialists' Collaboration 2003); consequently, current guidelines aim for a reduction of systolic blood pressure to ≤140 mmHg and of diastolic blood pressure to ≤ 90 mmHg (Mancia et al. 2007). The mode of treatment has also changed. Recognizing that most people require more than one drug to achieve adequate control, low-dose combinations of drugs from different drug classes are being used increasingly in order to maximize the common blood pressure-lowering effects while minimizing the class-specific side-effects, thereby increasing the likelihood of adherence (Ruschitzka 2011).

Organizationally, timely detection and treatment of hypertension is a challenging enterprise that requires much more than a sphygmomanometer and a prescription for drugs. A way needs to be found of reaching the large numbers of symptomless people with elevated blood pressure. In most countries, this is addressed through a proactive approach to the detection of hypertension, with measurement of blood pressure in patients consulting their doctors for other reasons. This has gradually become common practice in many high-income countries and is now included in many clinical practice guidelines. However, in addition, blood pressure measurements need to be carried out in a standardized way. Effective drugs need to be available to patients without financial barriers. Patients need to adhere to treatment and continue treatment for a long time, often lifelong. Also, regular monitoring is needed to see whether treatment goals are reached.

Realistically, this can only be done in primary care settings, but this places high demands on the system (MacMahon et al. 2008). Effective hypertension management programmes require protocols, record keeping, qualified personnel, patient education, appointment reminder systems and adequate financial incentives. A recent review concluded that primary care facilities need to have an organized system of regular follow-up and review of their hypertensive patients, that drug therapy should be implemented by means of a vigorous stepped care approach when patients do not reach target blood pressure levels, and that self-monitoring and appointment reminders may be useful adjuncts to improve blood pressure control (Glynn et al. 2010).

Successes and failures of hypertension detection and control

Trends in blood pressure and hypertension in Europe

Data on the detection, treatment and control of hypertension come from two complementary types of study: population-based surveys and surveys of those attending health facilities. Surveys undertaken in the population have the advantage of identifying those who may be unaware of having hypertension and of producing population-based measures of prevalence; however, while, if repeated, they can detect trends, they may be of limited value in explaining why those trends occurred. Facility-based surveys have the advantage of providing data on treatment patterns and quality of care, although they will miss those who are undiagnosed.

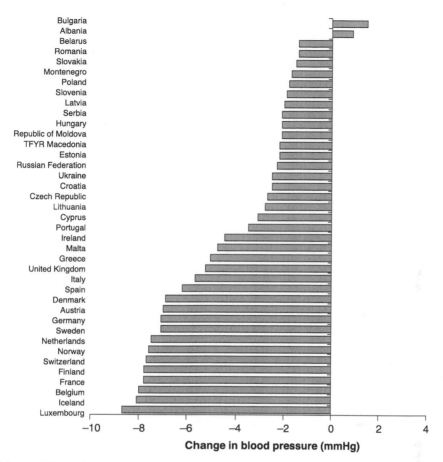

Figure 8.3 Reduction in average systolic blood pressure in men between 2008 and 1980

Source: Data compiled for the *Global Burden of Disease* study (Mathers et al. 2008), from national and regional surveys with measured blood pressure, and adjusted using complex algorithms (Danaei et al. 2011; web appendix, web table 4)
Note: TFYR Macedonia, the former Yugoslav Republic of Macedonia

Population-based surveys held over the period 1980–2005 show that average blood pressure levels have declined considerably in most western European countries, both among men and women. In most central and eastern European countries, however, trends have been less favourable, although seen over the whole period levels have declined (Figs 8.3 and 8.4) (Danaei et al. 2011). Among men in some central and eastern European countries, average blood pressure levels have risen in the most recent time period, and, as a result, total decline since 1980 has been modest (Danaei et al. 2011).

The reasons for these declines in blood pressure have been studied in only a few European countries, and the evidence for a role of improved treatment is not easy to interpret. Part of the decline is likely to be a result of reduced salt intake (see Chapter 4) and part from improved detection and treatment of

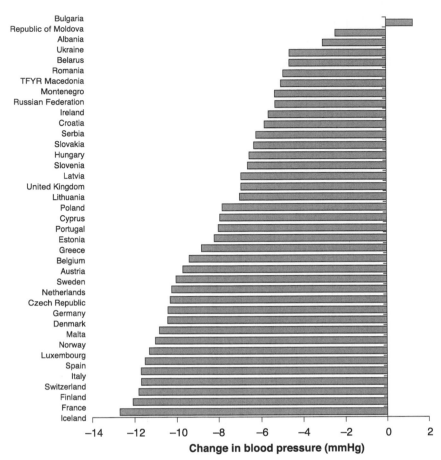

Figure 8.4 Reduction in average systolic blood pressure in women between 2008 and 1980

Source: Data compiled for the *Global Burden of Disease* study (Mathers et al. 2008), from national and regional surveys with measured blood pressure, and adjusted using complex algorithms (Danaei et al. 2011; web appendix, web table 4)
Note: TFYR Macedonia, the former Yugoslav Republic of Macedonia

hypertension. A population-based approach to evaluation of the effectiveness of hypertension management requires distinction of 'awareness' (the proportion of all patients with hypertension reporting to have a medical diagnosis of hypertension), 'treatment' (the proportion of patients with hypertension reporting receiving blood pressure-lowering medications) and 'control' (the proportion of patients with hypertension having an average blood pressure reading <140 mmHg systolic and <90 mmHg diastolic). Unfortunately, representative national data on these parameters over time are lacking in most countries and the evidence that exists is largely facility based.

It is widely believed that adherence to modern guidelines for the detection and treatment of hypertension has increased over the past decades, at least in western Europe, although longitudinal data are very limited. A study of outpatients with cardiovascular diseases in six western European countries (United Kingdom, France, Italy, Spain and Portugal) found that, even between as late as 1998 and 2006, the proportion of patients with hypertension who had their blood pressure controlled to below the 140/90 mmHg target increased considerably, from 27 to 49% (Steinberg et al. 2008).

England is one of the countries with longitudinal data. Compliance with guidelines was probably already comparatively high in the 1990s but it increased further after 1998. For example, between 1998 and 2005, the percentage of patients whose blood pressure had been recorded rose from 87% to 99%, blood pressure control at a 150/90 mmHg level rose from 48% to 82%, and prescription of beta-blockers as maintenance therapy increased from 47% to 80% (Campbell et al. 2007).

One of the very few longitudinal population-based studies was done in Belgium. Six regional and national surveys of systolic blood pressure conducted between 1967 and 1986 were analysed, and trends in blood pressure were compared between the growing group of people receiving treatment and the group of those not receiving treatment. More than half of the decline in average systolic blood pressure could be attributed to increased treatment (Joossens and Kesteloot 1991).

In Finland, longitudinal population-based studies have also shown remarkable declines in blood pressure, not only in North Karelia, where comprehensive community health promotion intervention was piloted (see Chapter 4), but also in the rest of the country (Vartiainen et al. 2010). This coincided with significant increases in awareness, treatment and control of hypertension. The reductions in average blood pressure were strongest among those receiving treatment for hypertension (Kastarinen et al. 2009). Although the decline in blood pressure in the population as a whole could partly be attributed to improved treatment, it was largely a result of the decline in salt consumption and an increase in physical exercise (Kastarinen et al. 2009).

These findings, and others, have led researchers to conclude that at least part of the decline in uncontrolled hypertension in western Europe can be ascribed to improved management (Primatesta and Poulter 2006; Falaschetti et al. 2009). However, all of these studies began several decades after safe and effective treatment for hypertension became available so they were beginning from a baseline at which many people were already being treated. It is important to recall that, prior to the early 1960s, no-one with hypertension was being controlled.

Despite these improvements, hypertension management is still far from optimal, as studies comparing western European countries with the United States have shown. Several facility-based studies have found consistently lower levels of control in western European countries than in the United States (Wolf-Maier et al. 2003; Wang et al. 2007) and surveys in the former USSR have demonstrated that many people who have been prescribed treatment take it only irregularly (Roberts et al. 2012).

In European facility-based surveys, the percentage of patients with known hypertension whose blood pressure is adequately controlled typically ranges between 30 and 50% (Banegas et al. 2011) (Fig. 8.5), and it is important to recall that these figures are almost certainly overestimates as they were obtained

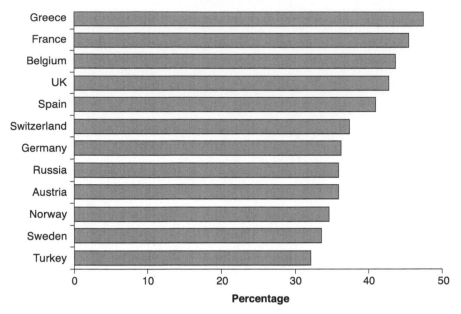

Figure 8.5 Percentage of patients whose blood pressure was controlled in the EURIKA study

Source: Banegas et al. 2011

from centres willing to engage in research. Consequently, the results from the Russian Federation seem inconsistent with population-level data on adherence to treatment (Roberts et al. 2010). It is clear that control has become much more widespread, although researchers often complain that blood pressure control is 'completely inadequate' (Kotseva et al. 2010), that resource-constrained health systems are unable to deliver care consistent with existing guidelines (Petursson et al. 2009), that many European physicians are not yet fully convinced that they should initiate treatment when blood pressure is above the threshold (Redon et al. 2011) and that more cases of stroke could be prevented if hypertension control was better (de Koning et al. 2004).

Trends in stroke incidence and mortality in Europe

One of the main aims of hypertension control is to prevent strokes. In recent years, stroke mortality has been declining in all European countries that have available data (Mirzaei et al. 2012). However, current levels of stroke mortality differ enormously between countries, and reflect the very different historical trajectories that countries have gone through. Some countries have had consistently declining stroke mortality since the 1950s, while others first saw their stroke mortality rise to a peak followed by a decline. The different moments in time at which mortality started to decline may be related to the implementation of various prevention strategies (Mirzaei et al. 2012).

As mentioned above, there are two main subtypes of stroke. Although these have separate diagnostic codes, a definitive diagnosis requires brain imaging, to which access varies considerably across Europe (Leys et al. 2007). Hence, in routinely collected mortality statistics it is impossible to distinguish reliably between ischaemic and haemorrhagic stroke. Studies that have been able to make this distinction, on the basis of more detailed clinical data, suggest that mortality trends have differed considerably between the two types. In England, mortality from haemorrhagic stroke, which used to be the most frequently occurring form of the disease, has declined precipitously since the 1940s, whereas mortality from ischaemic stroke has mirrored that of ischaemic heart disease (rising until the 1970s and then declining). As a result ischaemic stroke now accounts for the majority of deaths from stroke (McCarron et al. 2006). In Austria, while mortality from both types of stroke has declined, the decline from haemorrhagic stroke has accelerated since 2000 (Bajaj et al. 2010). The more rapid decline of haemorrhagic as opposed to ischaemic stroke is compatible with the hypothesis that much of the decline in stroke results from a declining prevalence of hypertension.

Detailed research in a limited number of countries has shown that declines in stroke mortality are mainly the result of declines in incidence. In the United States, for example, stroke mortality decline began around 1960 and has been found to be largely based on declines in incidence, although improvements in survival have also made a contribution (Benatru et al. 2006; Rautio et al. 2008). The declines in stroke incidence in the United States coincided with improved risk factor control, particularly improvements in detection and treatment of hypertension, declines in cholesterol and declines in smoking; the decline in incidence is, therefore, thought to be a result of these risk factor changes (Towfighi and Saver 2011).

Similar findings have been reported from a few western European countries, such as Finland (Lehtonen et al. 2004; Sivenius et al. 2004) where most of the decline in stroke mortality was the result of a decline in incidence. This is consistent with the hypothesis that improved detection and treatment of hypertension has contributed to the decline in stroke mortality. In contrast, some studies in other parts of Europe, such as northern Sweden (Stegmayr and Asplund 2003) and France (Benatru et al. 2006) have attributed reductions in mortality to improved management of stroke, a finding also obtained in studies undertaken in the central and eastern European countries that have recorded dramatic reductions in case fatality (Korv et al. 1996; Sienkiewicz-Jarosz et al. 2011). Although a European comparative study conducted in 2004–2006 in France, Italy, Lithuania, the United Kingdom, Spain and Poland found persisting worse outcomes in Lithuania than elsewhere (Heuschmann et al. 2011), other research has shown that declines in stroke mortality in Lithuania between 1986 and 2002 were a result of improved case fatality against a background of stable incidence in men and rising incidence in women (Rastenyte et al. 2006). This suggests that improved hypertension detection and treatment has not played a role in the decline of stroke mortality in Lithuania, and not perhaps in other eastern European countries.

We now turn to trends in stroke mortality in the different parts of Europe. As shown in Fig. 8.6, the Nordic countries, the United Kingdom and Ireland and the countries in the continental region have all seen their cerebrovascular

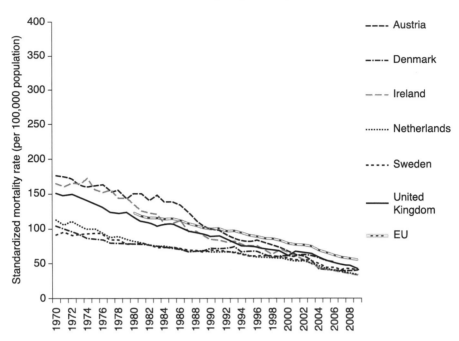

Figure 8.6 Trends in mortality from cerebrovascular disease in both sexes in north-western Europe, 1970–2009

Source: WHO Regional Office for Europe 2012

disease mortality decline in the last 40 years, and their mortality rates have converged to a level well below that of the EU as a whole. A study from England found that these declines were accompanied by reductions in the proportion of smokers, mean total cholesterol, mean systolic and diastolic blood pressures and major increases in premorbid treatment with antiplatelet, lipid-lowering and blood pressure-lowering drugs (Rothwell et al. 2004). Improved detection and treatment of hypertension has also contributed to the decline of ischaemic heart disease in north-west Europe. In England and Wales 10% of the decline between 1981 and 2000 was explained by declines in blood pressure (Unal et al. 2005). In Finland, similar results were found (Laatikainen et al. 2005).

Most countries in the south-west of Europe have experienced similar trends in stroke mortality as in northern and western Europe (Fig. 8.7). The main exception is Portugal, which had a much higher starting level of mortality and which, despite a substantial decline, still has a higher level of stroke mortality than the EU average. The Portuguese diet is traditionally very rich in salt, because salt was used for conservation, for example for the salted cod that is one of the pillars of Portuguese cuisine. Although the salt content of the Portuguese diet has been declining in recent decades, Portugal still has the highest rate of stroke mortality in western Europe. This is because of a high incidence, not because of high case fatality (Correia et al. 2004). The fact that a salty diet has lingered on for so much longer in Portugal may be related to the fact Portugal has long lagged behind other European countries in economic development,

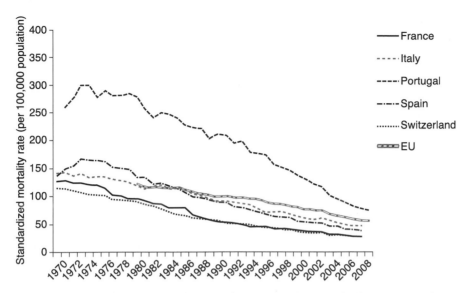

Figure 8.7 Trends in mortality from cerebrovascular disease in both sexes in southern Europe, 1970–2009

Source: WHO Regional Office for Europe 2012

which, in turn, reflects Portugal's relative isolation under the Salazar regime (Mackenbach 2009). At the same time, delays in introducing modern methods for hypertension management may also have played a role, with a study undertaken in 2003 finding that only 11% of those with hypertension were controlled (Macedo et al. 2005).

In contrast to other parts of Europe, mortality from stroke has first risen and then fallen in many central and eastern European countries (Fig. 8.8). In this region, stroke mortality only started to decline in the 1980s (e.g. Czech Republic, Hungary) or even later (e.g. Poland, Romania). This is likely to reflect high levels of uncontrolled hypertension (Balaz et al. 1980; Mark et al. 1991), a low priority placed on hypertension control by physicians (Mark et al. 1998) and delays in widespread prescribing of modern antihypertensive drugs.

In the USSR until 1990, access to modern antihypertensive drugs such as thiazide diuretics, beta-blockers and angiotensin-converting enzyme inhibitors was extremely limited, as was awareness among professionals and the general public of the benefits of regular treatment of asymptomatic individuals (Roberts et al. 2010). A survey undertaken in 2001 in eight countries of the former USSR (Armenia, Belarus, Georgia, Kazakhstan, Kyrgyzstan, the Republic of Moldova, the Russian Federation and Ukraine) revealed that only 26% of those who were aware of having hypertension took their prescribed drugs daily (Roberts et al. 2010). The situation had improved only slightly in 2010, despite improvements in the supply of drugs and better knowledge among physicians (Roberts et al. 2012). This suggests, as noted above for Lithuania, that most of the decline in stroke mortality in the former USSR must be from improved treatment of stroke, not improved detection and treatment of hypertension.

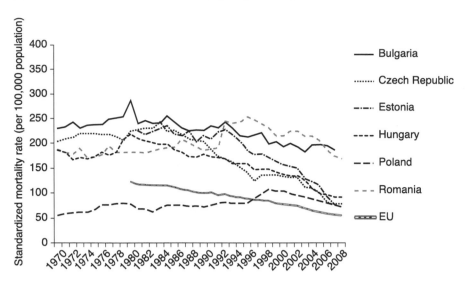

Figure 8.8 Trends in mortality from cerebrovascular disease in males in central and eastern Europe, 1970–2009

Source: WHO Regional Office for Europe 2012

The fluctuations seen in stroke mortality in the Russian Federation (Fig. 8.9) mirror those of total mortality, with peaks in 1994 and in 2003, suggesting that stroke mortality rose and fell with the economy. Whether the economy exerted its influence through fluctuations in excessive alcohol consumption or through fluctuations in access to adequate prevention and treatment for

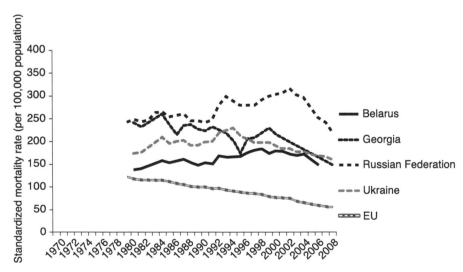

Figure 8.9 Trends in mortality from cerebrovascular disease in males in the former USSR, 1970–2009

Source: WHO Regional Office for Europe 2012

hypertension and stroke is difficult to say. Other causes of death amenable to medical intervention fluctuated in the same way, suggesting that access to adequate health care did indeed play a role (Andreev et al. 2003).

As a result of these divergent trends, inequalities in stroke mortality within Europe have risen dramatically: in 2009 stroke mortality in the Russian Federation was more than four times higher than the EU average.

Support for the suggestion that declines in stroke mortality partly reflect improvements in the management of hypertension comes from the fact that declines in stroke mortality have generally been larger in countries with stronger declines in average systolic blood pressure, although correlations are weak (0.22 for men and 0.27 for women) (Fig. 8.10).

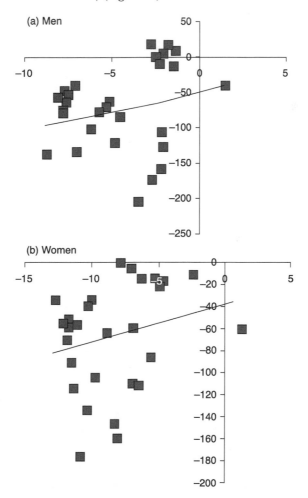

Figure 8.10 Association between decline in average systolic blood pressure (SBP) and decline in stroke mortality, 2008–1980

Source: Based on data from Fig. 8.3 and WHO Regional Office for Europe (2012)
Note: Change in systolic blood pressure, in mmHg, on x-axis and in stroke mortality, in deaths/100,000, on y-axis.

Discussion and conclusions

The evidence reviewed in this chapter is much less clear than was expected when the review was commenced. Consequently, it is appropriate to summarize the undisputed facts before speculating what they, collectively, indicate. First, clinical trials demonstrate convincingly that control of hypertension reduces the incidence of complications of high blood pressure, the most important of which is stroke. Second, death rates from stroke have been falling markedly in most European countries for several decades. Third, from a situation in the early 1960s where none of the 30–60% of the population with hypertension was receiving any treatment, up to half of these are now being treated and their blood pressure controlled. Fourth, despite the improvements in blood pressure management that have been made, there is still a long way to go.

However, there are also many gaps in our knowledge. First, although the expansion of stroke registers in recent years has vastly increased our knowledge of the epidemiology of this condition, there are few longitudinal data on incidence. Second, what data are available to link incidence to mortality provide conflicting results from different places. For example, in some places, the observed decline in mortality seems to have been driven largely by falling incidence while in others improved outcomes of established strokes appear to be responsible. However, this research almost entirely stems from a period long after effective treatment became available, so it is possible that the major gains from lowering blood pressure had already occurred. This is consistent with evidence that more intensive management of the acute stroke, particularly that informed by acute brain imaging, was introduced long after antihypertensive drugs became available.

While any conclusion must, of necessity, be somewhat speculative, some sense can be made of these superficially contradictory findings. Detection and treatment of hypertension is an effective strategy to prevent the cardiovascular complications of hypertension, including stroke. Compliance by health professionals with modern guidelines for the detection and treatment of hypertension has increased considerably in western Europe. Simultaneously, awareness, treatment and control of hypertension in the population have increased. We consider it likely that this has played a significant role in the decline of hypertension and in stroke mortality in the populations of western Europe, although the decline in hypertension has also benefited from declines in salt intake, and the decline in stroke mortality from a more intensive approach to management in the acute phase. Yet, detection and control of hypertension is still far from adequate, particularly in eastern Europe, and this is probably one of the factors behind the persisting higher prevalence of hypertension and stroke mortality in these countries.

References

Andreev, E.M., Nolte, E., Shkolnikov, V.M. et al. (2003) The evolving pattern of avoidable mortality in Russia, *International Journal of Epidemiology*, 32(3):437–46.

Bajaj, A., Schernhammer, E.S., Haidinger, G. and Waldhor, T. (2010) Trends in mortality from stroke in Austria, 1980–2008, *Wiener klinische Wochenschrift*, 122(11–12):346–53.

Balaz, V., Rywik, S., Bederova, A. and Wagrowska, H. (1980) Prevalence of ischaemic heart disease risk factors in male populations aged 45–54 years in Warsaw and Bratislava. Part II: hypertension, *Cor Vasa*, 22(3):140–6.

Banegas, J.R., Lopez-Garcia, E., Dallongeville, J. et al. (2011) Achievement of treatment goals for primary prevention of cardiovascular disease in clinical practice across Europe: the EURIKA study, *European Heart Journal*, 32(17):2143–52.

Benatru, I., Rouaud, O., Durier, J. et al. (2006) Stable stroke incidence rates but improved case-fatality in Dijon, France, from 1985 to 2004, *Stroke*, 37(7):1674–9.

Blood Pressure Lowering Treatment Trialists' Collaboration (2003) Effects of different blood-pressure-lowering regimens on major cardiovascular events: results of prospectively-designed overviews of randomised trials, *Lancet*, 362(9395):1527–35.

Campbell, S., Reeves, D., Kontopantelis, E. et al. (2007) Quality of primary care in England with the introduction of pay for performance, *New England Journal of Medicine*, 357(2):181–90.

Correia, M., Silva, M.R., Matos, I. et al. (2004) Prospective community-based study of stroke in northern Portugal: incidence and case fatality in rural and urban populations, *Stroke*, 35(9):2048–53.

Danaei, G., Finucane, M.M., Lin, J.K. et al. (2011) National, regional, and global trends in systolic blood pressure since 1980: systematic analysis of health examination surveys and epidemiological studies with 786 country-years and 5.4 million participants, *Lancet*, 377(9765):568–77.

Falaschetti, E., Chaudhury, M., Mindell, J. and Poulter, N. (2009) Continued improvement in hypertension management in England: results from the Health Survey for England 2006, *Hypertension*, 53(3):480–6.

Glynn, L.G., Murphy, A.W., Smith, S., Schroeder, K. and Fahey, T. (2010) Interventions used to improve control of blood pressure in patients with hypertension, *Cochrane Database of Systematic Reviews*, (2):CD005182.

Hajjar, I., Kotchen, J.M. and Kotchen, T.A. (2006) Hypertension: trends in prevalence, incidence, and control, *Annual Review of Public Health*, 27:465–90.

Hamilton, M., Thompson, E.M. and Wisniewski, T.K. (1964) The role of blood-pressure control in preventing complications of hypertension, *Lancet*, 1(7327):235–8.

Heuschmann, P.U., Wiedmann, S., Wellwood, I. et al. (2011) Three-month stroke outcome: the European Registers of Stroke (EROS) investigators, *Neurology*, 76(2):159–65.

INTERSALT (1988) INTERSALT: an international study of electrolyte excretion and blood pressure. Results for 24 hour urinary sodium and potassium excretion. Intersalt Cooperative Research Group, *British Medical Journal*, 297(6644):319–28.

Joint National Committee on Prevention, Detection, Evaluation and Treatment of High Blood Pressure (2004) *The Seventh Report of the Joint National Committee on Prevention, Detection, Evaluation, and Treatment of High Blood Pressure: Complete Report of the National High Blood Pressure Education Program*. Bethesda, MD: National Institutes of Health, National Heart, Lung, and Blood Institute.

Joossens, J.V. and Kesteloot, H. (1991) Trends in systolic blood pressure, 24-hour sodium excretion, and stroke mortality in the elderly in Belgium, *American Journal of Medicine*, 90(3A):5S–11S.

Kastarinen, M., Antikainen, R., Peltonen, M. et al. (2009) Prevalence, awareness and treatment of hypertension in Finland during 1982–2007, *Journal of Hypertension*, 27(8):1552–9.

Kearney, P.M., Whelton, M., Reynolds, K. et al. (2005) Global burden of hypertension: analysis of worldwide data, *Lancet*, 365(9455):217–23.

de Koning, J.S., Klazinga, N.S., Koudstaal, P.J. et al. (2004) Quality of care in stroke prevention: results of an audit study among general practitioners, *Preventive Medicine*, 38(2):129–36.

Korv, J., Roose, M. and Kaasik, A.E. (1996) Changed incidence and case-fatality rates of first-ever stroke between 1970 and 1993 in Tartu, Estonia, *Stroke*, 27(2): 199–203.

Kotseva, K., Wood, D., de Backer, G. et al. (2010) EUROASPIRE III. Management of cardiovascular risk factors in asymptomatic high-risk patients in general practice: cross-sectional survey in 12 European countries, *European Journal of Cardiovascular and Preventive Rehabilitation*, 17(5):530–40.

Laatikainen, T., Critchley, J., Vartiainen, E., Salomaa, V., Ketonen, M. and Capewell, S. (2005) Explaining the decline in coronary heart disease mortality in Finland between 1982 and 1997, *American Journal of Epidemiology*, 162(8):764–73.

Lehtonen, A., Salomaa, V., Immonen-Raiha, P. et al. (2004) Declining incidence and mortality of stroke in persons aged ≥75 years in Finland; the FINSTROKE study, *European Journal of Cardiovascular and Preventive Rehabilitation*, 11(6):466–70.

Leys, D., Ringelstein, E.B., Kaste, M. and Hacke, W. (2007) Facilities available in European hospitals treating stroke patients, *Stroke*, 38(11):2985–91.

Macedo, M.E., Lima, M.J., Silva, A.O. et al. (2005) Prevalence, awareness, treatment and control of hypertension in Portugal: the PAP study, *Journal of Hypertension*, 23(9):1661–6.

Mackenbach, J.P. (2009) Bacalhao under the Ponte 25 de Abril: impressions from Lisbon, *European Journal of Public Health*, 19(1):1.

MacMahon, S., Alderman, M.H., Lindholm, L.H. et al. (2008) Blood-pressure-related disease is a global health priority, *Lancet*, 371(9623):1480–2.

Mancia, G., de Backer, G., Dominiczak, A. et al. (2007) 2007 Guidelines for the management of arterial hypertension: the Task Force for the Management of Arterial Hypertension of the European Society of Hypertension (ESH) and of the European Society of Cardiology (ESC), *European Heart Journal*, 28(12):1462–1536.

Mark, L., Katona, A. and Deli, L. (1991) An attempt to evaluate the risk factors related to coronary heart disease in Hungary, *Cor Vasa*, 33(4):265–72.

Mark, L., Nagy, E., Kondacs, A. and Deli, L. (1998) The change of attitude of Hungarian physicians towards the importance of risk factors of coronary heart disease over the period 1985–1996, *Public Health*, 112(3):197–201.

Mathers, C., Boerma, T. and Fat, D.M. (2008) *The Global Burden of Disease 2004 Update*. Geneva: World Health Organization.

McCarron, M.O., Davey Smith, G. and McCarron, P. (2006) Secular stroke trends: early life factors and future prospects. *Quarterly Journal of Medicine*, 99(2):117–22.

Medical Research Council (1985) MRC trial of treatment of mild hypertension: principal results. Medical Research Council Working Party, *British Medical Journal (Clinical Research Edition)*, 291(6488):97–104.

Mirzaei, M., Truswell, A.S., Arnett, K. et al. (2012) Cerebrovascular disease in 48 countries: secular trends in mortality 1950–2005, *Journal of Neurology, Neurosurgery and Psychiatry*, 83(2):138–45.

Musini, V.M., Tejani, A.M., Bassett, K. and Wright, J.M. (2009) Pharmacotherapy for hypertension in the elderly, *Cochrane Database of Systematic Reviews*, (4):CD000028.

Petursson, H., Getz, L., Sigurdsson, J.A. and Hetlevik, I. (2009) Current European guidelines for management of arterial hypertension: are they adequate for use in primary care? Modelling study based on the Norwegian HUNT 2 population, *BMC Family Practice*, 10:70.

Primatesta, P. and Poulter, N.R. (2006) Improvement in hypertension management in England: results from the Health Survey for England 2003, *Journal of Hypertension*, 24(6):1187–92.

Rastenyte, D., Sopagiene, D., Virviciute, D. and Jureniene, K. (2006) Diverging trends in the incidence and mortality of stroke during the period 1986–2002: a study from the stroke register in Kaunas, Lithuania, *Scandinavian Journal of Public Health*, 34(5):488–95.

Rautio, A., Eliasson, M. and Stegmayr, B. (2008) Favorable trends in the incidence and outcome in stroke in nondiabetic and diabetic subjects: findings from the Northern Sweden MONICA Stroke Registry in 1985 to 2003, *Stroke*, 39(12):3137–44.

Redon, J., Erdine, S., Bohm, M. et al. (2011) Physician attitudes to blood pressure control: findings from the Supporting Hypertension Awareness and Research Europe-wide survey, *Journal of Hypertension*, 29(8):1633–40.

Roberts, B., Stickley, A., Balabanova, D. and McKee, M. (2010) Irregular treatment of hypertension in the former Soviet Union, *Journal of Epidemiology, Community Health*, 64:902–7.

Roberts, B., Stickley, A., Balabanova, D., Haerpfer, C. and McKee, M. (2012) The persistence of irregular treatment of hypertension in the former Soviet Union, *Journal of Epidemiology and Community Health*, 66:1079–82.

Rodgers, A., Ezzati, M., van der Hoorn, S. et al. (2004) Distribution of major health risks: findings from the Global Burden of Disease study, PLoS *Medicine*, 1(1):e27.

Rothwell, P.M., Coull, A.J., Giles, M.F. et al. (2004) Change in stroke incidence, mortality, case-fatality, severity, and risk factors in Oxfordshire, UK from 1981 to 2004 (Oxford Vascular Study), *Lancet*, 363(9425):1925–33.

Ruschitzka, F. (2011) Evidence for improvement in survival with antihypertensive combination treatment, *Journal of Hypertension*, 29(suppl 1):S9–14.

Sienkiewicz-Jarosz, H., Gluszkiewicz, M., Pniewski, J. et al. (2011) Incidence and case fatality rates of first-ever stroke: comparison of data from two prospective population-based studies conducted in Warsaw, *Neurologia i Neurochirurgia Polska*, 45(3):207–12.

Sivenius, J., Tuomilehto, J., Immonen-Raiha, P. et al. (2004) Continuous 15-year decrease in incidence and mortality of stroke in Finland: the FINSTROKE study, *Stroke*, 35(2):420–5.

Stegmayr, B. and Asplund, K. (2003) Stroke in northern Sweden, *Scandinavian Journal of Public Health Supplement*, 61:60–69.

Steinberg, B.A., Bhatt, D.L., Mehta, S. et al. (2008) Nine-year trends in achievement of risk factor goals in the US and European outpatients with cardiovascular disease, *American Heart Journal*, 156(4):719–27.

Towfighi, A. and Saver, J.L. (2011) Stroke declines from third to fourth leading cause of death in the United States: historical perspective and challenges ahead, *Stroke*, 42(8):2351–5.

Unal, B., Critchley, J.A. and Capewell, S. (2005) Modelling the decline in coronary heart disease deaths in England and Wales, 1981–2000: comparing contributions from primary prevention and secondary prevention, *British Medical Journal*, 331(7517): 614.

Vartiainen, E., Laatikainen, T., Peltonen, M. et al. (2010) Thirty-five-year trends in cardiovascular risk factors in Finland, *International Journal of Epidemiology*, 39(2):504–18.

Wang, Y.R., Alexander, G.C. and Stafford, R.S. (2007) Outpatient hypertension treatment, treatment intensification, and control in Western Europe and the United States, *Archives of Internal Medicine*, 167(2):141–7.

Wolf-Maier, K., Cooper, R.S., Banegas, J.R. et al. (2003) Hypertension prevalence and blood pressure levels in 6 European countries, Canada, and the United States, *Journal of the American Medical Association*, 289(18):2363–9.

WHO Regional Office for Europe (2012) *European Health for All Database (HFA-DB)*. Copenhagen: WHO Regional Office for Europe, http://data.euro.who.int/hfadb/ (accessed 4 June 2012).

World Health Organization (2009) *Global Health Risks: Mortality and Burden of Disease Attributable to Selected Major Risks*. Geneva: World Health Organization.

Wright, J.M. and Musini, V.M. (2009) First-line drugs for hypertension, *Cochrane Database of Systematic Reviews*, (3):CD001841.

chapter nine

Cancer screening

Ahti Anttila and Jose M. Martin-Moreno

Introduction

Cancer is a relatively common and often devastating group of diseases. In Europe as a whole, the yearly number of new cases of cancer is 3.4 million, and the yearly number of cancer deaths is 1.9 million (IARC 2008). Over the past decades, the incidence of cancer in Europe has been rising, but age-standardized death rates have fallen slightly, reflecting advances in the detection and management of the disease. The main policy options are primary prevention (by reducing exposure to risk factors for cancer), secondary prevention (by early detection and treatment) and treatment. This chapter deals with the second option and will highlight the main successes and failures of cancer screening in Europe in the past decades.

The ultimate purpose of cancer screening is to reduce cancer mortality in the population. By detecting cancer or preinvasive disease in an early stage – earlier than it would otherwise be diagnosed through usual clinical practice – treatment may be less aggressive and may achieve a better outcome than when cancer is diagnosed at a more advanced stage, leading to better quality of life and a longer survival. Cervical cancer screening exemplifies this; it is possible to detect and treat a preinvasive form of the disease and, under optimal conditions, to prevent the development of malignant disease.

Balanced against this, screening and the activities involved in subsequent diagnosis and treatment can also give rise to adverse effects. A 'positive' screening test simply identifies people who are at increased likelihood of having the condition, and further investigation is required to confirm the diagnosis. The adverse effects include psychosocial morbidity in women screened positive or subsequently given a diagnosis of cancer, as well as the complications and long-term consequences of cancer treatment (IARC 2002, 2005; Perry et al. 2006; Arbyn et al. 2008; Segnan et al. 2010).

Recognizing that the overall benefits should outweigh any harms that may result from screening, the EU Council has recommended population-based screening for breast, cervical and colorectal cancers on the basis of the available evidence of effectiveness, subject to implementation of appropriate quality assurance systems (Council of the European Union 2003). WHO has endorsed these recommendations for its 53 Member States in the European Region (WHO Regional Office for Europe 2011). Based on current projections, well over 500 million screening examinations for breast, cervical and/or colorectal cancer will be performed in publicly mandated programmes in the EU alone between 2010 and 2020 (von Karsa et al. 2008).

The three cancers covered by these recommendations account for almost one-fifth, or 400,000, of the 1.8 million cancer deaths in the European Region (IARC 2008). This is despite the fact that organized screening programmes for the first two have been in use for decades, with the techniques involved being implemented opportunistically even earlier. Organized cervical cancer screening has been undertaken in Finland since 1963. Breast cancer screening programmes began to be implemented in the late 1980s. Colorectal cancer screening programmes, however, have only been established in the 2000s and still cover a small part of Europe only (von Karsa et al. 2008).

Because it is too early to assess success and failure for colorectal cancer screening, this chapter will mainly focus on cervical and breast cancer screening. The analysis will show, for both cervical and breast cancer, that large variations exist in the availability of well-organized, population-based screening services in Europe, both within and outside the EU, and these are reflected in variations in population health outcomes.

Effectiveness of cancer screening

Cervical cancer screening

The available evidence suggests that well-organized screening programmes for cervical cancer reduce incidence and mortality from this disease by 80% or more (IARC 2005) (Table 9.1). Randomized controlled trials have not been performed, but prospective cohort studies, population-based trend studies and long-term observational evaluations of early screening programmes clearly support this claim.

The ultimate impact of cervical cancer screening on mortality in the general population is difficult to assess. Precancerous lesions take, on average, 10–12 years to become malignant (Gustafsson and Adami 1989; van Oortmarssen and Habbema 1991), and even invasive cancers do not lead to death until several years have passed. Moreover, roll-out of the screening programme is usually gradual, and, therefore, the full impact of cervical cancer screening is not apparent until decades after programme implementation has begun. Finally, trends in mortality are also determined by other factors, such as the underlying rate of infection with the causal agent, human papilloma virus.

Table 9.1 Effectiveness of cancer screening

Site, sex and test	Target age (years)	Screening interval (years)	Expected mortality outcome among invited (% reduction)	Source
Cervix, females, Pap smear	25 or 30 to 64	3–5	≥80	IARC 2005
Breast, females, mammography	50–69	2	25	IARC 2002
Colorectum, males and females, faecal occult blood tests	50–74	2	16	Hewitson et al. 2007

Breast cancer screening

Effectiveness of screening for breast cancer has been assessed by means of randomized controlled trials with long-term follow-up (IARC 2002). It has been estimated that bi-annual mammography screening programmes for breast cancer in women aged 50 to 69 years decrease mortality from the disease by approximately 25% among invited women (IARC 2002) (Table 9.1). The estimate includes deaths from those cancers that have been diagnosed during the randomisation period. Observational evaluations of routine screening programmes, carried out mainly in the Nordic countries where the attendance rates are usually very high (Olsen et al. 2005; Swedish Organised Service Screening Evaluation Group 2006; Sarkeala et al. 2008), are consistent with it being effective in lowering mortality, although it is important to note that there is persisting controversy about its effectiveness (Gotzsche et al. 2012).

The assessment of the impact of breast cancer screening on mortality in the general population is hampered by problems similar to those noted for cervical cancer screening. It is increasingly recognized that the term breast cancer includes a wide variety of tumour types, which progress with varying degrees of rapidity; consequently, some are very aggressive and may lead to death within a few years, while with others, the disease may progress very slowly, with deaths continuing to occur even 15–20 years after diagnosis. However, it is apparent that the reductions in mortality, typically of the order of 25%, seen in randomized controlled trials are not replicated in routine statistics on breast cancer mortality, where the reductions are more often in the range 5–15% in the general female population 15–20 years after full roll-out of the programme (Hristova and Hakama 1997; Anttila et al. 2008). In routine mortality statistics age at diagnosis is not taken into account, eg if the cancer leading to death had occurred before the start of the screening programme. The ultimate magnitude of the impact on overall breast cancer mortality in the whole female population depends on the age bands included in the screening policy, the time since onset of screening and the time since full population coverage has been reached. Simultaneously, other factors affect breast cancer mortality trends, including changes in exposure to risk factors (e.g. changes in reproductive history, diet and physical exercise; use of hormone replacement therapies; and alcohol consumption), changes in awareness of breast cancer and access to diagnosis and treatment outside the screening programme and improvements in breast cancer diagnosis and treatment. Therefore, the impact of screening as such is difficult to measure from trend studies; breast cancer mortality trends in the whole female population reflect the overall control of breast cancer rather than the impact of screening *per se*. Effectiveness evaluation requires higher-precision cohort linkage studies in randomized or non-randomized settings).

Colorectal cancer screening

Randomized controlled trials have shown that bi-annual screening for colorectal cancer with traditional guaiac-based faecal occult blood tests among those aged 50–74 years can reduce mortality from colorectal cancer by approximately 16% (Hewitson et al. 2007) (Table 9.1). Although colorectal cancer screening is now officially recommended by international agencies, the cost-effectiveness of population-based screening programmes for colorectal cancer remains somewhat contested (Hakama et al. 2005; Sigurdsson et al. 2012).

Assessing the impact of colorectal cancer screening programmes on mortality in the general population will probably be beset with the same difficulties as those encountered in cervical and breast cancer screening.

Successes and failures of cancer screening in Europe

Implementation of cancer screening in Europe

About one-fifth of the target population in the EU is covered by population-based cervical cancer screening (Table 9.2). Almost a third of the EU population resides in countries or regions where planning, piloting or roll-out of cervical cancer screening is still ongoing. Finally, there is also considerable screening activity with opportunistic testing alone (von Karsa et al. 2008). Non-population-based policies from previous decades are often still in place, and so screening may include only women with health insurance, or high-risk patients. Clearly, this situation is far from satisfactory.

The actual policies on cervical cancer screening also vary significantly between European countries (see Table 9.3 for some examples). Striking differences are found in the target age groups and the recommended screening interval; as a result, the total number of smears a woman is expected to undergo during her lifetime varies between 7 and more than 50. High-intensity screening policies such as those in Austria and Germany are not evidence based and are likely to have an unfavourable balance between benefits and harms. In addition, there are also differences in test methods, quality assurance practices and monitoring and evaluation of the screening programmes.

While some countries have more intensive screening practices than those prescribed by current EU recommendations (Arbyn et al. 2008), there are also countries where the capacity for testing and subsequent confirmation and treatment are insufficient – particularly in eastern Europe and in the CIS.

Table 9.2 Implementation of cancer screening in the European Union, 2007

Cancer type	Percentage of population covered			
	Population based, complete	Population based: planning, piloting, rollout	Non-population based only	No programme or no data
Cervix	22	29	47	3
Breast	41	50	6	4
Colon and rectum	0	43	27	30

Source: von Karsa et al., 2008

Table 9.3 Examples of variation in recommended cervical cancer screening policies in selected countries in Europe in 2007

	Target age (years)[a]	Screening interval (years)	Smears per woman lifetime	Population based	Coverage of smear tests for the 3- or 5-yearly period (%)
Austria	18+	1	50+	No	N/A
Belgium	25–64	3	14	No	67
Finland	(25)30–60(65)	5	7–9	Yes	90
Germany	20+	1	50+	No	N/A
Lithuania	30–60	3	11	No	53
The Netherlands	30–60	5	7	Yes	77
Poland	25–59	3	12	Yes	N/A
Romania	25–65	5	9	Yes	10
Slovenia	20–64	3	15	Yes	68
Sweden	23–60	3 or 5	12	Yes	73
United Kingdom (England)	(20)25–(60)64	3 or 5	10–16	Yes	74

Source: Anttila et al. 2009
Notes: N/A, not available
[a]Variation within the country on age indicated in parentheses

As a result of these variations in policy, the estimated costs per life-year gained vary significantly between countries. The unit costs per screen are usually lower in population-based programmes because they are organized in a more efficient way and prices are negotiated centrally. With more intensive policies (i.e. widening the target age group to include younger women and/or shortening the screening interval), the incremental cost-effectiveness ratio rises to very high costs per life-year gained, because the incremental effects diminish rapidly while the costs continue to go up (Arbyn et al. 2009a).

For breast cancer screening, the coverage of population-based screening programmes is somewhat larger than for cervical cancer screening (more than 40%). Many countries are planning, piloting or rolling out screening programmes, and the data suggest that in a few years 90% of the target population in Europe will be covered by population-based breast cancer screening programmes.

Impact of screening on the burden of mortality from cervical cancer in Europe

Although, as explained above, conclusions on the impact of screening on mortality in the general population (relative to other factors) will probably remain elusive, we will now describe the development of cervical cancer mortality in Europe and relate it to the implementation of cervical cancer screening.

Figure 9.1 shows trends of cervical cancer mortality in selected European countries as recorded in the WHO mortality database. The countries were selected based on the availability and quality of the cause-of-death information; see Arbyn et al. (2009b) for a discussion on the coding practices of the cause-of-death data. Among western European countries, Denmark, Finland, Sweden and the United Kingdom have had population-based programmes since the 1960s (although in the United Kingdom the programme was opportunistic until the late 1980s). Austria, Ireland, Norway and Switzerland, by comparison, have mainly had non-population-based screening activity. Mortality from cervical cancer has declined in all these countries, but the decrease is most consistent in countries with long-lasting population-based programmes (see data for Denmark, Finland, Sweden and the United Kingdom). In several countries, the historical decrease in cervical cancer mortality had already started before the year 1970, reflecting a combination of opportunistic screening, earlier diagnosis and better treatment; therefore, it is difficult to estimate the isolated effect of the screening programme from the trend observed in the figure. However, there is no evidence of similar decreases in cervical cancer mortality in central and eastern Europe or in the CIS, which is likely to be due at least in part to the absence of organized cervical cancer screening programmes.

Every year, there are approximately 54,500 new incident cases of cervical cancer and 24,900 deaths in Europe (IARC 2008). Of these, 31,000 incident cases and 13,400 deaths are in the EU. While still high, these figures represent a significant improvement from past decades. Mortality decreased by over 50% in the EU-15 between 1970–1974 and 2000–2004 (Arbyn et al. 2009b). Importantly, about 60% of this decrease has been attributed to cancer screening, translating into approximately 35,000 fewer incident cases and 15,000 fewer deaths per year in these countries (Ronco and Anttila 2009).

Compared with the potential long-term reduction of over 80% that could be reached with optimal screening policies, there is still considerable room for improvement. Incidence and mortality could realistically be halved in most countries by organizing services better, by introducing systematic quality assurance, by monitoring and evaluating outcomes and by increasing coverage.

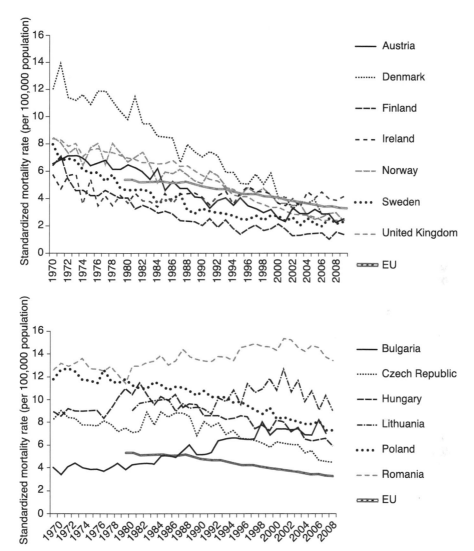

Figure 9.1   Cervical cancer mortality rates in selected countries in Europe, adjusted for age to the European standard population

Source: WHO Regional Office for Europe 2012

In central and eastern Europe, the potential benefit is even larger because no similar historical decrease in the disease burden has yet taken place.

Screening and mortality trends from breast cancer in Europe

Mortality from breast cancer has decreased in many European countries since the mid-1990s according to data in the WHO mortality database (Fig. 9.2). In

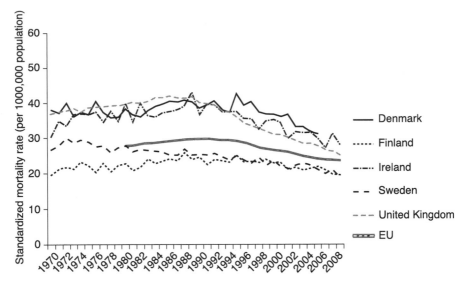

Figure 9.2 Breast cancer mortality trends in selected European countries in 1970–2009, adjusted for age to the European standard population

Source: WHO Regional Office for Europe 2012

addition to cancer screening programmes, such as those in place since the late 1980s in the Netherlands, Sweden and the United Kingdom, improvements in treatment have also contributed to these favourable trends, as explained above. In general, decreases in mortality have been strongest in western Europe.

In several countries in central and eastern Europe and the former USSR, mortality from breast cancer is still increasing (Bulgaria, the Republic of Moldova and the Russian Federation) or is stable at best. In these countries the burden of this disease – which was historically lower than that in western Europe – is increasing because of rising exposure to risk factors and more intense diagnostic activity (Hirte et al. 2007). Population-based screening programmes are not yet in place. There is a clear need to consider how to improve breast cancer control strategies in these countries, including strengthening of primary prevention, improving awareness of breast cancer, improving availability of diagnostic and treatment services for symptomatic patients and – if resources are available – considering organized screening.

The impact of breast cancer screening on mortality in the general population can best be seen in the age groups targeted by screening (Fig. 9.3). It is interesting to note that among women under 55 years of age (who were mostly diagnosed with breast cancer before they were eligible for screening), there has been a large decrease in breast cancer mortality in most European countries, much of which is likely to reflect improvements in treatment. At the same time, trends in mortality from breast cancer in older women (aged 55–69 and 70–84 years), where screening programmes may have had an effect, show contrasting developments between European countries. Some countries with population-based screening programmes in western Europe (such as Sweden

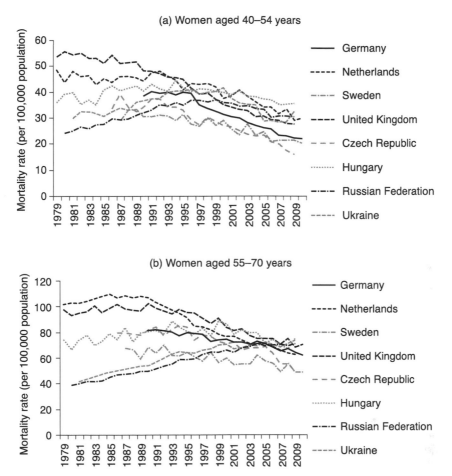

Figure 9.3 Breast cancer mortality trends in selected European countries, by age at death

Source: World Health Organization 2012

and the United Kingdom) show decreasing trends, whereas in other countries this is less obvious or the timing of the decrease is variable. However, in these age groups, it is difficult to differentiate the effects of screening and treatment; a modelling study undertaken using data from the United States estimated that the former accounted for a decline in mortality of 12.4% and the latter a decline of 14.6% between 1975 and 2000 (Mandelblatt et al. 2006).

Discussion and conclusions

Obstacles in cancer screening: the example of cervical cancer

Because effective cervical cancer screening has been available in many countries for more than half a century, these programmes can serve as a good way to understand the difficulties that are encountered when rolling out a successful population-based programme. Indeed, there are still many populations and regions where optimal results have not yet been achieved. This is because the management of a population-based programme is more complex than mere service provision: if societal aspects (e.g. awareness-raising activities) are not consistent with screening services, the outcomes may be suboptimal despite widespread availability of services.

In high-income settings, some population groups overuse screening services while others do not use them at all. At the same time, lack of monitoring, evaluation and quality assurance undermine programme effectiveness (Arbyn et al. 2009a). In contrast, in lower-income countries in Europe, the lack of sustainable financial and human resources is still a major obstacle. More collaboration between those involved in delivering a service can help to remove financial and human barriers, and to improve the quality and cost-effectiveness of screening. This is particularly important in the context of fiscal austerity policies being adopted by governments during the ongoing financial crisis (Martin-Moreno et al. 2012).

Countries with limited resources often face weaknesses in the capacity to plan services as well as a scarcity of resources for implementation of effective and affordable organization of screening. For example, in the new Member States of the EU, large numbers of cervical smears have been recommended, but little effort has been invested in coordination, integrated systems of quality assurance or cancer registration, and thus evaluation of the programme (Nicula et al. 2009; Anttila et al. 2010). In such settings, it may be better to reduce the frequency of screening and invest the resources in better management. The generally accepted recommendation to screen women from the age of 25–30 years until the age of 60–65 years, with a 3- to 5-year interval, yields approximately 7–15 tests in a lifetime per woman. In low-resource settings or during programme roll-out, it may be acceptable to plan for a smaller number of tests (e.g. five or fewer per lifetime).

The consequences of poor planning can be dramatic: if there is no screening register, for example, it is not possible to undertake linkage studies showing whether cervical cancer incidence and the subsequent burden of mortality have decreased among women who have participated in screening. There may be extensive screening activity that does not translate into reductions in the cervical cancer burden in the target population; such activity will not be cost-effective and may produce overall harm for women using the services (Anttila et al. 2010). Unfortunately, in many settings, there is a poor understanding of the effectiveness of different organizational and financing models for screening (Todorova et al. 2006; Nicula et al. 2009; Valerianova et al. 2010).

Poor coordination and organization of services may be manifest in a number of ways. Invitation procedures may not follow the recommendations for best practice (Veerus et al. 2010), leading to attendance rates as low as 10–30% among those invited (Anttila et al. 2009; Nicula et al. 2009; Veerus et al. 2010). Non-validated, non-standardized sampling or testing methods may be used that are incapable of recognizing precancerous lesions effectively (Viberga et al. 2010). Failure to specify responsibility for follow-up may lead to women with a positive test falling through the net and so denied appropriate diagnosis and treatment (Ronco and Anttila 2009).

New methods, new programmes

The science of cervical screening is changing rapidly, with manual examination of cervical smear slides giving way to automated liquid-based cytology (Cox 2004), while interest is growing in the potential of high-throughput detection of human papilloma virus (Arbyn et al. 2010; Micalessi et al. 2012). Furthermore, in time, the costs and benefits of screening are likely to change following the widespread introduction of vaccines for the human papilloma virus (European Centre for Disease Prevention and Control 2008; Bonanni et al. 2011). It will be important for those responsible for screening programmes to monitor these developments closely. Unfortunately, evaluation of these new methods in Europe has taken place mainly in wealthy settings and not always within a population-based public-health programme. One consequence of this is that the evidence may be difficult to apply directly in low-resource settings. This is unfortunate because there is scope to achieve a remarkable impact on disease prevention with very few tests over the course of a woman's life, for example the number of lifetime tests needed could be much smaller with human papilloma virus testing than with the current cytological testing.

It is essential that new screening programmes are evaluated in randomized controlled trials. These evaluations should include long-term follow-up of mortality as well as investigations of quality of life, potential adverse effects, costs and the feasibility of implementation. The decision to introduce a new population-based cancer screening programme should only be made after these very thorough multifaceted analyses have been carried out and when a broad consensus among stakeholders has emerged.

At present, randomized controlled trials have been completed or are ongoing for screening of several other common cancers, including prostate and lung cancers. Current evidence for these screening tests does not yet indicate that an appropriate balance between the benefit and harm of screening can be achieved in a population-based programme, so none of these is currently recommended for general introduction (Hakama et al. 2008; Martin-Moreno et al. 2009; Schroder et al. 2009; National Lung Screening Trial Research Team 2011). There may be a need to develop better test methods, diagnostic markers and treatments before large-scale cancer screening programmes for these cancer sites can be recommended. For now, these new screening methods simply represent the promise of the future, when cancer screening will detect a wide range of common neoplasms in time for patients to be treated effectively, successfully and at a minimal cost to health systems.

References

Anttila, A., Sarkeala, T., Hakulinen, T. and Heinavaara, S. (2008) Impacts of the Finnish service screening programme on breast cancer rates, *BMC Public Health*, 8:38.

Anttila, A. and Ronco, G. for the Working Group on the Registration and Monitoring of Cervical Cancer Screening Programmes in the European Union, within the European Network for Information on Cancer (EUNICE) (2009) Description of the national situation of cervical cancer screening in the member states of the European Union, *European Journal of Cancer*, 45(15):2685–2708.

Anttila, A., Arbyn, M., Veerus, P. et al. (2010) Barriers in cervical cancer screening programs in new European Union member states, *Tumori*, 96(4):515–16.

Arbyn, M., Anttila, A., Jordan, J. et al. (eds) (2008) *European Guidelines for Quality Assurance in Cervical Cancer Screening*. Luxembourg: Office for Official Publications of the European Communities.

Arbyn, M., Rebolj, M., de Kok, I.M. et al. (2009a) The challenges of organising cervical screening programmes in the 15 old member states of the European Union, *European Journal of Cancer*, 45(15):2671–8.

Arbyn, M., Raifu, A.O., Weiderpass, E., Bray, F. and Anttila, A. (2009b) Trends of cervical cancer mortality in the member states of the European Union, *European Journal of Cancer*, 45(15):2640–8.

Arbyn, M., Anttila, A., Jordan, J. et al. (eds) (2010) *European Guidelines for Quality Assurance in Cervical Cancer Screening*, second edition: summary document, *Annals in Oncology*, 21(3):448–58.

Bonanni, P., Levi, M., Latham, N.B. et al. (2011) An overview on the implementation of HPV vaccination in Europe, *Human Vaccination*, 7(suppl):128–35.

Council of the European Union (2003) *Council Recommendation of 2 December 2003 on Cancer Screening (2003/878/EC) OJ L 327:34–38*. Brussels: European Council.

Cox, J.T. (2004) Liquid-based cytology: evaluation of effectiveness, cost-effectiveness, and application to present practice, *Journal of the National Comprehensive Cancer Network*, 2(6):597–611.

European Centre for Disease Prevention and Control (2008) *Guidance for the Introduction of HPV Vaccines in EU Countries*. Stockholm: European Centre for Disease Prevention and Control.

Gotzsche, P.C., Jorgensen, K.J., Zahl, P.H. and Maehlen, J. (2012) Why mammography screening has not lived up to expectations from the randomised trials, *Cancer Causes and Control*, 23(1):15–21.

Gustafsson, L. and Adami, H.O. (1989) Natural history of cervical neoplasia: consistent results obtained by an identification technique, *British Journal of Cancer*, 60(1):132–41.

Hakama, M., Hoff, G., Kronborg, O. and Pahlman, L. (2005) Screening for colorectal cancer, *Acta Oncologica*, 44(5):425–39.

Hakama, M., Coleman, M.P., Alexe, D.-M. and Auvinen, A. (2008) Cancer screening, in M.P. Coleman, D.-M. Alexe, T. Albreht and M. McKee (eds) *Responding to the Challenge of Cancer in Europe*. Ljubljana: Institute of Public Health of the Republic of Slovenia, pp. 69–92.

Hewitson, P., Glasziou, P., Irwig, L., Towler, B. and Watson, E. (2007) Screening for colorectal cancer using the faecal occult blood test, Hemoccult, *Cochrane Database of Systematic Reviews*, (1):CD001216.

Hirte, L., Nolte, E., Bain, C. and McKee, M. (2007) Breast cancer mortality in Russia and Ukraine 1963–2002: an age-period-cohort analysis, *International Journal of Epidemiology*, 36(4):900–6.

Hristova, L. and Hakama, M. (1997) Effect of screening for cancer in the Nordic countries on deaths, cost and quality of life up to the year 2017, *Acta Oncologica*, 36(suppl 9):1–60.

IARC (2002) *Breast Cancer Screening*. Lyon, France: International Agency for Research on Cancer.

IARC (2005) *Cervix Cancer Screening*. Lyon, France: International Agency for Research on Cancer.

IARC (2008) The GLOBOCAN Project [website]. Lyon, France: International Agency for Research on Cancer, http://globocan.iarc.fr (accessed 4 June 2012).

von Karsa, L., Anttila, A., Ronco, G. et al. (2008) *Cancer Screening in the European Union. Report on the Implementation of the Council Recommendation on Cancer Screening.* Luxembourg: European Commission and International Agency for Research on Cancer.

Mandelblatt, J., Schechter, C.B., Lawrence, W., Yi, B. and Cullen, J. (2006) The SPECTRUM population model of the impact of screening and treatment on US breast cancer trends from 1975 to 2000: principles and practice of the model methods, *Journal of the National Cancer Institute Monographs*, (36):47–55.

Martin-Moreno, J.M., Harris, M., Garcia-Lopez, E. and Gorgojo, L. (2009) *Fighting Against Cancer Today: A Policy Summary.* Ljubljana: Institute of Public Health of the Republic of Slovenia.

Martin-Moreno, J.M., Anttila, A., von Karsa, L., Alfonso-Sanchez, J.L. and Gorgojo, L. (2012) Cancer screening and health system resilience: Keys to protecting and bolstering preventive services during a financial crisis, *European Journal of Cancer*, Epub ahead of print (PMID: 22424881).

Micalessi, I.M., Boulet, G.A., Bogers, J.J., Benoy, I.H. and Depuydt, C.E. (2012) High-throughput detection, genotyping and quantification of the human papillomavirus using real-time PCR, *Clinical Chemistry and Laboratory Medicine*, 50(4):655–61.

National Lung Screening Trial Research Team (2011) Reduced lung-cancer mortality with low-dose computed tomographic screening, *New England Journal of Medicine*, 365(5):395–409.

Nicula, F.A., Anttila, A., Neamtiu, L. et al. (2009) Challenges in starting organised screening programmes for cervical cancer in the new member states of the European Union, *European Journal of Cancer*, 45(15):2679–84.

Olsen, A.H., Njor, S.H., Vejborg, I. et al. (2005) Breast cancer mortality in Copenhagen after introduction of mammography screening: cohort study, *British Medical Journal*, 330(7485):220.

van Oortmarssen, G.J. and Habbema, J.D. (1991) Epidemiological evidence for age-dependent regression of pre-invasive cervical cancer, *British Journal of Cancer*, 64(3):559–65.

Perry, N., Broeders, M., de Wolf, C. et al. (eds) (2006) *European Guidelines for Quality Assurance in Breast Cancer Screening and Diagnosis.* Luxembourg: Publication Office of the European Communities.

Ronco, G. and Anttila, A. (2009) Cervical cancer screening in Europe: changes over the last 9 years, *European Journal of Cancer*, 45(15):2629–31.

Sarkeala, T., Heinavaara, S. and Anttila, A. (2008) Breast cancer mortality with varying invitational policies in organised mammography, *British Journal of Cancer*, 98(3):641–5.

Schroder, F.H., Hugosson, J., Roobol, M.J. et al. (2009) Screening and prostate-cancer mortality in a randomized European study, *New England Journal of Medicine*, 360(13):1320–8.

Segnan, N., Patnick, J. and Karsa, L. (eds) (2010) *European Guidelines for Quality Assurance in Colorectal Cancer Screening.* Luxembourg: Publication Office of the European Union.

Sigurdsson, J.A., Getz, L., Sjonell, G., Vainiomaki, P. and Brodersen, J. (2012) Marginal public health gain of screening for colorectal cancer: modelling study, based on WHO and national databases in the Nordic countries, *Journal of Evaluation of Clinical Practice*, Epub ahead of print (PMID: 22519671).

Swedish Organised Service Screening Evaluation Group (2006) Reduction in breast cancer mortality from organized service screening with mammography. 1. Further confirmation with extended data, *Cancer Epidemiology and Biomarkers in Prevention*, 15(1):45–51.

Todorova, I.L., Baban, A., Balabanova, D., Panayotova, Y. and Bradley, J. (2006) Providers' constructions of the role of women in cervical cancer screening in Bulgaria and Romania, *Social Science and Medicine*, 63(3):776–87.

Valerianova, Z., Panayotova, Y., Amati, C. for the EUROCHIP Working Group (2010) Cervical cancer screening in Bulgaria: past and present experience, *Tumori*, 96(4):538–44.

Veerus, P., Arbyn, M., Amati, C. for the EUROCHIP Working Group (2010) Impact of implementing a nationwide cervical cancer screening program on female population coverage by Pap-tests in Estonia, *Tumori*, 96(4):524–8.

Viberga, I., Engele, L., Baili, P. for the EUROCHIP Working Group (2010) Past, present and future of the cervical cancer screening in Latvia, *Tumori*, 96(4):529–37.

WHO Regional Office for Europe (2011) *Regional Committee for Europe: Action Plan for Implementation of the European Strategy for the Prevention and Control of Noncommunicable Diseases 2012–2016*. [Resolution EUR/RC61/12, Baku, Azerbaijan, 15 September 2011.] Copenhagen: WHO Regional Office for Europe.

WHO Regional Office for Europe (2012) *European Health for All Database (HFA-DB)*. Copenhagen: WHO Regional Office for Europe, http://data.euro.who.int/hfadb/ (accessed 4 June 2012).

World Health Organization (2012) *Mortality Database*. Geneva: World Health Organization, http://www.who.int/healthinfo/morttables/en/ (accessed 4 June 2012).

ten

Mental health

Ionela Petrea and Andrew McCulloch

Introduction

Psychiatric symptoms are widely distributed in the population and their degree and nature vary. For many mental disorders, the duration and severity of symptoms are key to diagnosis; consequently, mental illness can be thought of as one end of a spectrum of health experience. However, key thinkers in mental health, such as Keyes (2005), now use a two-dimensional model of mental health, recognizing that the absence of mental illness does not imply good mental health and that (albeit perhaps more rarely) the presence of a specific mental illness does not always imply bad mental health, a situation analogous with physical health. From a policy point of view, it is, therefore, important to recognize that the burden created by poor mental health includes both mental illness and poor mental health without a diagnosable mental illness – as both can adversely affect family, social and economic functioning. Since the late 1980s, some countries have started to include mental health promotion in their mental health policy, which has been driven historically by the need to respond to (severe) mental illness.

Mental illness can be divided into five main groups, as shown in Table 10.1. This indicates the relative prevalence and impact of each disease group and notes some distinctive policy issues relating to each of them.

Additionally, it must be recognized that the prevalence, presentation and impact of mental illness varies with age, gender, culture and social variables.

Age. Childhood disorders are quite different from those in adults and present much more behaviourally; similarly patterns of illness vary across adult life. Severe disorders generally appear and are at their worst in young adulthood; common mental disorders are most common in mid-life and dementias in old age.

Table 10.1 Groups of mental disorders

Groups	Example	Prevalence	Impact	Specific issues
Common mental disorders	Depression	Typically 10% of the population each year	Highest, important cause of suicide	Treatment rates, access, ability of primary care to treat
Severe mental disorders	Schizophrenia	Typically ≤1% of the population over the life course	High, important cause of mortality and disability	Deinstitutionalization, access to the required range of services, employment
Eating disorders	Anorexia nervosa	Least common group, but not uncommon in young women	Medium, but causes high mortality in sufferers	Specialist, evidence-based treatment
Personality disorders	Borderline personality disorder	Controversial but may be 3–4% of the population	High social impact from the criminal subgroup of this population	Treatment, diagnosis, access to appropriate services, links with criminal justice
Dementias	Alzheimer's disease	1 in 4–5 over 85 years, prevalence builds from middle age	Highest with the common disorders	Huge social and nursing care and family burden; these disorders are not dealt with in this chapter

Sources: Alonso et al. 2004a,b; McCulloch 2006; McGrath et al. 2008; McCulloch and Muijen 2011

Gender. Common mental disorders appear to be more common in women, and the presentation or impact of severe disorders and personality disorders is arguably more severe in men, although this may reflect other aspects of masculinity rather than the course of the disorder.

Culture. Illnesses are interpreted differently and responded to differently in different cultural, ethnic and religious groups.

Social variables. Patterns of substance misuse and indeed a whole myriad of other social variables impact on mental health.

Scale of the problem

In the EU, at least 165 million people (38%) have mental health problems at any one time (Wittchen et al. 2011). The most common is anxiety, experienced by 14% of the adult population, but these figures cover a wide range of diagnoses in children, adults and older people (Fig. 10.1).

The most recent available data show that neuropsychiatric disorders are the second largest cause of DALYs lost in Europe and account for 19% of the total, only 4% less than the leading cause, cardiovascular diseases (Mathers et al. 2008). They are among the top ten conditions in all European countries,

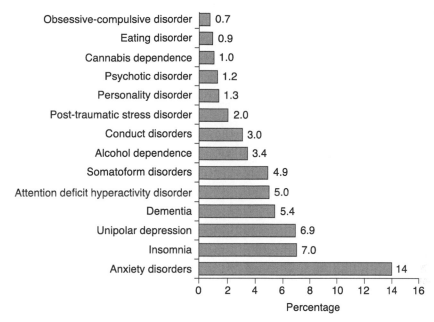

Figure 10.1   Prevalence of mental disorders in Europe 2010

Source: Wittchen et al. 2011

typically ranking first or second in EU Member States, third or fourth in south-eastern European countries and fifth or sixth in the CIS (Lopez 2006; Mathers et al. 2008). Mental disorders are by far the largest contributor to chronic conditions afflicting people in Europe, accounting for 40% of all years lived with disability.

Scope of mental health policy

Mental health policies are multifaceted, ranging from the promotion of mental health and the prevention of mental illness and of suicides, to the provision of mental health interventions in primary health care and deinstitutionalization, and to the prevention of stigma and discrimination and the protection of human rights and empowerment of people with mental health problems.

Mental health has been described as a 'wicked' public policy issue that requires detailed coordination of efforts across many government departments or ministries (Muijen and McCulloch 2009). This is because, if people with severe or persistent mental health problems are to recover their functioning, these individuals require coordinated support across housing, employment, social care, education, employment and welfare, in addition to health care. Many countries struggle to develop truly cross-governmental mental health policies, let alone to coordinate their implementation over time. This impacts on population mental health outcomes as health care cannot deliver alone. This, in turn, often means that governments only monitor health care or institutional indicators, or single outcome indicators such as suicide. While these measures may be all that is available, it is important to recognize that they do not give a balanced view of national performance on improving mental health.

Mental health outcomes

Evaluating the impact of mental health policies is challenging. Outcome indicators remain poorly defined compared with those for physical health. Ideally, outcome indicators for mental health would focus not on mortality (although suicide and excess deaths from physical causes are important indicators) but on improvements in symptoms, behaviour, functioning/impairment and social integration. However, few countries have systems in place for collecting data on such outcomes. Where such systems are operational, the validity of data is often questioned. Service users, carers and professionals attach different meanings to outcome measures in mental health, and often the measurements made by these groups differ significantly. Professionals often lack incentives to collect data, as results are rarely fed back into their practice; outcome assessment is primarily used to measure performance, with a potential punitive impact on poor performers and sometimes perverse financial incentives. Box 10.1 illustrates some innovative approaches in the Netherlands and England.

Over time, there have been many international initiatives, sponsored by WHO, OECD, the European Commission and the Council of Europe, to identify internationally standardized outcome indicators (Lavikainen et al. 2006; Mattke et al. 2006; WHO Regional Office for Europe 2008; Pincus and Naber 2009; Spaeth-Rublee et al. 2010; OECD 2011). These initiatives have been largely unsuccessful, but have raised awareness about the vulnerability of decision-makers who continue to rely primarily on input measures in formulating their policy decisions. A recent example is an OECD project that reviewed mental health outcome indicators in OECD Member States. It sought to identify indicators that had wide coverage, were routinely collected and were readily linked to activity data and time series (Spaeth-Rublee et al. 2010). After a thorough review of the available data, the authors only managed to identify one such indicator for which data were available in a range of countries (12): unplanned hospital re-admissions for mental disorders, defined as the number of re-admissions per 100 patients with a diagnosis of schizophrenia or bipolar disorder (OECD 2011). However, no historical data are available and, therefore, progress over time cannot be defined.

The human rights perspective

A human rights perspective has been a key driver in service improvement for people with mental health problems (Jenkins et al. 2002). Three international human rights treaties have been particularly influential in this regard: the *Universal Declaration of Human Rights* (United Nations General Assembly 1948), the *International Covenant on Economic, Social and Cultural Rights* (United Nations General Assembly 1966a) and the *International Covenant on Civil and Political*

Box 10.1   Development of outcome indicators

The Netherlands

In the Netherlands, service providers, together with psychiatrist and psychologist associations, agreed in 2009 to introduce a nationally standardized system for 'routine outcome monitoring' (GGZ Nederland 2012). The declared objectives were to facilitate shared decision-making by clients and professionals; professional reflection within teams, departments and/or providers; (scientific) research at regional and national levels; transparency in respect of the relevance and effectiveness of treatments and guidelines; and transparency in respect of the effectiveness of providers and mental health care organizations at national level. From 2011 onwards, all providers have to gather data from at least 20% of their clients at the beginning and the end of their treatment. Annually, this number will increase to 50% in 2014. From 2014 onwards, more than 500,000 clients and 20,000 professionals should be using 'routine outcome monitoring' on a daily basis. If providers do not meet the agreed targets, the penalty (or fine) will be a budget cut of 1.5–3.0%. This is equivalent to €200 million nationwide. Providers and insurers established a 'trusted third party' to collect and analyse outcome data and to present reliable benchmarks to facilitate the purchasing process of insurers. The client organizations are part of the board, and the professional associations participate in the scientific council.

England

In England, the Health of the Nation Outcome Scale has been built into the new 'payment by results' regime as the main measure in mental health, which means that all service providers have to measure outcomes across a broad range of conditions. The Outcome Scale is included into the Mental Health Minimum Data Set, which was mandatory since 2003 and covers behaviour, function/impairment, symptoms and social items. Research into its psychometric properties showed that they have adequate or good validity, reliability, sensitivity to change and acceptability. However, its results are often not consistent with findings of user-rated instruments (Jacobs 2009) and providers are finding it difficult to operationalize the new scheme in practice as the symptom and treatment clusters may not be robust.

Rights (United Nations General Assembly 1966b). The following core rights, derived from these and other sources, have had a major impact on shaping mental health and related legislation in Europe: the right to liberty, freedom from torture and inhuman treatment; the right to privacy; and the right to non-discrimination. However, there is still a long way to go in some countries (Guterman and McKee 2012).

This framework has been built upon in the last 20 years with a number of global and European statements specifically about the human rights of people with mental health problems. Governments have tended to view adherence with these frameworks as a key indicator of their performance on mental health and of their ability to deliver patient satisfaction and well-being, although enforcement of basic human rights is only one step towards delivering effective mental health services. However, the human rights agenda is a very useful policy lever, and adherence to basic human rights is an important quality indicator for mental health services.

The remainder of this chapter will address two areas of mental health policy where some comparable data exist within Europe, prevention of suicide and anti-stigma programmes.

Suicide

Trends in suicide in Europe

In 2009, 120,447 Europeans committed suicide, 46,839 in high-income countries and 73,608 in low- and middle-income countries (WHO Regional Office for Europe 2012a). This equates to 330 suicides every single day, every one both avoidable and unnecessary. These premature deaths accounted for 2% of the total disease burden (Mathers et al. 2008). Until very recently, the story of suicide in Europe appeared to be one of qualified success (Fig. 10.2). Deaths

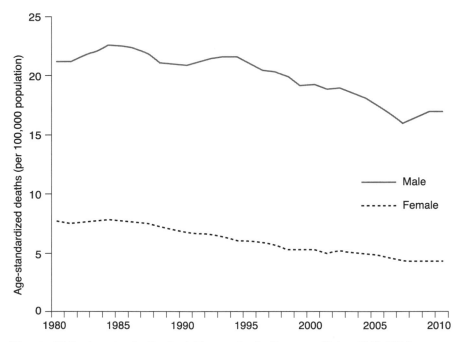

Figure 10.2 Age-standardized suicide rates in the European Union 1980–2010

Source: WHO Regional Office for Europe 2012b

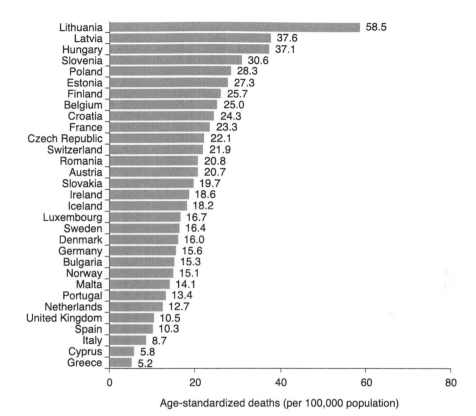

Figure 10.3   Age-standardized suicide rates, 2010 or nearest year

Source: WHO Regional Office for Europe 2012b

among men had fallen by 25% and among women by 43%. Unfortunately, these gains have not been sustained and, since 2008, the trends have reversed.

However, these figures combine data from 27 different countries, each with their own experience of suicide. For example, suicide rates vary more than ten-fold between Greece with the lowest rate (5.2 per 100,000 population) to Lithuania with the highest rate (58.5 per 100,000)(Fig. 10.3).

Trends have also varied considerably in recent decades (Fig. 10.4).

Before seeking to interpret these data, it is first necessary to assess their validity. In some societies, suicide is highly stigmatized. For example, church authorities, viewing suicide as a mortal sin, historically refused to bury suicide victims in consecrated grounds, potentially giving rise to reluctance by physicians to record suicide as the cause of death. As Durkheim and Buss (2006) originally noted, religious belief may influence the acceptability of suicide as a 'solution' to one's problems. More recent empirical research suggests that it is the degree of religious commitment that is important rather than the denominational affiliation (Stack and Lester 1991; Stack and Kposowa 2011).

Another factor that influences the validity of routinely registered suicide data is the amount of evidence required to designate a death as suicide. For example,

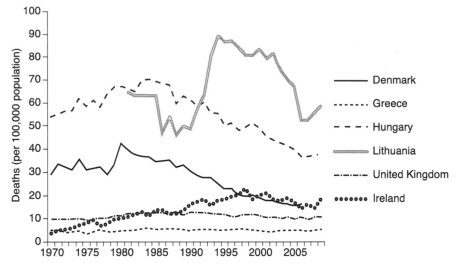

Figure 10.4 Trends in age-standardized suicide rates in selected countries

Source: WHO Regional Office for Europe 2012b

in Luxembourg, a suicide note is required while in the United Kingdom intent is determined by a legally qualified assessor (a coroner) (Chishti et al. 2003). Sensitivities or uncertainties about recording a death as suicide may be manifest in higher than expected use of the label 'death of undetermined cause'. Cross-national comparisons suggest that this may contribute to observed differences at a point in time and to observed trends over time. For example, the observed increase in suicides from the 1970s onward in Ireland (Fig. 10.4) was accompanied by a decline in deaths of undetermined cause. However, this could explain at most 46% of the change, indicating that at least part of the increase was real (Kelleher et al. 1997). A detailed analysis of rates in the EU-15 likewise concluded that some of the variation could result from differences in recording deaths of undetermined cause, but only a small proportion (Chishti et al. 2003).

A recent systematic review identified only few detailed evaluations of the reliability of suicide data (Tollefsen et al. 2012). This has led to other pragmatic approaches, such as the 2:20 rule, whereby countries are deemed to meet a quality benchmark for suicide data if they report fewer than 2.0 undetermined deaths per 100,000 population and if the proportion of undetermined deaths to suicides is 0.20 (Varnik et al. 2011). On this basis, the following countries satisfied the benchmark: Greece, Norway, Spain, the Netherlands, Luxembourg, France, Austria, Italy, Romania, Hungary, Ireland and Finland. Among the remaining countries, the Baltic states had particularly high death rates from undetermined causes, and Portugal, the United Kingdom, Slovakia and Poland had high ratios of undetermined causes to suicides. The remaining countries were just outside the benchmark. Consequently, caution is required in interpreting the data.

It is also important to understand some of the basic demographic features of suicide. As already noted, it is much more common in men than in women,

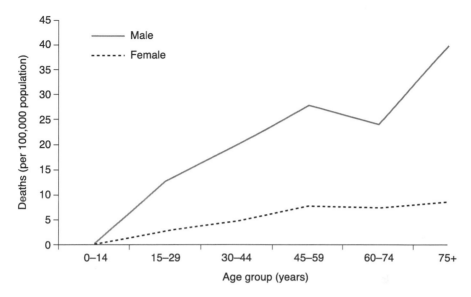

Figure 10.5   Suicide rates by age and sex in the European Union, 2010 or latest available year

and this is true at all ages (Fig. 10.5). Suicides also increase with age, particularly among men. Divorced and widowed men are about twice as likely to commit suicide as those who are married, but there is no difference by marital status among women (Kposowa 2000).

The act of suicide is influenced by factors acting at three levels, each of which gives rise to potential opportunities to intervene (Nordentoft 2007). These are, first, measures that promote resilience, thereby enabling individuals to deal better with crises that may afflict them. Second, there are measures that address specific risk factors and groups at risk of suicidal behaviour. Third, there are measures directly aimed at the process of suicide. This chapter will consider each in turn.

Promoting resilience

The recent upturn in suicides in some European countries, reversing a long-term downward trend, has coincided with a massive financial crisis in which unemployment in many countries has soared, in some cases to 25% of the population (and 50% of young people) (Stuckler et al. 2011). While it is too early to assess the precise association between the economy and suicide during the present crisis, largely because of the absence of timely mortality data from all countries, there are some important pointers from previous economic crises. A study of mortality trends in 30 western European countries between 1970 and 2007 found that every 1% increase in unemployment was associated with a 0.79% rise in suicides at ages younger than 65 years (Stuckler et al. 2009). This was consistent with findings from previous crises, such as the Great Depression in the 1920s and 1930s (Stuckler et al. 2012). However, the study of European countries also showed that this association was not inevitable. For example, suicide rates increased markedly in Spain in the recession in the late 1980s, falling back once recovery was underway. In contrast, in Sweden and Finland, which also experienced a major recession a few years later, suicide rates continued a long-term steady decline while unemployment rates rose. The researchers identified the presence of active labour market programmes in which governments invested in a range of activities designed to get people back into work, such as retraining and provision of information on vacancies, as a possible explanation. They calculated that expenditure (in 2003 terms) of US$ 190 per capita on such programmes could entirely decouple the observed association between unemployment and suicides.

Intervening with those at risk

Systematic reviews have identified the measures most likely to reduce suicides as training of general practitioners to recognize and treat depression and risk of suicide, and improving accessibility of care for those at risk, as well as reductions in access to the means of suicide (see below) (Mann et al. 2005; van der Feltz-Cornelis et al. 2011).

The role of antidepressant medication is less clear. Unlike a number of its neighbours in central Europe, Hungary has experienced a sustained decline in suicides for several decades, despite many adverse economic factors. The reasons are not known for certain, but it has been suggested that this reflects a large increase in the prescription of antidepressants (Rihmer 2009). In contrast, a study in Spain found no association between trends in antidepressant consumption and suicides (Arias et al. 2010). Research in the Nordic countries has been inconclusive. One study found some short-lived reductions in suicides around the time that selective serotonin reuptake inhibitors were being introduced, but, in general, the declines preceded their introduction (Reseland et al. 2006). A more recent study found no significant association with increased prescribing (Zahl et al. 2010). These findings are consistent with a 2007 systematic review concluding that there was limited but inconsistent evidence to support the hypothesis that increased prescribing of antidepressants reduced suicide risk at the population level (Baldessarini et al. 2007).

Intervening in the process of suicide

There is some evidence that suicides can be facilitated by greater ease of access to the means of killing oneself and can be prevented by making it more difficult to access these means (Sarchiapone et al. 2011). For example, the increased use of coal gas in England and Wales from the middle of the 19th century until the 1970s was associated with an increase in suicides using this means, with no corresponding decline from other means (Thomas and Gunnell 2010). A very specific example is the decision, made in the light of evidence that 84% of suicides by Israeli soldiers involved their personal weapons, to reduce access to these weapons at weekends. There was a subsequent 40% reduction in army suicides (Lubin et al. 2010). Danish research on the means of suicide in Denmark between 1970 and 2000 identified substantial declines in the use of those means that had become less accessible (Nordentoft et al. 2006). These included various drugs, such as barbiturates and certain analgesics, and carbon monoxide, because of the withdrawal of coal gas for domestic heating and the installation of catalytic converters in cars. The authors calculated that reduction in means of suicide was associated with a 55% reduction in overall suicides.

Other evidence is, however, less convincing. In 1998, the United Kingdom Government introduced regulations to limit the number of paracetamol tablets in a pack in an attempt to reduce deaths from intentional overdose. This was, in part, based on the observation that deaths from paracetamol poisoning were less common in France, where pack sizes were already limited (Chan 2000). The death rate from paracetamol poisoning did fall subsequently but at a similar rate to suicides using other drugs not covered by the regulations, and most researchers have concluded that it is not possible to discern any specific effect of this measure (Hawkins et al. 2007; Morgan et al. 2007). This conclusion is supported by a comparison of the United Kingdom and Ireland, where legislation requiring somewhat smaller pack sizes than in the United Kingdom was implemented in 2001 (Hawton et al. 2011). This found no difference in the amounts of paracetamol ingested, although in Ireland this required more packs. Similarly, research in the Nordic countries found no association between reductions in prescribing tricyclic antidepressants, which are potentially fatal in overdose, and suicide rates (Zahl et al. 2010), although earlier research in the United States had found a geographical association between prescribing tricyclic antidepressants and suicides in rural areas (Gibbons et al. 2005). However, a very recent study examined the impact of removing co-proxamol (paracetamol and dextropropoxyphene) from sale in England and Wales in 2005 (Hawton et al. 2012). This is a combination analgesic widely prescribed and implicated in large numbers of suicides. Over the following six years, suicides involving this substance fell by over 60%, with no corresponding increase in suicides using other analgesics.

Box 10.2 describes the measures taken to tackle suicide rates in England.

Anti-stigma and non-discrimination

Prevalence of stigma

Mental illness continues to be stigmatized in many societies, just as some physical diseases such as cancer once were. This can easily act as a barrier to successful treatment and rehabilitation if not tackled effectively.

Findings of a survey of 14 countries coordinated by a patient-driven pan-European organization (the GAMIAN-Europe study) showed that over 40% of the mental health service users with a diagnosis of schizophrenia or other psychotic disorder surveyed experienced moderate or high levels of self-stigma, and almost 70% moderate or high perceived discrimination (Brohan et al. 2010). Another European study among people with schizophrenia in 27 countries found that stigma and discrimination have a negative impact on

Box 10.2   Case study: Measures to tackle suicide rates in England

Suicide rates in the United Kingdom have long been below the EU average, although they did increase in the 1970s and 1980s among men, before falling in the 1990s and after 2000. However, rates in 2009 were still 6% higher than in 1970. Over the same period, suicide rates among women have decreased steadily since 1980 and are now less than 50% of what they were in 1970. Measures to reduce suicide have evolved over many years. Until the 1990s, the approach was piecemeal but there were many initiatives including the creation of a national befriending service (the Samaritans), run by a non-governmental organization. There was also evidence that reduced access to the means of suicide, albeit as a consequence of other policies, was effective, including the replacement of coal gas (containing carbon monoxide) by natural gas (methane) and the introduction of catalytic converters in cars.

During the 1980s and 1990s, a more strategic approach began to emerge combining the following features:

- public information
- training of general practitioners in suicide awareness
- reduction in access to the means of suicide
- focus on at-risk groups (e.g. farmers, young men, inpatients).

During this time, it became apparent from the international literature that training of general practitioners and reductions in access to the means of suicide were the most likely to yield results, coupled with outreach to young people (Gunnell and Frankel 1994; Mann et al. 2005).

In 1999, suicide prevention was made a key part of national mental health policy, set out in the National Service Framework for Mental Health (Department of Health 1999). It remains a priority in mental health policy (Department of Health 2011; HM Government 2011). The English anti-suicide strategy is broad based, embracing the following six key areas: (1) reduction of risk in high-risk groups; (2) tailored approaches to improve the mental health of such groups; (3) reduction in access to means; (4) providing better information and support to those bereaved by suicide; (5) working with the media; and (6) supporting research, data collection and monitoring.

Particular areas where progress has been noted include:

- significant reductions in suicide rates in inpatient units and prisons by reducing means of suicide and by education of staff
- reductions in suicide by young men (although now threatened by the economic crisis)
- physician education (e.g. the Royal College of Psychiatrists' Defeat Depression campaign and subsequent work)
- work on suicide clusters, media guidelines, etc.

However, there remain areas that require further attention, including the mental health and support needs of older men.

both private life (making or keeping friends, intimate or sexual relationships) and social integration (finding and keeping a job; applying for work, training or education) of these service users, and as many as 70% of them reported that they felt the need to conceal their diagnosis (Thornicroft et al. 2009; Ucok et al. 2012).

Besides self-reported experiences of stigma, an indirect indicator of stigma and social distance is given by public attitudes towards people with mental health problems. Findings of the 2010 *Eurobarometer 345: Mental Health* showed that a substantial proportion of European citizens would find it hard just to talk to people with significant mental health problems (European Commission 2010). Interestingly, there is a strong statistical correlation ($r = 0.59$) between these attitudes and the suicide rates among men in these countries (Fig. 10.6).

What works

There are strong theoretical reasons to suggest that national commitment to tackle stigma is a necessary backdrop to allow other initiatives to flourish. Stigma has a major negative impact on the realization of mental health policy both by discouraging access to effective services, limiting their development,

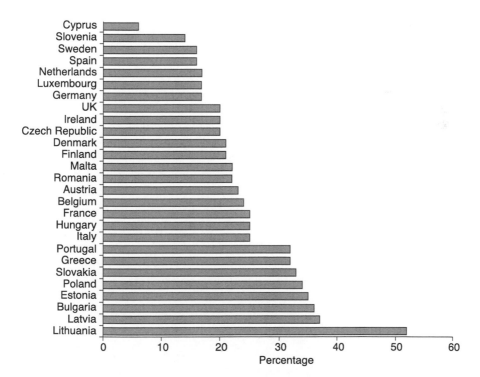

Figure 10.6   Proportion of people who would find it difficult talking to someone with significant mental health problems

Source: European Commission 2010

and by preventing recovery. Many service users report that the impact of stigma is worse than the direct psychiatric symptoms (Thornicroft 2006). Yet there is even less research to guide policies to reduce stigma than there is to reduce suicides.

At the same time, there is evidence that specific interventions can work, such as experiential training or exposure to people with mental illness and interventions with specific populations. The existing research shows that three main methods of anti-stigma intervention are most often considered to be effective: protest, contact and education (Corrigan and Penn 1999; Corrigan et al. 2001; Penn and Corrigan 2002; Corrigan and Gelb 2006; Mental Health Foundation 2012). A comprehensive and sustained approach is likely to be most effective, although gains cannot yet be quantified. However, theoretical and practical arguments are clear.

Current status of implementation across European countries

Most European countries (83%) report that they have implemented some programmes and/or activities to tackle stigma and discrimination against people with mental health problems (WHO Regional Office for Europe 2008). They vary from international programmes (e.g. the World Psychiatric Association *Schizophrenia: Open the Doors* anti-stigma programme) to national campaigns and local initiatives. However, few of these initiatives have been evaluated, so their outcomes are often unclear.

Outcomes of policies and programmes

There are different ways of assessing outcomes of anti-stigma policies and programmes: evaluations of anti-stigma campaigns, self-reported experiences of stigma from cross-sectional surveys of patients and surveys of public opinion regarding attitudes to people with mental illness. Data are limited to those countries that have actively pursued specific interventions and programmes in this area. Box 10.3 presents two such campaigns, in Germany and in Scotland. Figure 10.7 illustrates survey results of attitudes to mental health problems in Scotland.

In conclusion, as these findings show, there is still a long way to go in reducing the stigma associated with mental illness in Europe and a continued failure to do so is likely to be a barrier to effective treatment and rehabilitation of those affected.

Discussion and conclusions

Mental health services in transition

Countries differ in the way in which policy-makers undertake the development and implementation of policy. This is because countries have dissimilar

Box 10.3   Outcomes of anti-stigma programmes in two countries

---

Germany

The World Psychiatric Association global programme to reduce stigma and discrimination because of schizophrenia, *Schizophrenia: Open the Doors* (Sartorius 1997), was implemented in six German cities between 2001 and 2004 and aimed to 'improve knowledge, attitudes and behaviour, in the general public and specific target groups, increase social acceptance of people with schizophrenia and their families, and improve the course of illness and quality of life for people suffering from schizophrenia' (p. 16). The programme was evaluated using pre- and post-implementation surveys. The evaluation showed that the impact of the programme on the general population was positive – that is, there was a significant decrease in social distance in relation to people with schizophrenia – but the authors noted that improvements were small. The evaluation covered an awareness programme aimed at raising the early recognition, stereotypes, attitudes and beliefs related to people with schizophrenia (Baumann et al. 2007).

Scotland

The *See me* anti-stigma campaign in Scotland (Davidson et al. 2009; Myers et al. 2009) had five core objectives:

- to tackle stigma and discrimination by raising public awareness of how both affect individuals with mental health problems, and by improving the public understanding of mental health
- to challenge individual incidents of stigma and discrimination
- to involve people in anti-stigma activities across Scotland at national and local levels and across sectors and communities of interest
- to ensure that the voices and experiences of people with mental health problems and their carers are heard
- to promote a culture of learning and evaluation through all its work, so that effectiveness can be demonstrated and lessons shared.

The evaluation, carried out four years into the implementation of the campaign, used qualitative and quantitative research methods and approached both the general population and specific target groups (e.g. young people). It found that 'see me' was a 'ground breaking campaign', particularly successful in stimulating a wide range of connected activities. It also led to tangible changes in media reporting of mental illness, making it 'increasingly unacceptable to use derogative terms or negative story lines'. However, the changes in public perceptions, although in the desired direction, were quite limited (Davidson et al. 2009; Myers et al. 2009) (see Fig. 10.7).

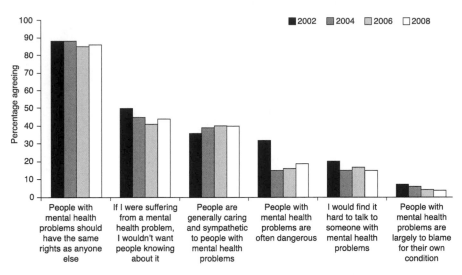

Figure 10.7 Attitudes to mental health problems in Scotland 2002–2008

Source: Davidson et al. 2009

governing cultures and, from country to country, policy-makers develop policies with quite different mind-sets and expectations for their implementation and accountability. National mental health policies have had a decidedly stronger impact in countries where adoption of policy documents results in unambiguous expectations that commitments will be made and that the targets and milestones that have been set will be met (e.g. the United Kingdom's *National Service Framework for Mental Health*; Department of Health 1999). An additional precondition for the success of national policies is that decision-makers and relevant stakeholders are held accountable for the progress achieved during the time frame set for the implementation of that policy.

In countries from western and northern Europe, the transformation of mental health services has occurred in part because of the new therapeutic options becoming available (Cowen 1996; Owens 1996) and the emergence of critiques of traditional psychiatric practice (Szasz 2001), but also because the magnitude of the problem and its major economic implications became apparent at this time, leading to an acute need for solutions. However, the shift towards 'not just bricks and mortar' (Burns et al. 1998) took time, while policy-makers often underestimated the need for support required by the people who previously lived in asylums, particularly those who were severely disabled.

In 1977, a working group appointed by the WHO Regional Office for Europe (1978), with experts from nine countries from across the European Region, stated that the main constraints to development of mental health services (some of which are still valid today) included lack of adequate information about the size and the nature of mental health problems and resources available to cope with them; lack of national mental health policy; unavailability and inaccessibility of services; inadequacy of staffing; lack of financial resources; ineffective coordination and administration of resources; outdated and inappropriate legislation; lack of relevant research; lay and professional bias against people with a mental illness (i.e. stigma and discrimination); resistance to change; and lack of political will. It is, however, the presence of bias, prejudice, fear and ignorance among the public, mental health professionals and decision-makers, that has been identified as the root cause of inertia and even resistance to provision of adequate mental health services. This leads to low levels of investment in mental health, which constrains progress. The report concluded that the 'greatest impediment to progress lay in the minds of men rather than in their pockets and purses'. At the same time, moving to provision of community-based services is dependent on investments in mental health, as demonstrated by the correlation between mental health budgets as a proportion of the total health budget and the availability of community-based services.

In many countries from the former communist bloc in central eastern and south-eastern Europe, the recent adoption of mental health policies and practices nationally was rarely rooted in local processes, and consequently achieved insufficient ownership from key stakeholders and decision-makers. These policies were adopted primarily as a response to international pressures and, at the same time, as a means of formally satisfying vocal requests for action from national champions, even if there was no intention to pursue their implementation. Significant progress was generally achieved only when political commitment increased, stimulated by international pressure in response to reports of human rights violations, as well as by international funding for implementation of reforms, political support and the potential for inclusion in different 'clubs' of countries (e.g. the EU). Further on, where financial investments were made, they led to improvements in mental health facilities, to improved infrastructure in mental hospitals and the setting up of pilot community services. However, 'mainstreaming' community services is vulnerable to a failure to engage psychiatrists and managers of existing services in the process of change. Setting up isolated pilot initiatives on the outskirts of the mental health system, driven by foreign donors and isolated national experts, while motivated by a genuine desire to induce change, has proved to be relatively ineffective. While some engagement from professionals in these initiatives is often achieved through training, career or income opportunities, they can often remain 'orphan' initiatives if there is no clear strategic context or mechanism for taking them to scale.

Conclusions

The data presented in this chapter show the difficulties in measuring progress in terms of health outcomes for people with mental health problems. Investments in mental health remain low, disproportionately so given the burden of disease posed by mental health problems. Fundamentally, this reflects the stigma and lack of hope and expectations surrounding mental ill health. We can, however, draw some conclusions from the limited available evidence.

Rates of suicide have fallen across Europe, in some cases substantially, and while there are many concerns about the quality of the data, the observed changes are, to some extent, likely to be real. However, the reasons for these declines are not fully understood. There is some evidence that countries that provide greater support at times of hardship, specifically active labour market programmes, are able to decouple the adverse effects of unemployment on suicide. There is also some evidence that reduction in access to the means of suicide has played a role in some countries, although it is difficult to make linkages to specific policies. There are, however, worrying signs that suicides are increasing in many parts of Europe at a time when governments are imposing severe austerity regimes.

The stigma associated with mental illness remains a barrier to effective treatment and rehabilitation. The observed association between perceived stigma and suicide rates deserves further investigation. Unfortunately, only a few countries seem to be addressing the stigma associated with mental illness explicitly, and even those that have done so have achieved quite limited results.

Above all, this chapter has highlighted the weak research base on which to develop effective policies on mental health in Europe. Although, over several decades, things have improved, at least in terms of the most severe outcome, suicide, it is still not entirely clear how this was achieved.

References

Alonso, J., Angermeyer, M.C., Bernert, S. et al. (2004a) Prevalence of mental disorders in Europe: results from the European Study of the Epidemiology of Mental Disorders (ESEMeD) project, *Acta Psychiatrica Scandinavica Supplement* 420:21–7.

Alonso, J., Angermeyer, M.C., Bernert, S. et al. (2004b) Use of mental health services in Europe: results from the European Study of the Epidemiology of Mental Disorders (ESEMeD) project, *Acta Psychiatrica Scandinavica Supplement* 420:47–54.

Arias, L.H., Lobato, C.T., Ortega, S. et al. (2010) Trends in the consumption of antidepressants in Castilla y Leon (Spain). Association between suicide rates and antidepressant drug consumption, *Pharmacoepidemiology and Drug Safety*, 19(9):895–900.

Baldessarini, R.J., Tondo, L., Strombom, I.M. et al. (2007) Ecological studies of antidepressant treatment and suicidal risks, *Harvard Review of Psychiatry*, 15(4):133–45.

Baumann, A., Zaske, H., Decker, P. et al. (2007) [Changes in the public's social distance toward individuals with schizophrenia in six German cities. Results of representative pre- and postinterventional telephone surveys from 2001 to 2004] *Nervenarzt*, 78(7):787–8, 790–5.

Brohan, E., Elgie, R., Sartorius, N. and Thornicroft, G. (2010) Self-stigma, empowerment and perceived discrimination among people with schizophrenia in 14 European countries: the GAMIAN–Europe study, *Schizophrenia Research*, 122(1–3):232–8.

Burns, T., Gargan, L., Walker, L. et al. (1998) Not just bricks and mortar: report of the Royal College of Psychiatrists Working Party on the size, staffing, structure, siting, and security of new acute adult psychiatric in-patient units, *Psychiatric Bulletin*, 22:465–6.

Chan, T.Y. (2000) Improvements in the packaging of drugs and chemicals may reduce the likelihood of severe intentional poisonings in adults, *Human Experimental Toxicology*, 19(7):387–91.

Chishti, P., Stone, D.H., Corcoran, P., Williamson, E. and Petridou, E. (2003) Suicide mortality in the European Union, *European Journal of Public Health*, 13(2):108–14.

Corrigan, P. and Gelb, B. (2006) Three programs that use mass approaches to challenge the stigma of mental illness, *Psychiatr Services*, 57(3):393–8.

Corrigan, P.W. and Penn, D.L. (1999) Lessons from social psychology on discrediting psychiatric stigma, *American Psychologist*, 54(9):765–76.

Corrigan, P.W., River, L.P., Lundin, R.K. et al. (2001) Three strategies for changing attributions about severe mental illness, *Schizophrenia Bulletin*, 27(2):187–95.

Cowen, P.J. (1996) Advances in psychopharmacology: mood disorders and dementia, *British Medical Bulletin*, 52(3):539–55.

Davidson, S., Sewel, K., Tse, D., Mori, I. and O'Connor, R. (2009) *Well? What Do You Think? 2008: The Fourth National Scottish Survey of Public Attitudes to Mental Wellbeing and Mental Health Problems*. Edinburgh: Scottish Government Social Research.

Department of Health (1999) *National Service Framework for Mental Health*. London: The Stationery Office.

Department of Health (2011) *No Health Without Mental Health*. London: The Stationery Office.

Durkheim, E. and Buss, R. (2006) *On Suicide*. London: Penguin.

European Commission (2010) *Special Eurobarometer 345: Mental Health*. Brussels: European Commission.

van der Feltz-Cornelis, C.M., Sarchiapone, M., Postuvan, V. et al. (2011) Best practice elements of multilevel suicide prevention strategies: a review of systematic reviews, *Crisis*, 32(6):319–33.

GGZ Nederland (2012) *Routine Outcome Monitoring in Dutch Mental Healthcare*. Amersfoort: GGZ Nederland.

Gibbons, R.D., Hur, K., Bhaumik, D.K. and Mann, J.J. (2005) The relationship between antidepressant medication use and rate of suicide, *Archives of General Psychiatry*, 62(2):165–72.

Gunnell, D. and Frankel, S. (1994) Prevention of suicide: aspirations and evidence, *British Medical Journal*, 308(6938):1227–33.

Guterman, L. and McKee, M. (2012) Severe human rights abuses in healthcare settings, *British Medical Journal*, 344:e2013.

Hawkins, L.C., Edwards, J.N. and Dargan, P.I. (2007) Impact of restricting paracetamol pack sizes on paracetamol poisoning in the United Kingdom: a review of the literature, *Drug Safety*, 30(6):465–79.

Hawton, K., Bergen, H., Simkin, S. et al. (2011) Impact of different pack sizes of paracetamol in the United Kingdom and Ireland on intentional overdoses: a comparative study, *BMC Public Health*, 11:460.

Hawton, K., Bergen, H., Simkin, S. et al. (2012) Six-year follow-up of impact of co-proxamol withdrawal in England and Wales on prescribing and deaths: time-series study, PLoS *Medicine*, 9(5):e1001213.

HM Government (2011) *Consultation on Preventing Suicide in England*. London: The Stationery Office.

Jacobs, R. (2009) *Investigating Patient Outcome Measures in Mental Health*. York: Centre for Health Economics, University of York.

Jenkins, R., McCulloch, A., Friedli, L. and Parker, C. (2002) *Developing a National Mental Health Policy*. [Maudsley Monograph.] London: Psychology Press.

Kelleher, M.J., Keeley, H.S. and Corcoran, P. (1997) The service implications of regional differences in suicide rates in the Republic of Ireland, *Irish Medical Journal*, 90(7):262–4.

Keyes, C.L. (2005) Mental illness and/or mental health? Investigating axioms of the complete state model of health, *Journal of Consulting and Clinical Psychology*, 73(3):539–48.

Kposowa, A.J. (2000) Marital status and suicide in the National Longitudinal Mortality Study, *Journal of Epidemiology and Community Health*, 54(4):254–61.

Lavikainen, J., Fryers, T. and Lehtinen, V. (2006) *Improving Mental Health Information in Europe*. Helsinki: Stakes and European Union.

Lopez, A.D. (2006) *Global Burden of Disease and Risk Factors*. New York: Oxford University Press for the World Bank.

Lubin, G., Werbeloff, N., Halperin, D. et al. (2010) Decrease in suicide rates after a change of policy reducing access to firearms in adolescents: a naturalistic epidemiological study, *Suicide and Life Threatening Behavior*, 40(5):421–4.

Mann, J.J., Apter, A., Bertolote, J. et al. (2005) Suicide prevention strategies: a systematic review, *Journal of the American Medical Association*, 294(16):2064–74.

Mathers, C., Boerma, T. and Fat, D.M. (2008) *The Global Burden of Disease 2004 Update*. Geneva: World Health Organization.

Mattke, S., Epstein, A.M. and Leatherman, S. (2006) The OECD Health Care Quality Indicators Project: history and background, *International Journal of Quality of Health Care*, 18(suppl 1):1–4.

McCulloch, A. (2006) Understanding mental health and mental illness, in C. Jackson and K. Hill (eds) *Mental Health Today: A Handbook*. Brighton: Pavilion.

McCulloch, A. and Muijen, M. (2011) Mental health, in K. Walshe and J. Smith (eds) *Health Care Management*. Maidenhead: McGraw-Hill, pp. 235–56.

McGrath, J., Saha, S., Chant, D. and Welham, J. (2008) Schizophrenia: a concise overview of incidence, prevalence, and mortality, *Epidemiology Reviews*, 30:67–76.

Mental Health Foundation (2012) *Reducing Stigma. A Policy Brief on Stigma and Discrimination for States of Guernsey*. London: Mental Health Foundation.

Morgan, O.W., Griffiths, C. and Majeed, A. (2007) Interrupted time-series analysis of regulations to reduce paracetamol (acetaminophen) poisoning, PLoS *Medicine*, 4(4):e105.

Muijen, M. and McCulloch, A. (2009) Public policy and mental health, in M. Gelder, N. Andreasen, J. Lopez-Ibor and J. Geddes (eds) *New Oxford Textbook of Psychiatry*. Oxford: Oxford University Press, pp. 1425–502.

Myers, F., Woodhouse, A., Whitehead, I. et al. (2009) *Evaluation of 'see me': the National Scottish Campaign Against the Stigma and Discrimination Associated with Mental Ill-Health*. Edinburgh: Scottish Government Social Research.

Nordentoft, M. (2007) Prevention of suicide and attempted suicide in Denmark. Epidemiological studies of suicide and intervention studies in selected risk groups, *Danish Medical Bulletin*, 54(4):306–69.

Nordentoft, M., Qin, P., Helweg-Larsen, K. and Juel, K. (2006) Time-trends in method-specific suicide rates compared with the availability of specific compounds. The Danish experience, *Nordic Journal of Psychiatry*, 60(2):97–106.

OECD (2011) *Health at a Glance 2011: OECD Indicators*. Paris: Organisation for Economic Co-operation and Development.

Owens, D.G. (1996) Advances in psychopharmacology: schizophrenia, *British Medical Bulletin*, 52(3):556–74.

Penn, D.L. and Corrigan, P.W. (2002) The effects of stereotype suppression on psychiatric stigma, *Schizophrenia Research*, 55(3):269–76.

Pincus, H.A. and Naber, D. (2009) International efforts to measure and improve the quality of mental healthcare, *Current Opinion in Psychiatry*, 22(6):609.

Reseland, S., Bray, I. and Gunnell, D. (2006) Relationship between antidepressant sales and secular trends in suicide rates in the Nordic countries, *British Journal of Psychiatry*, 188:354–8.

Rihmer, Z. (2009) Suicide, what policy can do about it, in *Thematic Conference under the European Pact for Mental Health and Well-being: Prevention of Depression and Suicide – Making it Happen*, Budapest.

Sarchiapone, M., Mandelli, L., Iosue, M., Andrisano, C. and Roy, A. (2011) Controlling access to suicide means, *International Journal of Environmental Research and Public Health*, 8(12):4550–62.

Sartorius, N. (1997) Fighting schizophrenia and its stigma: a new World Psychiatric Association educational program, *British Journal of Psychiatry*, 170:297.

Spaeth-Rublee, B., Pincus, H.A. and Huynh, P.T. (2010) Measuring quality of mental health care: a review of initiatives and programs in selected countries, *Canadian Journal of Psychiatry*, 55(9):539–48.

Stack, S. and Kposowa, A.J. (2011) Religion and suicide acceptability: a cross-national analysis, *Journal of Scientific Study and Religion*, 50(2):289–306.

Stack, S. and Lester, D. (1991) The effect of religion on suicide ideation, *Social Psychiatry and Psychiatric Epidemiology*, 26(4):168–70.

Stuckler, D., Basu, S., Suhrcke, M., Coutts, A. and McKee, M. (2009) The public health effect of economic crises and alternative policy responses in Europe: an empirical analysis, *Lancet*, 374(9686):315–23.

Stuckler, D., Basu, S., Suhrcke, M., Coutts, A. and McKee, M. (2011) Effects of the 2008 recession on health: a first look at European data, *Lancet*, 378(9786):124–5.

Stuckler, D., Meissner, C., Fishback, P., Basu, S. and McKee, M. (2012) Banking crises and mortality during the Great Depression: evidence from US urban populations, 1929–1937, *Journal of Epidemiology and Community Health*, 66(5):410–19.

Szasz, T. (2001) Mental illness: psychiatry's phlogiston, *Journal of Medical Ethics*, 27(5):297–301.

Thomas, K. and Gunnell, D. (2010) Suicide in England and Wales 1861–2007: a time-trends analysis, *International Journal of Epidemiology*, 39(6):1464–75.

Thornicroft, G. (2006) *Actions Speak Louder: Tackling Discrimination Against People with Mental Illness*. London: Mental Health Foundation.

Thornicroft, G., Brohan, E., Rose, D., Sartorius, N. and Leese, M. (2009) Global pattern of experienced and anticipated discrimination against people with schizophrenia: a cross-sectional survey, *Lancet*, 373(9661):408–15.

Tollefsen, I.M., Hem, E. and Ekeberg, O. (2012) The reliability of suicide statistics: a systematic review, *BMC Psychiatry*, 12(1):9.

Ucok, A., Brohan, E., Rose, D. et al. (2012) Anticipated discrimination among people with schizophrenia, *Acta Psychiatrica Scandinavica*, 125(1):77–83.

United Nations General Assembly (1948) *Universal Declaration of Human Rights*. [Resolution 217 A (III).] New York: United Nations.

United Nations General Assembly (1966b) *International Covenant on Civil and Political Rights*. [Resolution 2200A (XXI).] New York: United Nations.

United Nations General Assembly (1966a) *International Covenant on Economic, Social and Cultural Rights*. [Resolution 2200A (XXI).] New York: United Nations.

Varnik, P., Sisask, M., Varnik, A. et al. (2011) Validity of suicide statistics in Europe in relation to undetermined deaths: developing the 2–20 benchmark. *Injury Prevention*, Epub before print (doi:10.1136/injuryprev-2011-040070).

WHO Regional Office for Europe (1978) *Constraints in Mental Health Services Development*. [Report on a Working Group, Cork, 28 June – 1 July 1977.] Copenhagen: WHO Regional Office for Europe.

WHO Regional Office for Europe (2008) *Policies and Practices for Mental Health in Europe*. Copenhagen: WHO Regional Office for Europe.

WHO Regional Office for Europe (2012a) *European Mortality Database*. Copenhagen: WHO Regional Office for Europe, http://data.euro.who.int/hfamdb/ (accessed 10 July 2012).

WHO Regional Office for Europe (2012b) *European Health for All Database (HFA-DB)*. Copenhagen: WHO Regional Office for Europe, http://data.euro.who.int/hfadb/ (accessed 4 June 2012).

Wittchen, H.U., Jacobi, F., Rehm, J. et al. (2011) The size and burden of mental disorders and other disorders of the brain in Europe 2010, *European Neuropsychopharmacology*, 21(9):655–79.

Zahl, P.H., De Leo, D., Ekeberg, O., Hjelmeland, H. and Dieserud, G. (2010) The relationship between sales of SSRI, TCA and suicide rates in the Nordic countries, *BMC Psychiatry*, 10:62.

chapter eleven

Road traffic injuries

Dinesh Sethi and Francesco Mitis

Introduction

Burden of disease

In 2008, there were 120,000 road traffic fatalities and 2.4 million non-fatal injuries in the 53 countries of the WHO European Region (WHO Regional Office for Europe 2009). Road Traffic Injuries (RTIs) are the leading cause of death in young people aged 5–29 years and are concentrated among males, who account for 80% of deaths. Societal losses are substantial, and estimates suggest that these amount to between 1 and 3% of a country's GDP (Sethi 2007).

Within Europe, however, there are large variations in the burden of disease from RTIs. In low- and middle-income countries, RTI mortality rates are twice as high as in high-income countries (18.7 versus 7.9 deaths per 100,000 population); consequently, 80% of RTI deaths occur in low- and middle-income countries (WHO Regional Office for Europe 2009). While in Europe as a whole 53% of RTI deaths occur among occupants of motorized four-wheelers (mainly cars) and 39% among vulnerable road users (with pedestrians (28%) as the largest group), the proportion of pedestrians is much higher in the CIS (37%). Road safety policies, therefore, should take into account the needs of vulnerable road users and not just the needs of motorized four-wheelers (OECD 1998; Ameratunga et al. 2006). Similarly there are large inequalities in RTI mortality rates between socioeconomic groups; for example, child pedestrian and cyclist deaths are considerably higher among the more deprived than among the better off (Roberts and Power 1996; Edwards et al. 2006).

Progress in road safety

Many high-income countries in Europe, such as the Nordic countries, the United Kingdom and the Netherlands, have achieved improved levels of safety through the development and sustained implementation of road safety policies and programmes. These interventions involve a combination of legislation, regulation, enforcement, engineering and education. Substantial improvements in mortality and morbidity have been achieved mainly by reducing the severity of crashes, rather than the number of crashes, through safer road behaviour and improvements in the design and safety of vehicles, equipment and road environments (Racioppi 2004). In contrast, many low- and middle-income countries have not yet achieved comparable levels of road safety because of weak or very recent policy development and implementation. Improvements in road infrastructure and vehicle safety, regulatory practices and modification of driver behaviour have not kept pace with the rapid motorization and urbanization in these countries (McKee et al. 2000; Peden 2004; Racioppi 2004; Sethi 2006).

This chapter will examine successful and less successful road safety policies in European countries, starting with a short review of the evidence for the effectiveness of specific policies.

Effectiveness of road traffic safety policies

A *public health approach to road safety*

A World Health Assembly resolution on *Road Safety and Health* called on WHO Member States to include RTI prevention in their public health plans and to implement evidence-based actions as outlined in the *World Report on Road Traffic Injury Prevention* (Peden 2004). At the level of the EU, the European Commission developed a *Road Safety Action Programme* in 2003, which called on EU Member States to develop road safety plans with targets to halve RTI fatalities by 2010 compared with 2000 figures (European Commission 2003). These international policies have all emphasized the need for greater commitment and multisectoral action by governments.

The *World Report on Road Traffic Injury Prevention* (Peden 2004) and the accompanying WHO European Region report (Racioppi 2004) emphasized a public health approach to RTI prevention. One of the fundamental principles of this approach is that, while crashes cannot be entirely prevented, the severity of crashes can be minimized in order to reduce the severity of injuries and fatalities. Other elements of this approach include the following.

- There is a well-established and growing evidence base for interventions that have been identified as effective and that should be implemented in countries throughout Europe.
- There are a large number of risk factors and exposures that road safety policies and plans need to tackle. These require uniquely different approaches based upon the local contexts and priorities. Road safety policies, consequently, have to consist of several programmes, which may be implemented concurrently to tackle the different risks.
- The traffic environment is a complex one and caters for a large variety of road users, ranging from occupants of lorries, buses and cars to more vulnerable road users such as motorized two-wheelers, cyclists and pedestrians. Exposure

to different risks will vary with geography, motor car ownership, private car usage, and so on.

- Transport and fiscal policy and the availability of efficient public transport alternatives will influence motor car usage and are, therefore, a potential target for policies to reduce RTIs. Measures such as congestion charges, user fees and taxation may discourage car use, thereby reducing exposure.
- Road safety policies and legislative changes to mitigate risks require proper enforcement if these are to succeed and will be unsuccessful if inadequately implemented. The same policies may result in very different outcomes if not properly implemented and enforced.
- The prevention of RTIs requires multisectoral action and a central coordinating body for road safety, with political support and resources necessary for it to succeed. In those countries where there is a lack of political will to implement policies or where governance structures are not in place or weak, then road safety policies will be less likely to succeed.

The *World Report on Road Traffic Injury Prevention* identified the following factors as key areas for preventive intervention (Peden 2004):

- controlling speed
- stopping driving when under the influence of alcohol
- enforcing use of safety equipment such as motorcycle and cycle helmets and seat-belts
- increasing conspicuousness
- improving vehicle crash protection
- making infrastructural changes to road design to ensure that speed is controlled and that vulnerable road users are not exposed to unnecessary risk by mixing them with motorized traffic.

Both the *World Report on Road Traffic Injury Prevention* (Peden 2004) and the accompanying WHO European Region Report (Racioppi 2004) have usefully synthesized the evidence on the effectiveness of various programmes for prevention.

The evidence base

Speed is a major risk factor for all road users, increasing the likelihood of death or serious injury. Vulnerable road users, such as pedestrians, are more at risk from speeding vehicles; pedestrians have a 50% chance of surviving if hit by vehicles travelling at speeds of 45 km/h but this rises to 90% at speeds of 30 km/h (Pasanen 1991). Nearly half the deaths on the roads in children under 15 years are as pedestrians (Peden 2004). Legislative measures are considered comprehensive if the urban speed limit is less than or equal to 50 km/h and if local authorities are allowed to reduce speed limits to adapt these to local conditions (WHO Regional Office for Europe 2009). Various strategies for reducing speed exist, ranging from reducing speed limits to less than 30 km/h near schools and residential areas, reducing speed limits on hazardous roads, enhanced enforcement with radar detectors, electronic signs providing feedback on speeds and using speed cameras. Existing research consistently shows that speed cameras are an effective intervention in reducing road traffic collisions and related casualties (DiGuiseppi et al. 1998). Other approaches include area-wide traffic calming measures (Bunn et al. 2003). As in other fields of public health, structural measures such as these are more effective than relying on education of drivers or pedestrians (Duperrex et al. 2002). Road function, traffic composition, types of road user and road design all need to be considered when determining speed limits (Peden 2004; Sethi et al. 2007). Speed control also has positive impacts on other consequences of road transport by virtue of reduced congestion, air pollution and noise.

Consuming alcohol before driving increases the risk of a crash as well as the likelihood that death or serious injury will result. In the EU, it is estimated that driving while under the influence of alcohol contributes annually to at least 10,000 deaths and is implicated in 30–40% of driver deaths (European Transport Safety Council 2003). There is a strong evidence base for effective interventions (Anderson 2009). Passing a drinking and driving law and enforcing it can reduce the number of road deaths by around 20% (Peden 2004; World Health Organization 2007a). Random breath testing is the primary drinking and driving law enforcement tool and is thought to be most effective. With random breath testing, the police can stop and perform a breath test on a driver at any time, irrespective of their driving behaviour. The combination of highly visible sites to conduct sobriety testing with media campaigns that support enforcement is most effective. Evaluation of random breath testing has shown long-term reductions in alcohol-related crashes. The recommended safe upper limit for blood alcohol concentration of 0.5 g/l has been taken up by most countries (exceptions are the United Kingdom and Malta, which have 0.8 g/l and CIS countries which have 0.0 g/l); a special blood alcohol maximum of 0.2 g/l for young and novice drivers has been taken up by fewer countries. It is most often the young inexperienced drivers who are most likely to be affected harmfully by drinking and who pose the main danger, rather than those who are chronic abusers. One of the key measures in combating drink driving is the implementation of police enforcement measures and increasing drivers' perception of the risk of being detected for excess alcohol (Peden 2004; Goss et al. 2008; Anderson 2009).

Safety equipment, such as helmets and seat-belts, are also highly effective. Research has shown that correctly wearing a motorcycle helmet can cut the risk of death by 40% and reduce the risk of serious head injuries by 70% (World Health Organization 2006; Liu et al. 2008). Wearing a cycle helmet is known to be protective in reducing the severity of head injury (Thompson et al. 2000). Research has shown that legislation increases cycle helmet wearing and that this is associated with a decrease in head injuries (Karkhaneh et al. 2006). However, there is some unresolved controversy about making the wearing of cycle helmets compulsory because of concerns that it will reduce the amount of cycling, and thus physical activity (Rissel and Wen 2011). Wearing a seat-belt reduces the risk of being ejected from a vehicle and suffering serious or fatal injury by 40–50% among front seat passengers and by 25–75% among rear-seat occupants (Elvik and Vaa 2004; WHO Regional Office for Europe 2009). Successful policies are those that have involved both social marketing campaigns and stringent enforcement, with high fines.

Improved conspicuousness and visibility through the use of street lighting is of some benefit in preventing road traffic crashes (Beyer and Ker 2009). Drivers of motorcycles wearing reflective clothing have a 37% reduced risk of crash-related injuries and those using daytime headlights have a 27% reduced risk. Reductions in RTIs have also been attributed to the use of compulsory daytime lights for motor vehicles and motorized two-wheelers (Elvik and Vaa 2004). The wearing of reflective strips and walking in well-lit streets facing traffic improves detection by drivers (Kwan and Mapstone 2006).

Infrastructural measures can also be highly effective. For example, motor-ways are much safer than conventional two-lane roads. Detailed studies using geographical data have shown how vehicle crashes are concentrated in places where the road infrastructure is unsafe (Flahaut 2004). Speed control can be effectively achieved by area-wide traffic calming. Measures such as speed bumps, 30 km/h zones and road closures have been shown to reduce traffic speed and RTIs. In London, this achieved a reduction in speeds by an average of 15 km/h and a reduction of serious or fatal RTIs by 53% (Webster and Layfield 2003). Roundabouts are one way of slowing traffic flows and are more effective in reducing the severity of crashes than ordinary junctions and stop signs. Marked cycle lanes, school crossing patrols and safe routes to schools all show varying degrees of efficacy. One study of roads in England and Wales found that, after adjusting for other factors, areas with more curves on roads had lower rates of crashes than those where more roads were straight, possibly because drivers paid less attention on the latter (Haynes et al. 2007). There is also some evidence that the layout of urban areas may influence rates of crashes, with the 'loops and lollipops' model, characterized by sweeping loops and cul-de-sacs, used in many residential areas since the 1970s being safer than the traditional gridiron or parallel models of the past (Rifaat et al. 2010). Road design and environmental adaptation, therefore, has a critical role to play in modifying speed and in protecting vulnerable road users by ensuring that they are protected by limiting their exposure to traffic of high kinetic energy (Roberts et al. 1995; OECD 1998; Sonkin et al. 2006). However, this is an area that has been the subject of relatively little research, leaving the authors of a Cochrane review to conclude that the evidence was promising but the available studies were very heterogeneous (Bunn et al. 2003).

Post-crash care policies may also help to reduce RTI mortality and other adverse health outcomes (Noland and Quddus 2004). Important factors in reducing death and adverse consequences of crashes include having one universal prehospital care access telephone number, such as 112, the optimal organization of the trauma services and the quick arrival of emergency response teams (Mock et al. 2004; Mock 2009). However, the main focus of this chapter is on prevention and, therefore, policies for the organization of prehospital and trauma care have not been considered.

Evidence on costs and benefits of policies

The evidence base for road safety interventions is well developed compared with that for other causes of injury (Peden 2004; Sethi 2006). The financial savings to society from selected road safety interventions are presented in Table 11.1. Although the precise magnitude of the cost–benefit ratio may be country specific, these measures are of proven value for money (Institute for Road Safety Research 2001; European Transport Safety Council 2003; Elvik and Vaa 2004). For example, for every €1 spent on random breath testing for alcohol control, there is a saving of €36. The savings include reductions in health care costs as well as in costs of material damage and economic productivity. The strength of the evidence warrants that there should be more widespread implementation of these road safety measures and highlights the need for greater political commitment to implement road safety policies.

Table 11.1 Financial savings to society from selected road safety interventions

Measure on which €1 could be spent	Savings (€)
Road design to minimize exposure to high risk scenarios	
Simple road markings	1.5
Upgrading marked pedestrian crossings	14
Pedestrian bridges or underpasses	2.5
Guard rails along the roadside	10.4
Removal of roadside obstacles	19.3
Median guard rail	10.3
Signing of hazardous curves	3.5
Cycle lanes	9.7
Area-wide speed and traffic management	9.7
Roundabouts (4 leg)	9.3
Speed control	
Speed enforcement	1.5
Speed cameras	2.1
Lowering speed limit on hazardous roads	14.3
Conspicuousness	
Daytime running lights (normal bulbs)	4.4
Roadside lighting	10.7
Seat belt	
Seat-belt reminders	6
Child restraints	32
Seat-belt enforcement	2.4
Alcohol control	
Random breath testing	36
Helmets	
Cycle helmets	29
Motorcycle helmets	16

Sources: Institute for Road Safety Research 2001; European Transport Safety Council 2003; Elvik and Vaa 2004

Successes and failures of road traffic safety policy

Implementation of road safety policies in Europe

To monitor progress in implementing the recommendations of the *World Report on Road Traffic Injury Prevention,* WHO conducted a global survey for the *Global Status Report on Road Safety* with the participation of 49 countries of the European Region ((WHO Regional Office for Europe 2009). Only 33% of these countries have comprehensive laws relating to five key risks: speeding, drinking and driving, and the non-use of helmets, seat-belts and child restraints. In addition, legislation will only be effective if enforced, and few countries report that legislation is effectively enforced in all areas. It is clear, therefore, that there is a need for improved implementation of road safety policy in Europe. Specific examples of insufficient implementation of effective road safety policies include the following.

Only two-thirds of European countries have an urban speed limit of less than 50 km/h; CIS countries have an urban limit of 60 km/h, or more (WHO Regional Office for Europe 2009). One-fifth of countries do not allow local adaptation of speed limits. Enforcement of speed limits is a key issue and most countries report that this could be improved.

Only half of the countries have a law requiring comprehensive helmet use for all riders of two-wheelers irrespective of age, religion or engine size. There is concern that enforcement practices and safety standards for helmets are poorly implemented. Routine data on helmet wearing show that there is an association between helmet wearing and deaths in motorcycle riders, implying that European countries with more successful implementation of this policy save lives (Fig. 11.1).

As noted above, there is a reluctance to legislate for compulsory wearing of cycle helmets lest this deter cycling and the benefits of physical activity would be lost (Hagel and Pless 2006). Many countries, however, require that children wear cycle helmets. Affordability of safety equipment is also an important issue, as use of the equipment will not only be influenced by disposable income for different social groups but also by the price of safety equipment relative to income, particularly in middle-income countries (Hendrie et al. 2004). Community-based programmes consisting of a combination of education and subsidies for safety equipment, such as helmets, to ensure access and affordability are also promising. These can be targeted to at risk groups such as youth in deprived areas.

All countries in the European region have legislation mandating the use of seat-belts, but 10% of countries have not mandated the compulsory use of seat-belt use in the rear of vehicles. When examined at a European level, there is a strong correlation between front seat-belt wearing and mortality in car occupants adjusted for car ownership (Fig. 11.2). These data imply that successful implementation of this policy saves lives.

In order to improve conspicuousness, several EU Member States now require that anyone providing roadside assistance or leaving a stranded vehicle should always wear a reflective vest. Spain and Italy were pioneer countries and others are following suit.

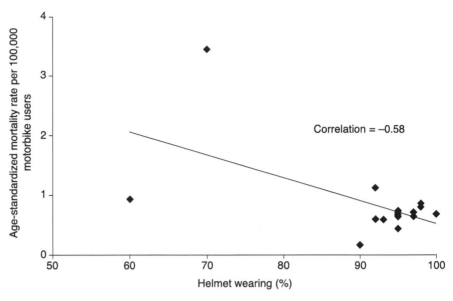

Figure 11.1 Mortality in motorcycle riders and helmet wearing in 16 European countries

Source: Calculated from data provided by WHO Regional Office for Europe (2009)

Case studies from north-western Europe

Some of the safest countries in the world are in north-western Europe (Fig. 11.3). Many of these countries have over the past few decades had a sustained approach to road safety. Sweden, the Netherlands and the United Kingdom have very much led the field (UK Department of Transport 2000; Koornstra 2002; Racioppi 2004).

In Sweden, an ambitious Road Traffic Safety Bill was passed by a large majority in the Riksdag (the Swedish Parliament) in October 1997. The basis of the Bill was Vision Zero, a policy document from the Swedish Government setting out a strategy to achieve zero deaths or serious injuries within the road transport system (Swedish Government 1997). It is based on the principle that, while crashes are always likely to happen, serious injuries and deaths can be avoided if the amount of kinetic energy to which road users are exposed is minimized (Haddon 1995; Belin et al. 2011). It represents a paradigm shift from a reactive to a proactive road safety policy. To achieve this, it called for a partnership between designers, road users, employers and police, whereby designers should design roads, vehicles and safety equipment to ensure that serious crashes and injuries do not occur, and road users should follow rules to ensure safety for themselves and other road users. The police have an obligation to enforce rules such as speed limits, drink driving, seat-belt use and following the Highway Code. Organizations (both private and public) are required to demonstrate corporate responsibility by ensuring safe driver behaviour. Environmental concerns are also addressed, as less-aggressive driving leads to less fuel

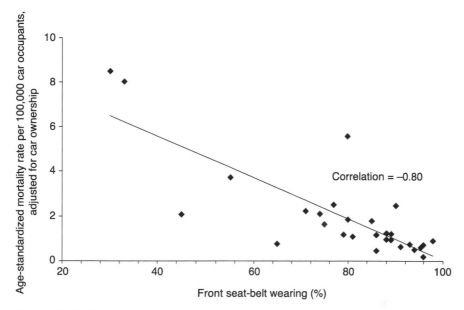

Figure 11.2 Mortality in car occupants and wearing a seat-belt in the front seats in 29 European countries

Source: Calculated from data provided by WHO Regional Office for Europe (2009)

consumption and emission of gases. The emergency services and health sector are tasked with ensuring efficient transportation and quality emergency trauma care to minimize fatality and long-term disability. The Bill has been considered a huge success and since its introduction there has been a three-fold reduction in the number of deaths from RTIs. Sweden's roads are considered among the safest in the world.

In the Netherlands, a *Sustainable Safety* strategy was developed in the 1990s and modified in 1998, with targets to reduce deaths by 50% and serious injuries by 40% in 2010 compared with 1998. This was linked to the development of better road infrastructure (separating vehicles according to their mass, speed and direction), to the development of safer vehicles and to modifications of road user behaviour (Schermers 1999). Attention was paid to the protection of vulnerable road users, in particular cyclists and pedestrians (Koornstra 2002; Racioppi 2004). Other notable interventions were the introduction of 30 km/h zones and ensuring safer infrastructure among other routes. Interventions and policies implemented since the early 1980s are shown in Fig. 11.4, together with the trend in RTI mortality rate. The road safety measures implemented as part of the *Sustainable Safety* strategy have been evaluated, and for the period 1998–2007 were shown to have had a positive road safety effect. They were estimated to having resulted in a 32% reduction in traffic fatalities, exceeding the targets, and having had a cost–benefit ratio of 1:3.6 (Weijermars and van Schagen 2009).

In the United Kingdom, there is a comprehensive approach in *Tomorrow's Roads: Safer for Everyone*, with a strategy to reduce road deaths and serious

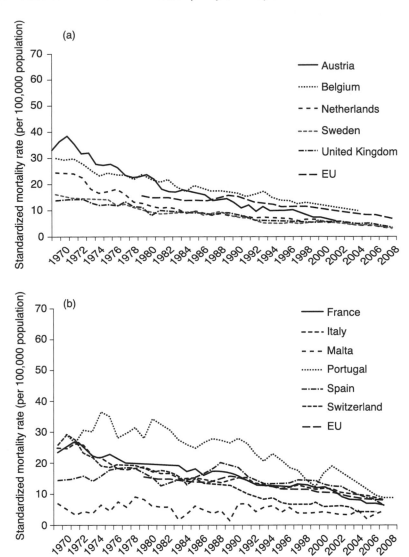

Figure 11.3 Trends in age-standardized death rates from road traffic injuries in north-western (a) and south-western (b) Europe, 1970–2008

Source: WHO Regional Office for Europe 2012a

injuries by 40% and deaths and serious injuries among children by 50% by 2010 (UK Department of Transport 2000; Koornstra 2002; Racioppi 2004). Legislation in the United Kingdom requiring the compulsory wearing of seat-belts was introduced in 1983 for front seat passengers and in 1989 and 1991 for child and adult rear passengers, respectively. The passage of the law concerning front seat-belts through Parliament took ten years because of resistance by a leading motoring organization and by groups opposed to what they described

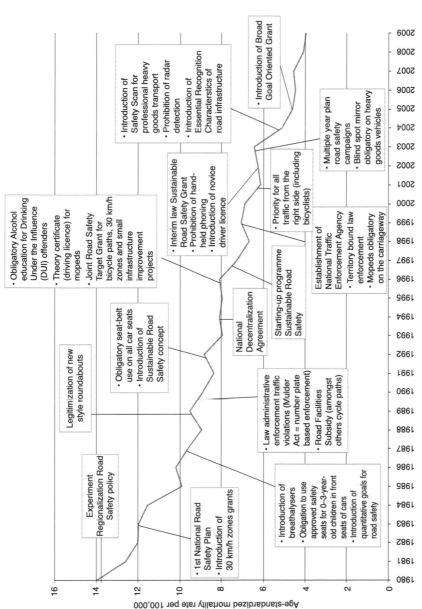

Figure 11.4 Trend in the age-standardized death rate from road traffic injuries in the Netherlands in relation to the main interventions to improve road safety, 1980–2009

Sources: WHO Regional Office for Europe (2012a) and data from national informants

as a 'nanny state' (Breen 2004). Once implemented, however, the law has led to 60,000 lives being saved and 600,000 fewer serious injuries over a 25-year period, and it has been hailed as a great success by the UK Department of Transport (Avery 1984). Legislation and enforcement, with powerful media campaigns at repeated intervals, have been effective in achieving high compliance. This has been reported as 94% for front seat users and 93% for rear seated children, but only 70% of adults are secured in the rear.

Case studies from south-western Europe

Some countries in south-western Europe have made substantial progress in the last decade or so (Fig. 11.5). Among these, France, Portugal and Spain attained

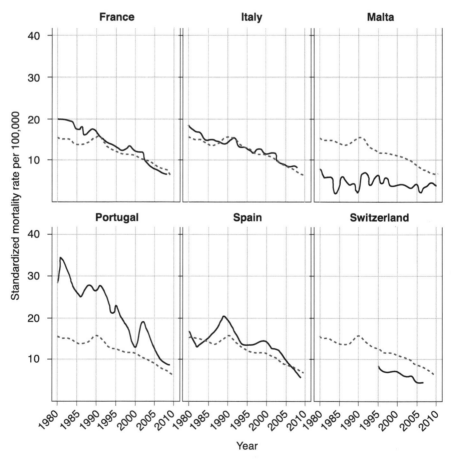

Figure 11.5 Trends in age-standardized death rates from road traffic injuries in south-western Europe, 1980–2010

Source: WHO Regional Office for Europe 2012a
Notes: Dark line, country trend; dashed line, average trend for European Union

the EU target of halving RTI deaths in 2010 compared with 2001 (European Traffic Safety Council 2011). The examples of France and Portugal are discussed in greater detail.

France has made great strides in reducing fatalities on its roads (Gerondau 2007). This has been the result of numerous factors, including adoption and enforcement of legislation on speeding, seat-belts and drink driving. Since 2002, a combination of factors has accelerated the rate of decrease in annual fatalities (Fig. 11.6). From the early 1970s to 2009, deaths have declined from more than 16,000 annually to just over 4000 annually. In the seven years from 2001 to 2009, success has been attributed to the high level of political commitment, intersectoral action, stricter enforcement, social marketing campaigns, blood alcohol concentration testing and the introduction of speed cameras to ensure compliance with speed limits (Gerondau 2007).

Portugal is another example of a country in south-west Europe that has made great strides since the mid-1970s (Fig. 11.7). From having one of the highest RTI mortality rates before joining the EU in 1986, the annual number of deaths has fallen from 2500 in 1988 to about 700 in 2010. Some road safety measures, such as helmets for motorcyclists, front seat-belts and drink driving legislation, had already been introduced prior to this, but a first comprehensive National Road Safety Plan was implemented in 2003. This included periodic technical inspections of vehicles; assessments of high-risk roads; mandatory use of child restraints, seat-belts and helmets; lower speed limits; measures to tackle drunk driving; higher fines' and stricter enforcement. Collectively, these have had a dramatic effect. On-the-spot penalty fines and greater enforcement by the police resulted in high compliance with seat-belt rules (86% use for front and 45% use for rear seats). Road layouts considered dangerous were reconstructed. The most marked effect has been on occupants of four-wheelers, although there has been a notable decrease in pedestrian fatalities as well (European Traffic Safety Council 2011). The country has practically met its target of halving the number of road fatalities in 2010 compared with 2001, and RTI mortality rates have fallen to near the EU average.

Another example comes from Italy where, from 2000 to 2010, a 34% increase in the wearing of front seat-belts was observed (ISS and Ministry of Infrastructure and Transport 2011), which was associated with a 53% decrease in deaths of car occupants (ISTAT 2011). Seat-belt wearing was thought to be an important contributory factor.

Case studies from central and eastern Europe

The majority of central and eastern European countries has made some progress over the last few decades (Fig. 11.8). Of note among these are the Baltic countries, which have shown the greatest declines in RTI mortality rates in the last few years. After peaks in the early 1990s, a result of the liberalization of traffic and rejection of state authority after the fall of communism, levels remained about double the EU average until the last few years, when greater priority was given to achieving better road safety levels. Membership of the EU and the EU target of halving road traffic deaths by 2010 compared with 2001 has had positive

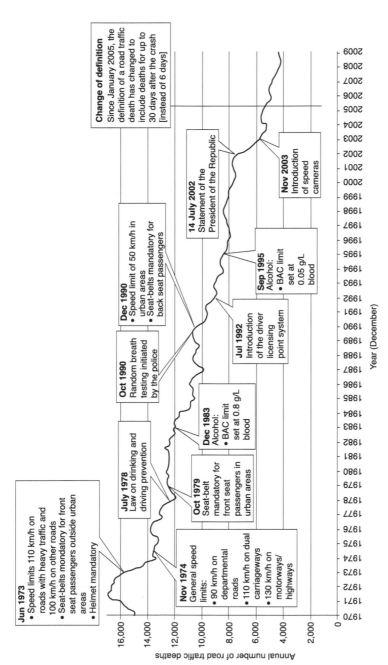

Figure 11.6 Trend in the number of deaths from road traffic injuries in metropolitan France in relation to the main interventions to improve road safety, 1970–2009

Source: Hanlon 2012

Note: BAC, blood alcohol concentration

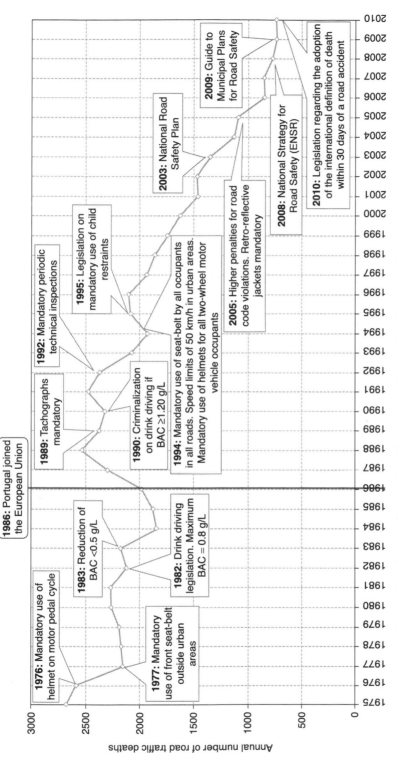

Figure 11.7 Trend in the number of deaths from road traffic injuries in Portugal in relation to the main interventions to improve road safety, 1975–2010

Sources: WHO Regional Office for Europe (2012a) and data from national informants

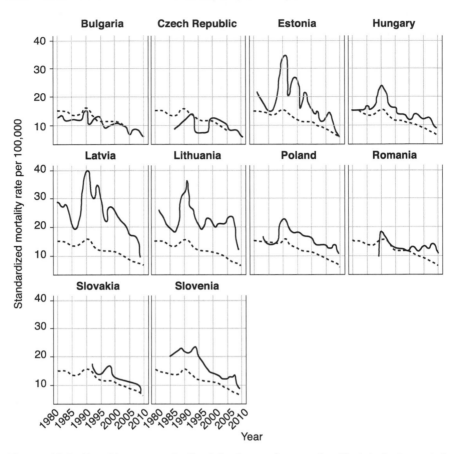

Figure 11.8 Trend in age-standardized death rates from road traffic injuries in central and eastern Europe, 1980–2010

Source: WHO Regional Office for Europe 2012a
Notes: Dark line, country trend; dashed line, average trend for European Union

effects, and the three Baltic countries and Slovenia are among the eight EU Member States to attain this target (European Traffic Safety Council 2011). However, some of the steep declines seen after 2008 may also reflect reduced vehicle use as a consequence of the global financial crisis (Stuckler et al. 2011).

The example of Latvia will be discussed in greater detail (Fig. 11.9). Road traffic deaths decreased from 997 in 1991 to 254 in 2009. From 1996 onwards, a series of road safety interventions, including urban speed limits and compulsory use of seat-belts and helmets, were introduced. New programmes in 1999 consisted of the compulsory use of headlights, child car seats, reflectors for pedestrians and winter tyres, and restricting mobile phone use. From 2004, the introduction of a penalty point system and far stricter enforcement, particularly for drunk driving and other traffic infringements, has contributed to a steeper fall in deaths (European Traffic Safety Council 2011). The third National

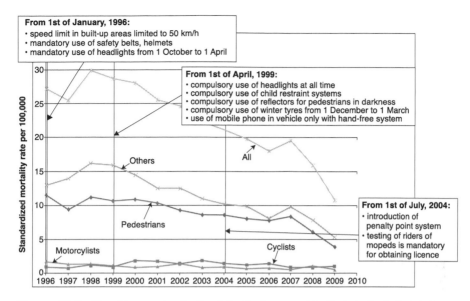

Figure 11.9   Trend in age-standardized deaths from road traffic injuries in Latvia in relation to the main interventions to improve road safety, 1996–2009, by road user type

Sources: WHO Regional Office for Europe (2012b) and data from national informants

Road Safety Plan 2007–2013 brought renewed focus on road safety as a priority. In addition to the large falls in four-wheeler occupant deaths, there has also been a large reduction in deaths of pedestrians. Although rates in Latvia are still higher than the EU average, Latvia has attained the EC target of halving the road traffic fatality rate by 2010. Pressing problems still exist, such as too few speed cameras, enforcing speed restrictions to protect pedestrians, improving the road network and renewing the car fleet: 70% of cars in use are more than ten years old.

Case studies from south-eastern Europe

Countries in south-eastern Europe mostly show a downward trend in the RTI mortality rate (Fig. 11.10). In some countries, such as Greece, however, progress has not been as marked as that of some other EU Member States such as Portugal and Spain. A few countries, such as Albania and Serbia, have shown a decline followed by an increase (European Traffic Safety Council 2011).

The example of Serbia will be considered in more detail (Fig. 11.11). In Serbia, the initial fall in RTI mortality from 1992 onwards can be explained by reduced motorcar usage because of the effect of the United Nations sanctions. Since about 2004, there has been an increase in RTI mortality for all types of road user. This was in spite of efforts to implement safety policies; these did not keep pace with the increased exposure resulting from rapid motorization. Renewed efforts are being made recently and a new Road Safety Law from 2009 is showing some early benefits.

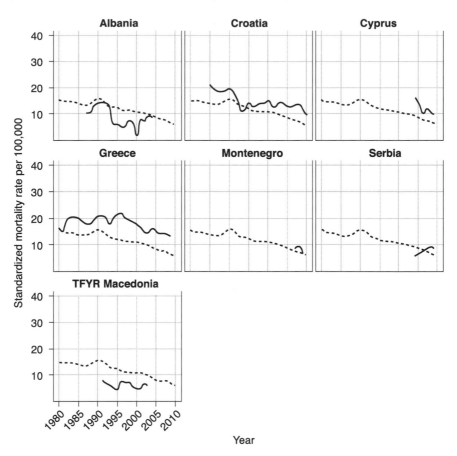

Figure 11.10 Trends in age-standardized death rates from road traffic injuries in south-eastern Europe, 1980–2010

Source: WHO Regional Office for Europe 2012a
Notes: Dark line, country trend; dashed line, average trend for European Union

Case studies from the Commonwealth of Independent States

The countries of the Caucasus (Armenia, Azerbaijan and Georgia) appear to have RTI mortality rates that are stable of late and lower than those of the EU. In contrast, the Russian Federation, Ukraine, Belarus and the Republic of Moldova have RTI mortality rates far higher than the EU. In the Russian Federation, there was a substantial rise of RTI mortality rates against a backdrop of a 260% increase in the car fleet since 1990, with a staggering 208,558 road crashes resulting in 34,506 deaths and 251,386 injured in 2004. The biggest problem was reported to occur in urban areas, with large numbers of deaths among both car occupants and pedestrians. This appeared to be linked to a range of circumstances, from unsafe infrastructure and high urban speeds to frequent drinking and driving and low penalties for traffic offences (European

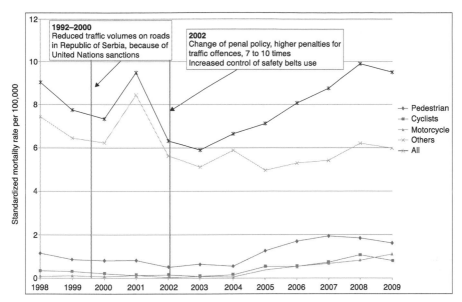

Figure 11.11 Trend in age-standardized deaths from road traffic injuries in Serbia in relation to the main interventions to improve road safety, 1996–2009, by road user type

Sources: WHO Regional Office for Europe (2012b) and data from national informants

Conference of Ministers of Transport 2006a,b). Much greater policy attention has been given to the issue of road safety lately, with commitment from the highest level. Measures are being taken to reduce the urban speed limit from 60 km/h to 50 km/h, and to have stricter enforcement of existing laws on seat-belts, speed and drinking and driving, plus investment in infrastructure. Recent reports show that there has been a fall in RTI deaths to 28,000 in 2010.

Discussion and conclusions

The approach undertaken in this chapter has been to identify evidence-based interventions in the literature and match these to actions undertaken during the period of observation. It has not been possible to undertake a formal trend analysis to determine whether the reductions in deaths can be causally attributed to the implementation of specific road safety policies. Nevertheless, the evidence strongly argues in favour of the successes of road safety policy in Europe in many countries.

This chapter has shown that there are numerous evidence-based policies in road safety but that there is considerable variation in the implementation of these policies within Europe. Where they have been implemented successfully, these policies appear to have led to a marked reduction in RTI mortality, as has been documented in Sweden, the Netherlands and the United Kingdom. In these countries, policies have been based on a systems approach whereby the road transport system, vehicles and individual behaviour are modified to ensure that if crashes occur the amount of kinetic energy transferred to individuals is minimized.

Successful policy implementation requires political commitment, good governance structures, intersectoral working, policies with targets, having a lead authority for road safety, strong capacity and civil society involvement in safety (Peden 2004). Road safety programmes require action by different sectors, emphasizing the need for leadership, commitment, clear communication and good coordination. Countries that have succeeded have used a science-based approach and have focused on having safer car design and road environment to protect all road users from serious injury, and on tackling the risk factors of speed, drink driving and using safety equipment. A science-based approach will also help to avoid negative policy outcomes. For example, legislation allowing those holding car driving licences to drive light motorcycles in Spain without having to take a special motorcycle driving test caused more harm than good, with an increase in the number of road injuries among these riders (Perez et al. 2009).

International agencies such as the United Nations, WHO and EU have helped to raise the public health priority given to road safety and have mandated the health sector to have a catalytic role in an area of health policy that would traditionally be led by the transport or justice sector. Not all countries, however, have been able to implement road safety policies, and some of the determinants of this have been previously described (World Health Organization 2007b; Sethi 2010). These include poor governance, weak legislation, inadequate enforcement, lack of a lead authority, not working across sectors, poor capacity, inadequate resources, lack of coordination and not having clearly defined roles and actions and targets.

The recent decline in vehicle use as a consequence of the financial crisis is likely to be transient; countries that have failed to respond to the long-term challenge of increasing road use by adopting road safety policies have witnessed a concomitant increase in road traffic casualties (Peden 2004). There is almost a ten-fold difference between the country with the highest and the country with the lowest rate in Europe. It has been suggested that if all countries in the WHO European Region had the same road traffic mortality rate as the country with the lowest rate (or safest country) in the Region, then an estimated 55,000 lives could be saved in one year (or 63% of all RTI deaths) (Sethi 2006).

The recent call by the EC for a 50% reduction in serious RTIs and fatalities in the decade from 2010 to 2020 in EU Member States (European Commission 2003) will refocus attention on the road safety problem. The United Nations' *Decade of Action for Road Safety* advocates for greater action by Member States, urging them to develop plans for the decade 2011–2020. In response, 27 countries from the European Region have held their own launches of the *Decade of Action* since 11 May 2011. Such advocacy and the implementation of science-informed road safety policy will help to reduce the relentless daily loss of lives on the roads.

Road transport is also linked to health effects other than just RTIs. These include air pollution leading to respiratory illness, cancer and cardiovascular diseases; noise causing psychological ill effects; over-reliance on car transportation, leading to a lack of physical activity causing obesity and cardiovascular diseases;

and the emission of greenhouse gases, climate change and the associated health ill effects (Racioppi 2004). Improvements in road safety will, therefore, also lead to these other environmental and health benefits (Woodcock et al. 2009). There are, therefore, opportunities for policy synergy with the global climate change and non-communicable disease agendas (WHO Regional Office for Europe 2011; World Health Organization 2011).

This chapter has shown that, although good progress is being made in road safety in Europe, many countries need to strive for more sustained implementation of these road safety policies. Many policies are transferable; the reasons for the successes and failures of implementation would be more obvious if data on reliable indicators were collected more systematically.

Acknowledgements

We are grateful to Dr Margaret Peden, Ms Francesca Racioppi and Dr Gauden Galea for their helpful comments.

References

Ameratunga, S., Jackson, R. and Norton, R. (2006) Death and injury on roads, *British Medical Journal*, 333(7558):53–4.

Anderson, P. (2009) *Reducing Drinking and Driving in Europe*. London: Institute of Alcohol Studies.

Avery, J.G. (1984) Seat belt success: where next? *British Medical Journal (Clinical Research Edition)*, 288(6418):662–3.

Belin, M.A., Tillgren, P. and Vedung, E. (2011) Vision Zero: a road safety policy innovation, *International Journal of Injury Control and Safety Promotion*, 9(2): 171–9.

Beyer, F.R. and Ker, K. (2009) Street lighting for preventing road traffic injuries, *Cochrane Database of Systematic Reviews*, (1):CD004728.

Breen, J. (2004) Road safety advocacy, *British Medical Journal*, 328(7444):888–90.

Bunn, F., Collier, T., Frost, C. et al. (2003) Area-wide traffic calming for preventing traffic related injuries, *Cochrane Database of Systematic Reviews*, (1):CD003110.

DiGuiseppi, C., Roberts, I., Li, L. and Allen, D. (1998) Determinants of car travel on daily journeys to school: cross sectional survey of primary school children, *British Medical Journal*, 316(7142):1426–8.

Duperrex, O., Bunn, F. and Roberts, I. (2002) Safety education of pedestrians for injury prevention: a systematic review of randomised controlled trials, *British Medical Journal*, 324(7346):1129.

Edwards, P., Roberts, I., Green, J. and Lutchmun, S. (2006) Deaths from injury in children and employment status in family: analysis of trends in class specific death rates, *British Medical Journal*, 333(7559):119.

Elvik, R. and Vaa, T. (2004) *Handbook of Road Safety Measures*. Amsterdam: Elsevier.

European Commission (2003) *European Road Safety Action Programme. Halving the Number of Road Accident Victims in the European Union by 2010: A Shared Responsibility*. Brussels: European Commission.

European Conference of Ministers of Transport (2006a) *Road Safety Performance. National Peer Review: Russian Federation*. Paris: European Conference of Ministers of Transport.

European Conference of Ministers of Transport (2006b) *Young Drivers. The Road to Safety*. Paris: European Conference of Ministers of Transport.

European Traffic Safety Council (2011) *2010 Road Safety Target Outcome: 100,000 fewer deaths since 2001.* [Fifth Road Safety PIN Report.] Brussels: European Traffic Safety Council.

European Transport Safety Council (2003) *Cost Effective EU Transport Safety Measures.* Brussels: European Transport Safety Council.

Flahaut, B. (2004) Impact of infrastructure and local environment on road unsafety. Logistic modeling with spatial autocorrelation, *Accident Analysis and Prevention*, 36(6):1055–66.

Gerondau, C. (2007) *Road Safety in France. Reflections on Three Decades of Road Safety Policy.* London: Foundation for the Automobile and Society.

Goss, C.W., van Bramer, L.D., Gliner, J.A. et al. (2008) Increased police patrols for preventing alcohol-impaired driving, *Cochrane Database of Systematic Reviews*, (4):CD005242.

Haddon, W., Jr. (1995) Energy damage and the 10 countermeasure strategies. 1973, *Injury Prevention*, 1(1):40–4.

Hagel, B.E. and Pless, B.I. (2006) A critical examination of arguments against bicycle helmet use and legislation, *Accident Analysis and Prevention*, 38(2):277–8.

Hanlon M. (2012) France's bold drink driving legislation: every car to carry a breathalyzer, *Gizmag*, 24 February, http://www.gizmag.com/france-breathalyzer-legislation/21541/ (accessed 10 July 2012).

Haynes, R., Jones, A., Kennedy, V., Harvey, I. and Jewell, T. (2007) District variations in road curvature in England and Wales and their association with road-traffic crashes, *Environment and Planning A*, 39(5):1222–37.

Hendrie, D., Miller, T.R., Orlando, M. et al. (2004) Child and family safety device affordability by country income level: an 18 country comparison, *Injury Prevention*, 10(6):338–43.

Institute for Road Safety Research (2001) *Cost–Benefit Analysis of Measures for Vulnerable Road Users.* Amsterdam: Institute for Road Safety Research.

ISS and Ministry of Infrastructure and Transport (2011) *Il sistema Ulisse per il monitoraggio dell'uso dei dispositivi di sicurezza in Italia [The System Ulysses for Monitoring the Use of Seat Belts and Helmets in Italy].* [Sicurezza Stradale: verso il 2020.] Rome: Istituto Superiore di Sanità e Ministero delle Infrastrutture e dei Trasporti.

ISTAT (2011) *Road Accidents Resulting in Deaths and Injuries.* Rome: Istituto nazionale di statistica.

Karkhaneh, M., Kalenga, J.C., Hagel, B.E. and Rowe, B.H. (2006) Effectiveness of bicycle helmet legislation to increase helmet use: a systematic review, *Injury Prevention*, 12(2):76–82.

Koornstra, M. (2002) SUNflower: a comparative study of the development of road safety in Sweden, the United Kingdom, and the Netherlands. Leidschendam: Dutch Institute of Road Safety Research.

Kwan, I. and Mapstone, J. (2006) Interventions for increasing pedestrian and cyclist visibility for the prevention of death and injuries, *Cochrane Database of Systematic Reviews*, (4):CD003438.

Liu, B.C., Ivers, R., Norton, R. et al. (2008) Helmets for preventing injury in motorcycle riders, *Cochrane Database of Systematic Reviews*, (1):CD004333.

McKee, M., Zwi, A., Koupilova, I., Sethi, D. and Leon, D. (2000) Health policy-making in central and eastern Europe: lessons from the inaction on injuries, *Health Policy Plan*, 15(3):263–9.

Mock, C. (2009) *Guidelines for Trauma Quality Improvement Programmes.* Geneva: World Health Organization.

Mock, C., Quansah, R., Krishnan, R., Arreola-risa, C. and Rivara, F. (2004) Strengthening the prevention and care of injuries worldwide, *Lancet*, 363(9427):2172–9.

Noland, R.B. and Quddus, M.A. (2004) Improvements in medical care and technology and reductions in traffic-related fatalities in Great Britain, *Accident Analysis and Prevention*, 36(1):103–13.

OECD (1998) *Safety of Vulnerable Road Users*. Paris: Organisation for Economic Co-operation and Development.

Pasanen, E. (1991) *Driving Speeds and Pedestrian Safety*. Espoo: Helsinki University of Technology Transportation Engineering.

Peden, M. (2004) *World Report on Road Traffic Injury Prevention*. Geneva: World Health Organization.

Perez, K., Mari-Dell'Olmo, M., Borrell, C. et al. (2009) Road injuries and relaxed licensing requirements for driving light motorcycles in Spain: a time-series analysis, *Bulletin of the World Health Organization*, 87(7):497–504.

Racioppi, F. (2004) Preventing road traffic injury: a public health perspective for Europe. Copenhagen: WHO Regional Office for Europe.

Rifaat, S.M., Tay, R. and de Barros, A. (2010) Effect of street pattern on road safety: are policy recommendations sensitive to aggregations of crashes by severity? *Transportation Research Record*, 2147:58–65.

Rissel, C. and Wen, L.M. (2011) The possible effect on frequency of cycling if mandatory bicycle helmet legislation was repealed in Sydney, Australia: a cross sectional survey, *Health Promotion Journal of Australia*, 22(3):178–83.

Roberts, I. and Power, C. (1996) Does the decline in child injury mortality vary by social class? A comparison of class specific mortality in 1981 and 1991, *British Medical Journal*, 313(7060):784–6.

Roberts, I., Norton, R., Jackson, R., Dunn, R. and Hassall, I. (1995) Effect of environmental factors on risk of injury of child pedestrians by motor vehicles: a case–control study, *British Medical Journal*, 310(6972):91–4.

Schermers, G. (1999) *Sustainable Safety: A Preventative Road Safety Strategy for the Future*. Rotterdam: Ministry of Transport; Transport Research Centre.

Sethi, D. (2006) *Injuries and Violence in Europe: Why They Matter and What Can Be Done*. Copenhagen: WHO Regional Office for Europe.

Sethi, D. (2007) *Youth and Road Safety in Europe*. Copenhagen: WHO Regional Office for Europe.

Sethi, D. (2010) *Preventing Injuries in Europe: From International Collaboration to Local Implementation*. Copenhagen: WHO Regional Office for Europe.

Sethi, D., Racioppi, F. and Bertollini, R. (2007) Preventing the leading cause of death in young people in Europe, *Journal of Epidemiology and Community Health*, 61(10):842–3.

Sonkin, B., Edwards, P., Roberts, I. and Green, J. (2006) Walking, cycling and transport safety: an analysis of child road deaths, *Journal of the Royal Society of Medicine*, 99(8):402–5.

Stuckler, D., Basu, S., Suhrcke, M., Coutts, A. and McKee, M. (2011) Effects of the 2008 recession on health: a first look at European data, *Lancet*, 378(9786):124–5.

Swedish Government (1997) *Vision Zero and the Traffic Safety Society*. [Bill 1996/97:137.] Stockholm: Swedish Government.

Thompson, D.C., Rivara, F.P. and Thompson, R. (2000) Helmets for preventing head and facial injuries in bicyclists, *Cochrane Database of Systematic Reviews*, (2):CD001855.

UK Department of Transport (2000) *Tomorrow's Roads: Safer for Everyone*. London: The Stationery Office.

Webster, D.C. and Layfield, R.E. (2003) *Review of 20 mph Zones in London Boroughs*. London: Transport for London.

Weijermars, W.A.M. and van Schagen, I.N.L.G. (2009) *Tien jaar Duurzaam Veilig: verkeersveiligheidsbalans 1998–2007 [Ten years of Sustainable Safety; Road Safety*

Assessment 1998–2007], Leidschendam: Stichting voor Wetenschappelijk Onderzoek Verkeersveiligheid.

Woodcock, J., Edwards, P., Tonne, C. et al. (2009) Public health benefits of strategies to reduce greenhouse-gas emissions: urban land transport, *Lancet*, 374(9705):1930–43.

WHO Regional Office for Europe (2009) *European Status Report on Road Safety*. Copenhagen: WHO Regional Office for Europe.

WHO Regional Office for Europe (2011) *Action Plan for Implementation of the European Strategy for the Prevention and Control of Noncommunicable Diseases 2012–2016*. Copenhagen: WHO Regional Office for Europe.

WHO Regional Office for Europe (2012a) *European Health for All Database (HFA-DB)*. Copenhagen: WHO Regional Office for Europe, http://data.euro.who.int/hfadb/ (accessed 4 June 2012).

WHO Regional Office for Europe (2012b) *European Mortality Database*. Copenhagen: WHO Regional Office for Europe, http://data.euro.who.int/hfamdb/ (accessed 10 July 2012).

World Health Organization (2006) Helmets: a road safety manual for decision-makers and practitioners. Geneva: World Health Organization.

World Health Organization (2007a) *Drinking and Driving. A Road Safety Manual for Decision-makers and Practitioners*. Geneva: World Health Organization.

World Health Organization (2007b) *Preventing Injuries and Violence: A Guide for Ministries of Health*. Geneva: World Health Organization.

World Health Organization (2011) *Health in the Green Economy*. Geneva: World Health Organization.

twelve

Air pollution

Johan Mackenbach, Susann Henschel,
Patrick Goodman, Sylvia Medina and
Martin McKee

Introduction

Outdoor air pollution poses a considerable threat to the environment as well as
to human health, leading to illness and premature death. Fortunately, considerable progress has been made over the past decades in reducing air pollution,
although important challenges remain. This chapter will review the main successes (and some failures) of these efforts to control air pollution, focusing on
their impact on human health.

Adverse effects of different pollutants on human health have been well
documented in Europe and other parts of the world (Katsouyanni et al. 2007;
Medina et al. 2009; WHO Regional Office for Europe 2004). Awareness of these
health effects was boosted by a number of disastrous events, particularly the
Great Smog in London in December 1952. Stagnant weather conditions caused a
sharp increase in the concentration of air pollutants, and more than three times
as many people died than would have been expected under normal conditions.
This and other similar events have led not only to advances in air pollution
control but also to research that has increased considerably our understanding
of the health effects of air pollution (Brunekreef and Holgate 2002).

Initially, research focused on sulphur dioxide and 'black smoke'. These are
released during the combustion of traditional fossil fuels such as coal and were
the main culprits of the London Great Smog. In the late 1970s, however, air
pollution from these sources had diminished greatly, at least in many parts of
western Europe, as a result of shifts to other fuels as well as effective abatement
measures (as noted below, Dublin was one exception; Kelly and Clancy 1984;
Clancy et al. 2002). Around that time other components of air pollution were
identified to be of concern and hence widely used to characterize air quality
(Brunekreef and Holgate 2002): nitrogen oxides (produced by the ever-rising
number of motor vehicles), ozone (produced by the action of sunlight on

nitrogen dioxide and hydrocarbons during warm and sunny weather) and small airborne particles (fine particulate matter: particulate matter of less than 10 μm (PM10) or even 2.5 μm (PM2.5); some emitted directly during combustion of diesel and other fuels and some formed in the atmosphere from oxidation and transformation of primary gaseous emissions). These three components now constitute the most problematic pollutants in terms of causing harm to health. The key emission sources are energy production in power plants, industry and households, and road transport.

Exposure to ambient air pollution has been linked to a number of different health outcomes. Most obviously, this affects the respiratory system but there is also growing evidence of effects on the cardiovascular system (Pelucchi et al. 2009; Brook et al. 2010). Both short- and long-term effects have been found. A selection of some of the most important health effects linked to specific pollutants is summarized in Table 12.1. Outdoor air pollution is estimated to account for 2.5% of deaths in high-income countries and 0.8% of DALYs (World Health Organization 2009).

One of the most important contributors to the overall health burden is long-term exposure to fine particulate matter. This has been estimated to reduce life expectancy by a year or more in the Netherlands, a country with particularly high exposure to this form of air pollution (Brunekreef 1997). In Europe as a whole (excluding the former USSR, but including the Baltic states), pollution

Table 12.1 A selection of important health effects linked to specific pollutants

Pollutant	Effects related to short-term exposure	Effects related to long-term exposure
Particulate matter	Lung inflammatory reactions, respiratory symptoms, adverse effects on the cardiovascular system, increase in medication usage, increase in hospital admissions, increase in mortality	Increase in lower respiratory symptoms, reduction in lung function in children and adults, increase in chronic obstructive pulmonary disease, reduction in life expectancy mainly from cardiopulmonary disorders and lung cancer
Ozone	Adverse effects on pulmonary function, lung inflammatory reactions, adverse effects on respiratory symptoms, increase in medication usage, increase in hospital admissions, increase in mortality	Reduction in lung function development
Nitrogen dioxide[a]	Effects on pulmonary function particularly in asthmatics, increase in airway allergic inflammatory reactions, increase in hospital admissions, increase in mortality	Reduction in lung function, increased probability of respiratory symptoms

Source: WHO Regional Office for Europe 2004
Note: [a]In ambient air, nitrogen dioxide serves as an indicator for a complex mixture of mainly traffic-related pollutants

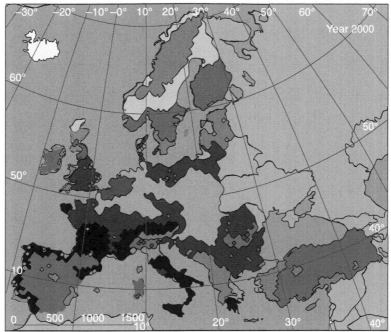

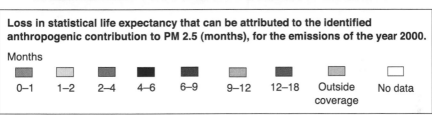

Figure 12.1   Loss of average life expectancy (in months) attributable to exposure to fine particulate matter (PM$_{2.5}$) in 2000

Source: European Environment Agency 2010a

by PM2.5 causes 500,000 premature deaths per year, corresponding to an estimated 5 million years of life lost (European Environment Agency 2010a). As Fig. 12.1 shows, reductions in life expectancy attributable to PM2.5 in air are concentrated in some of the most heavily urbanized and industrialized parts of Europe. Exposure to ozone concentrations exceeding critical levels for health is associated with more than 20,000 premature deaths in the EU-25 annually (European Environment Agency 2010a). Similar estimates are not available for nitrogen oxides or sulphur dioxide.

Children seem particularly sensitive to some pollutants. Other groups that are more sensitive include the elderly, those with cardiorespiratory disease and people in lower socioeconomic groups. Epidemiological studies have been unable to establish threshold levels below which no adverse health effects of air pollution occur (WHO Regional Office for Europe 2004).

Effectiveness of air pollution control policies

Emissions of air pollutants occur as a result of almost all economic and societal activities; consequently, increases in economic activity and population numbers are important drivers of increases in emissions. Over the past decades, however, it has been possible to partly decouple emission developments from economic growth, both by improving energy efficiency in the production of goods and services and by reducing emissions relative to the amount of energy consumed (European Environment Agency 2010b).

Emission reduction has been achieved by a variety of means and has depended, to a large extent, on international collaboration. Such collaboration has played a larger role in this area than in many other areas of health policy. The reasons are that both the health threats and the countermeasures transcend national borders. Air pollution from power plants drifts across country borders; vehicles that may or may not be subject to emission regulations are produced in one country and driven in another; and, in a globalizing world, industries demand a level playing field created by internationally agreed norms and regulations.

The main countermeasures taken in the period 1970–2010 are briefly summarized and their effectiveness in reducing the four main components of air pollution and their associated health impacts is reviewed.

Sulphur dioxide

Sulphur dioxide is emitted when fuels with a high sulphur content, such as coal and heavy fuel oils, are burnt. Emissions can be reduced by shifting to other fuels with lower sulphur content, such as natural gas, or by capturing sulphur dioxide before it is released into the air. The main source of sulphur dioxide emissions since the 1970s has been industry (including the energy sector).

In the 1970s, it became clear that countries' exposures to sulphur dioxide air pollution, for example in the form of 'acid rain', were strongly dependent on their neighbours' emissions and, in 1979, the United Nations Economic Commission for Europe established a *Convention on Long-range Transboundary Air Pollution*. Over the years, several protocols have been adopted to reduce sulphur emissions. In addition to these United Nations protocols, several EU Directives have been implemented on the regulation of sulphur emissions, focusing on ceilings for sulphur emissions during combustion of fuels in power plants and industry and on the sulphur content of fuels (Vestreng et al. 2007).

Within these agreements, countries also agreed to exchange harmonized information on their emissions and to have their data validated. Consequently, we are now rather well informed about trends, particularly since about 1980. Historical data show that, in Europe, total sulphur dioxide emissions rose steeply until 1980, when a peak was reached and an equally steep decline began (Fig. 12.2). In 2004, total emissions were less than a third of those in 1980. Three periods of emission reduction have been identified. The period 1980–1989 was characterized by low annual emission reductions for Europe as a whole, with emission reductions occurring mainly in western Europe. No international protocols were as yet in place, but western European countries

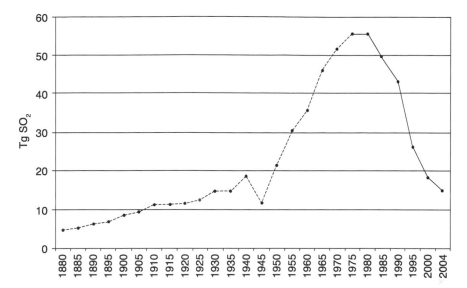

Figure 12.2   Historical development of sulphur dioxide emissions in Europe

Source: Vestreng et al. 2007

Note: Tg: teragram = 10^{12} gram = mega tonne

had already started to implement new technologies and fuels. In central and eastern Europe, emissions still were on the rise (Vestreng et al. 2007).

The period 1990–1999, by comparison, was characterized by large annual emission reductions for Europe as a whole, reflecting emission reductions in both western and central and eastern Europe. International protocols were in place that stimulated western European countries to continue their efforts to reduce pollutants. In central and eastern Europe, reductions occurred first as a result of the economic recession and the closing down of old heavy industries; when activity levels started to increase again, however, new technologies were implemented, which helped to keep emissions down. The annual emission reductions in the period 2000–2004 are again lower, with equally large reductions in both eastern and western countries (Vestreng et al. 2007). Since then emissions have continued to fall, although there is an increasing number of countries with year-to-year increases in sulphur emissions.

The effectiveness of these policies is evident from the fact that current sulphur dioxide emission levels are considerably below the level that would have been expected if they had been determined by trends in economic activity only, without concerted European policies. Reduced emissions have also led to reduced atmospheric concentrations of sulphur dioxide (European Environment Agency 2010a,b).

Particulate matter

The key anthropogenic sources of particulate matter and its precursors are road vehicles and industrial installations. Since 1990, the EU regulates exhaust emissions for both light- and heavy-duty vehicles and has gradually lowered the permissible emission limits. As a result, substantial declines in particulate matter emissions from vehicles have occurred since the end of the 20th century despite a large increase in the number of vehicles and total traffic activity over the same period. Emissions from industry of particulate matter and their precursors have also declined as a result of EU Directives on emissions (European Environment Agency 2011). In 2005, total road traffic particulate matter emissions were 63% lower than they would have been in the absence of EU standards, and a similar effect size was estimated for industry-related emissions-limiting directives (European Environment Agency 2010a,b).

Long-term trend data on particulate matter air concentrations are not available as methods of measurement have changed over time. Harmonized data covering Europe as a whole have only been available since 1999, and these data, surprisingly, show small and inconsistent reductions, perhaps as a result of measurement problems (European Environment Agency 2011). It is unclear, therefore, whether population health can have improved much as a result of measures to control particulate matter emissions.

Nitrogen oxides

Road transport has been the dominant source of nitrogen oxides emissions since the 1970s. Protocols and directives of the United Nations Economic Commission for Europe and the EU have set increasingly ambitious emissions ceilings for nitrogen oxides, both for individual vehicle types and at the national level. These stimulated the implementation of technological improvements to vehicles that can reduce emissions, such as improved combustion and the fitting of catalytic convertors.

Long-term trend data on nitrogen oxides emissions for Europe as a whole show a substantial increase during most of the 20th century until a major turning point was reached around 1990, after which emissions have declined (Fig. 12.3). Between 1950 and 1980, the steep rise in emissions was a result of a steep upward trend in liquid fuel use. Between 1980 and 1990, the rise in emissions became less steep, partly as a result of a slowing in the rate of growth of fuel consumption after the first oil crisis in western Europe, and of decreased fuel consumption in many central and eastern European countries.

It was only after 1990 that the effect of emission reduction policies set in. Improved vehicle technologies and stringent inspection systems reduced nitrogen oxides in road traffic emissions in the period 1990–2000 in western Europe, despite economic growth and increases in fuel consumption.

In central and eastern Europe, emissions declined in this period as well, but as a result of the economic crisis and of imports of cleaner cars from western Europe. After 2000, emissions in Europe as a whole continued to decrease, but less steeply because the economic recovery in eastern Europe increased emissions from road traffic in this region (Vestreng et al. 2009).

Long-term trend data on nitrogen oxides concentration in air are not available, but trends since 1999 show a consistent decline in average concentrations as well as in the proportion of urban populations exposed to limit levels set for protecting human health (European Environment Agency 2011).

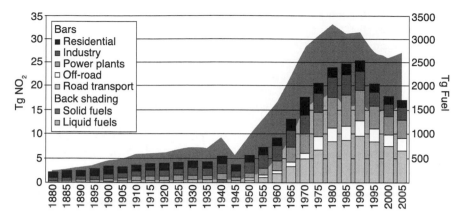

Figure 12.3   Historical trends of nitrogen oxides emissions in Europe (in teragrams)

Source: Vestreng et al. 2009

Note: Tg: teragram = 10^{12} gram = mega tonne

Ozone

Ground-level ozone is not directly emitted into the atmosphere but formed from a chain of chemical reactions following emissions of precursor gases, including nitrogen oxides (see above). Policy measures to reduce ozone concentrations mainly target emissions of these precursors, and many of the United Nations and EU Directives mentioned above are, therefore, also relevant for the reduction of ozone concentrations. In addition, the EU has set specific standards for exposure to ozone in its 2008 Air Quality Directive (European Environment Agency 2011).

Long-term trends of ozone concentrations can only be assessed for a limited number of European countries, mainly in western Europe. Since the early 1990s, when only a few measurement sites were available, the number of days in which ozone concentrations exceeded a maximum value (120 µg/m³) has declined in most of the sites. By the end of the 1990s, many more locations were producing data than in the earlier years and they covered a larger area of Europe. Since then, most stations reported fewer episodes when the daily threshold was exceeded, although some recorded an increase, mainly in southern and central Europe. Annual mean concentrations of ozone, however, do not show a consistent downward trend (European Environment Agency 2011).

Successes and failures of air pollution control in Europe

Health impacts

Estimates of the overall health impact of the measures described above are scarce. The massive reductions in sulphur dioxide concentrations must have had a positive impact on European population health, but the magnitude of this impact is not precisely known. This is because the reductions in sulphur dioxide have coincided with rising estimates of the impact of sulphur dioxide on health, suggesting that sulphur dioxide was a marker for other compounds that have changed over time (Brunekreef and Holgate 2002).

Within the Aphekom project (www.aphekom.org) a study undertaken in 20 cities across Europe, aiming to assess the impact of the implementation of EU legislation on sulphur content in certain liquid fuels over the period 1990–2004, it was found there was a general downward trend without any stepwise changes coinciding with the introduction of specific directives. Concentrations were relatively high in Athens and Budapest throughout the study period, but even in those cities concentrations declined substantially. In this project, no changes in the impact of sulphur dioxide on health outcomes over time were observed, and it was estimated that the reductions in sulphur dioxide levels prevented more than 2000 deaths per year in the 20 cities starting in the year 2000 compared with levels prior to October 1994 (A. Le Tertre et al. 2012 (manuscript submitted for publication).

Trends in air concentrations of particulate matter and ozone over the period 1970–2010 have been unclear, but air concentrations of nitrogen oxides have almost certainly decreased substantially. Taken together, there must have been a positive net effect on population health, even though its magnitude is not precisely known. It has been estimated that EU air emission policies reduced the negative health impact of the road transport sector in Europe as a whole (measured in terms of years of life lost) by 13% and 17% through reduced emissions of PM2.5 and ozone, respectively. Similarly, the negative health impact of the industrial sector was reduced by 60% by 2005 through reduced emissions of PM2.5 compared with a non-policy scenario (European Environment Agency 2010a,b).

Although many of the air pollution control policies were coordinated internationally, there have been considerable between-country differences in progress against these health hazards. A few of these specific successes will be highlighted, together with some international comparative data.

Selected national and local successes

The reunification of the German Democratic Republic and the Federal Republic of Germany in 1990 was accompanied by marked changes in the political environment, in socioeconomic structures and in air pollution controls (Henschel et al. 2012). Between 1989 and 1991, an immediate and remarkable fall in pollutant emissions was observed (Ebelt et al. 2001). These rapid and favourable trends continued throughout the 1990s as a result of a shift from brown coal to natural gas as the major energy source for industries, power plants and domestic space heating (Peters et al. 2009)l; there were also changes in the composition of the vehicle fleet, for example a shift from cars with a two-stroke motor to cars having three-way catalytic converters (Ebelt et al. 2001). Within a decade, ambient air pollution in the former German Democratic Republic converged with levels in the former Federal Republic of Germany (Sugiri et al. 2006). Although some studies were unable to find a short-term effect of improved air quality on mortality (Breitner et al. 2009; Peters et al. 2009), other studies found that differences in lung function among children aged five to seven years between cities of the former German Democratic Republic and the former Federal Republic of Germany vanished simultaneously with the reduction in air pollution (Sugiri et al. 2006), and that bronchitic symptoms decreased (Frye et al. 2003).

Dublin, the capital of Ireland, experienced extreme air pollution episodes during the 1980s, mainly through a shift from the use of oil for space heating to cheaper solid fuel, particularly bituminous coal and peat (Henschel et al. 2012). This shift occurred because of the policy of the Irish Government to reduce dependence on imported oil following the 1970 world oil crisis (Goodman and Clancy 2002). Marked increases in respiratory deaths at a main Dublin hospital in 1982 were associated with an extraordinarily severe episode (Kelly and Clancy 1984). Eventually the government had to take action to improve air quality; in September 1990 the marketing, sale and distribution of coal was banned in Dublin. An immediate fall in air pollution levels was observed with implementation of the ban (Medina et al. 2002, pp. 217–219), and mortality from respiratory and cardiovascular causes also declined substantially (Clancy et al. 2002). Following the success of this intervention, the ban was extended stepwise to 11 other Irish cities (Goodman et al. 2009). The first city to follow was Cork, and here too both air pollution and mortality levels declined simultaneously with implementation of the ban (Goodman et al. 2009; Rich et al. 2009).

London, one of the world's megacities, with approximately 8 million inhabitants, suffered from major traffic congestion from the 28 million journeys made on each day into and out of the city. On 17 February 2003, the traffic Congestion Charging Scheme was launched, with its main objective to reduce traffic congestion in the central area of the city by charging, initially, £5 (€6) daily, increased to £8 (€9.60) in 2005, for each four-wheeled vehicle entering the area on weekdays. At the same time, further measures were taken to improve traffic flow in London, such as bus network improvements and improvements of walking and cycling schemes (Transport for London 2006). After one year, a traffic volume reduction of 18% and a congestion reduction of 30% were observed (Transport for London 2004; Henschel et al. 2012). No clear changes in air quality were observed (Tonne et al. 2008; Kelly et al. 2011a). There were also some changes in the composition of PM10, such as lower levels of copper, zinc and bioavailable iron, thought to result from reductions in brake and tyre use (Kelly et al. 2011b). Some (small) health benefits are likely to have been achieved as well. The estimated years of life gained per 100,000 population were predicted to be 26 years for Greater London and 183 years for residents within the wards covered by the Congestion Charging Scheme (Tonne et al. 2008). There was also a suggestive decline in hospital admissions for bronchiolitis (Tonne et al. 2010).

In Stockholm, capital and largest city of Sweden, a similar congestion charging scheme trial was found to reduce air pollution levels in the inner city area. Taking nitrogen dioxide as a marker for traffic emissions, a population health impact of 206 years of life gained per 100,000 people for the area of Greater Stockholm over a 10-year period was calculated, assuming that the decrease of the exposure level would persist (Johansson et al. 2009).

Between-country variations

As shown in Table 12.2, there have been substantial differences between countries in the extent and timing of their sulphur dioxide emission reductions. In 2004,

Table 12.2 Sulphur dioxide emission trends in European countries, 1980–2004

Country	Sulphur dioxide emission (Gg)					
	1980	1985	1990	1995	2000	2004
Albania	72	73	74	14	32	32
Armenia	141	100	86	15	11	8
Austria	344	179	74	47	32	29
Azerbaijan	603	543	615	260	162	130
Belarus	740	690	888	344	162	97
Belgium	828	400	361	262	171	154
Bosnia and Herzegovina	482	483	484	360	420	427
Bulgaria	2,050	2,314	2,007	1,477	918	929
Croatia	150	164	178	70	60	85
Cyprus	28	35	46	41	51	45
Czech Republic	2,257	2,277	1,876	1,090	264	227
Denmark	450	333	176	133	27	23
Estonia	287	254	274	117	96	90
Finland	584	382	259	95	74	83
France	3,216	1,496	1,333	968	613	484
Georgia	230	273	43	6	7	5
Germany	7,514	7,732	5,289	1,708	630	559
Greece	400	500	487	536	493	537
Hungary	1,633	1,404	1,011	705	486	240
Iceland	18	18	9	9	9	9
Ireland	222	140	186	161	131	71
Italy	3,437	2,045	1,795	1,320	755	496
Kazakhstan	639	575	651	528	506	425
Latvia	96	97	97	47	10	4
Lithuania	311	304	263	92	43	40
Luxembourg	26	26	26	7	4	4
Malta	29	29	29	33	26	17
Netherlands	490	258	189	127	72	66
Norway	136	91	53	34	27	25
Poland	4,100	4,300	3,278	2,381	1,507	1,286
Portugal	266	198	317	332	306	203
Republic of Moldova	308	282	175	94	13	15
Romania	1,055	1,255	1,310	882	727	685

Country	Sulphur dioxide emission (Gg)					
	1980	1985	1990	1995	2000	2004
Russian Federation	7,323	6,350	6,113	3,101	2,263	1,858
Serbia and Montenegro	406	478	593	428	396	341
Slovakia	780	613	542	239	127	97
Slovenia	234	241	198	127	99	55
Spain	3,024	2,542	2,103	1,809	1,479	1,360
Switzerland	491	266	117	79	52	47
The former Yugoslavian Republic of Macedonia	107	109	110	93	90	87
Turkey	1,030	1,345	1,519	1,397	2,122	1,792
Ukraine	3,849	3,463	3,921	2,342	1,599	1,145
United Kingdom	4,838	3,714	3,699	2,343	1,173	833
Total	**55,340**	**48,448**	**42,896**	**26,282**	**18,263**	**15,162**

Source: Vestreng et al. 2007
Note: Gg: Gigagram = 10^9 grams

the grand total for all countries in the table was a reduction to 25% of the sulphur dioxide emissions in 1980; however, in several countries the reductions were considerably lower, such as Bulgaria, Croatia, Estonia, Portugal, Romania, the Russian Federation and Spain. Greece even saw its emissions increase over this period. While some of these developments are likely to reflect a catch-up in economic growth or in road traffic volume, the examples of the Czech Republic and Poland show that such growth can be combined with substantially reduced emissions (Vestreng et al. 2007).

Reductions in emissions of nitrogen oxides have also differed substantially among countries. Policy measures involved new standards for technological improvements to vehicles, and while the automobile industry has dutifully complied with these regulations, the speed with which they have impacted on actual pollution levels is largely dependent on the pace of turnover of the vehicle fleet. While average passenger car fleet emissions in Germany and Switzerland reached emission standards within five years of their introduction, Spain, with a rather old vehicle fleet, took more than ten years. A comparison of estimated nitrogen oxides emission between western and central and eastern Europe shows that the average passenger car in central and eastern Europe has up to ten times higher emissions than its equivalent in western Europe. Similar differences, but of a lesser magnitude, are found for light- and heavy-duty vehicles (Vestreng et al. 2009).

It is not surprising, therefore, that air pollution concentrations also differ substantially between European countries (Fig. 12.4). High concentrations of sulphur dioxide are mainly found in central and eastern Europe. High concentrations of particulate matter are found in these countries as well, but are also found in the north of Italy and in some urban and industrial centres in the rest of western Europe. High concentrations of nitrogen dioxide are found

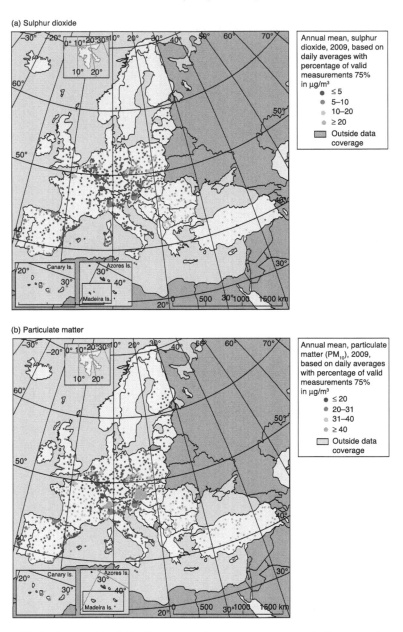

Figure 12.4 Geographical distribution of air pollutant exposure in Europe. (a) Sulphur dioxide. Dark orange dots refer to places where the limit value of 20 µg/m³ for protection of vegetation is exceeded. (b) Particulate matter (PM₁₀). Dark orange dots refer to places where the annual value of 40 µg/m³ set in the European Union 2005 Air Quality Directive is exceeded; light orange where the statistically derived 24-hour limit of 31 µg/m³ is exceeded; pale green where the WHO air quality guidance value for PM₅₀ of <50 µg/m³ is exceeded; and dark green where concentrations below the WHO air quality guidance value for PM₁₀ is achieved.

Source: European Environmental Agency 2011

(c) Nitrogen oxides

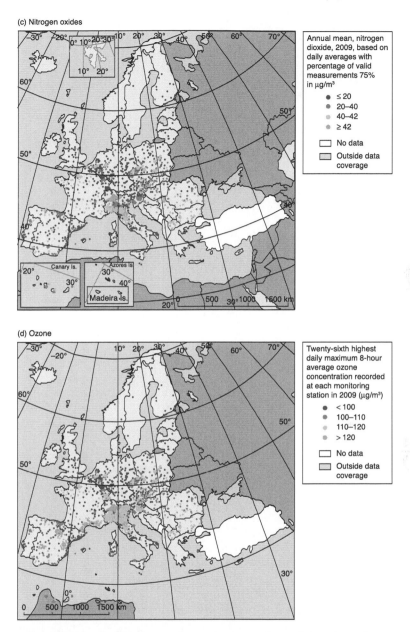

(d) Ozone

Figure 12.4 contd.   (c) Nitrogen oxides. Light orange dots refer to places that exceed the annual limit value of 40 μg/m³; dark orange where places exceed this limit plus the margin of tolerance (i.e. 42 μg/m³). (d) Ozone, as 8-hour average recorded values. Dots show the proximity to meeting the target value. Dark orange dots show the 26th highest daily values exceeding the 120 μg/m³ threshold, implying exceeding the target values

Source: European Environmental Agency 2011

in urban centres across Europe. High levels of ozone air pollution are found in a zone stretching from the east coast of Spain across the south of France and Italy into central and eastern Europe (European Environment Agency 2011).

Discussion and conclusions

Air pollution is one among many causes of cardiorespiratory disease. Unlike, say, cigarette smoking, where exposure can be measured relatively easily in terms of the number of packs smoked over a period of years, individual exposure to ambient air pollution is much more difficult to measure. Also, while there are extensive time-series data on some of the more visible pollutants, the dangers posed by invisible ones, such as fine particulate matter, have only been appreciated much more recently. Furthermore, and again unlike cigarette smoking, there are no specific health outcomes for air pollution, but these occur across a range of conditions and causes of death. Consequently, the health effects of air pollution control are difficult to quantify.

The picture painted in this chapter is a mixed one. There have been some clear successes, such as the reductions in sulphur dioxide and nitrogen oxides, which must have produced substantial health gains. Yet the situation with regard to particulate matter and ozone is less clear, although particulate matter concentrations are likely to have gone down considerably since the 1950s. The picture is also mixed geographically. Countries in western Europe have been much more successful in reducing emissions than those in central and eastern Europe, and at least some of the reductions in the latter countries are incidental to the closure of highly polluting factories on economic rather than health grounds.

Overall, emission levels are a product of the volume of material emitted into the atmosphere and the concentration of pollutants within it. The successes observed are primarily a result of technological advances, such as catalytic converters in motor vehicles, or changes in the type of fuel being used, rather than the amount of material being emitted, which has tended to increase with economic growth. This should give rise to concern for the future. Even leaving aside concerns about emissions of greenhouse gases, not considered in this chapter, the scope for further advances in cleaning the products of burning fossil fuels may be limited. It cannot, therefore, be assumed that the gains seen in recent decades will continue at the same pace.

There is an important lesson from these experiences. Air pollution is characterized by externalities, and those who produce the pollution do not normally have to pay for the damage it causes. Consequently, it is not possible to leave it to the market to control. As the examples in this chapter show, success has been brought about by regulation, frequently acting as a spur for technological innovation. Moreover, the cross-border nature of pollution means that this is not an issue that can be addressed by any country on its own. Although this is perhaps the most obvious example of where concerted international regulatory action is needed to safeguard health, it is not the only one, something that will be discussed in subsequent chapters.

Acknowledgements

Professor Bert Brunekreef and Professor Erik Lebret provided suggestions on how to approach this chapter.

References

Breitner, S., Stolzel, M., Cyrys, J. et al. (2009) Short-term mortality rates during a decade of improved air quality in Erfurt, Germany, *Environmental Health Perspectives*, 117(3):448–54.

Brook, R.D., Rajagopalan, S., Pope, C.A. et al (2010) Particulate matter air pollution and cardiovascular disease: an update to the scientific statement from the American Heart Association. *Circulation*, 121:2331–78.

Brunekreef, B. (1997) Air pollution and life expectancy: is there a relation? *Occupational and Environmental Medicine*, 54(11):781–4.

Brunekreef, B. and Holgate, S.T. (2002) Air pollution and health, *Lancet*, 360(9341):1233–42.

Clancy, L., Goodman, P., Sinclair, H. and Dockery, D.W. (2002) Effect of air-pollution control on death rates in Dublin, Ireland: an intervention study, *Lancet*, 360(9341):1210–14.

Ebelt, S., Brauer, M., Cyrys, J. et al. (2001) Air quality in postunification Erfurt, East Germany: associating changes in pollutant concentrations with changes in emissions, *Environmental Health Perspectives*, 109(4):325–33.

European Environment Agency (2010a) *The European Environment. State and Outlook 2010. Air pollution.* Copenhagen: European Environment Agency.

European Environment Agency (2010b) *Impact of Selected Policy Measures on Europe's Air Quality.* Copenhagen: European Environment Agency.

European Environment Agency (2011) *Air Quality in Europe: 2011 Report.* [EEA Technical Report.] Luxembourg: European Environment Agency.

Frye, C., Hoelscher, B., Cyrys, J. et al. (2003) Association of lung function with declining ambient air pollution, *Environmental Health Perspectives*, 111(3):383–7.

Goodman, P.G. and Clancy, L. (2002) Summary of the intervention to reduce particulate pollution levels in Dublin, in S. Medina, A. Plasència, L. Artazcoz et al. (eds) *APHEIS Health Impact Assessment of Air Pollution in 26 European Cities*. Paris: Institut de Veille Sanitaire, pp 101–4.

Goodman, P.G., Rich, D.Q., Zeka, A., Clancy, L. and Dockery, D.W. (2009) Effect of air pollution controls on black smoke and sulfur dioxide concentrations across Ireland, *Journal of Air Waste Management Association*, 59:207–13.

Henschel, S., Atkinson, R., Zeka, A. et al. (2012) Air pollution interventions and their impact on public health, *International Journal of Public Health*, 57(5):757–768.

Johansson, C., Burman, L. and Forsberg, B. (2009) The effects of congestions tax on air quality and health. *Atmospheric Environment*, 43:4843–54.

Katsouyanni K, Touloumi G, Spix C, Schwartz J, Balducci F, Medina S, Rossi G, Wojtyniak B, Sunyer J, Bacharova L, Schouten JP, Ponka A, Anderson HR. Short-term effects of ambient sulphur dioxide and particulate matter on mortality in 12 European cities: results from time series data from the APHEA project. Air Pollution and Health: a European Approach. *BMJ*. 1997 Jun 7; 314(7095):1658–63.

Kelly, I. and Clancy, L. (1984) Mortality in a general hospital and urban air pollution, *Irish Medical Journal*, 77:322–4.

Kelly, F., Anderson, H.R., Armstrong, B. et al. (2011a) *The Impact of the Congestion Charging Scheme on Air Quality in London. Part 2. Analysis of the Oxidative Potential of Particulate Matter.* [Research Report 155.] Boston, MA: Health Effects Institute, pp. 73–144.

Kelly, F., Anderson, H.R., Armstrong, B. et al. (2011b) *The Impact of the Congestion Charging Scheme on Air Quality in London. Part 1. Emissions Modelling and Analysis of Air Pollution Measurements.* [Research Report 155.] Boston, MA: Health Effects Institute, pp. 5–71.

Medina, S., Plasència, A., Artazcoz, L. et al. for the APHEIS Group (2002) *APHEIS Health Impact Assessment of Air Pollution in 26 European Cities. Second Year Report, 2000–2001.* Paris: Institut de Veille Sanitaire.

Medina S, Le Tertre A, Saklad M et al. for the APHEIS Group (2009) Air pollution and health. A European information system. *Air Qual Atmos Health,* 2:185–98.

Pelucchi, C., Negri, E., Gallus, S. et al. (2009) Long-term particulate matter exposure and mortality: a review of European epidemiological studies, *BMC Public Health,* 9:453.

Peters, A., Breitner, S., Cyrys, J. et al. (2009) The influence of improved air quality on mortality risks in Erfurt, Germany, *Research Reports of the Health Effects Institute,* 137:5–77; discussion 79–90.

Rich, D.Q., George, P., Goodman, P.G. et al. (2009) Effect of air pollution control on mortality in County Cork, Ireland, in *Health Effects Institute Annual Conference.* Boston, MA, Health Effects Institute.

Sugiri, D., Ranft, U., Schikowski, T. and Kramer, U. (2006) The influence of large-scale airborne particle decline and traffic-related exposure on children's lung function, *Environmental Health Perspectives,* 114(2):282–8.

Tonne, C., Beevers, S., Armstrong, B., Kelly, F. and Wilkinson, P. (2008) Air pollution and mortality benefits of the London congestion charge: spatial and socioeconomic inequalities, *Occupational and Environmental Medicine,* 65(9):620–7.

Tonne, C., Beevers, S., Kelly, F.J. et al. (2010) An approach for estimating the health effects of changes over time in air pollution: an illustration using cardio-respiratory hospital admissions in London, *Occupational and Environmental Medicine,* 67(6):422–7.

Transport for London (2004) *Central London Congestion Charging. Impacts Monitoring. Second Annual Report.* London: Transport for London.

Transport for London (2006) *Central London Congestion Charging. Impacts Monitoring. Fourth Annual Report.* London: Transport for London.

United Nations Economic Commission for Europe (1979) *Convention on Long-range Transboundary Air Pollution.* Geneva: United Nations Economic Commission for Europe.

Vestreng, V., Myhre, G., Fagerli, H., Reis, S. and Tarrason, L. (2007) Twenty-five years of continuous sulphur dioxide emission reduction in Europe, *Atmospheric Chemistry and Physics,* 7:5099–5143.

Vestreng, V., Ntziachristos, L., Semb, A. et al. (2009) Evolution of NO_x emissions in Europe with focus on road transport control measures, *Atmospheric Chemistry and Physics,* 9:1503–1520.

WHO Regional Office for Europe (2004) *Health Aspects of Air Pollution. Results of the WHO Project Systematic Review of Health Aspects of Air Pollution in Europe.* Copenhagen: WHO Regional Office for Europe.

World Health Organization (2009) *Global Health Risks: Mortality and Burden of Disease Attributable to Selected Major Risks.* Geneva: World Health Organization.

chapter thirteen

Comparative analysis of national health policies

Johan Mackenbach and Martin McKee

Introduction

The previous chapters have reviewed a number of health policies of proven effectiveness that have been implemented in European countries and have assessed what their population health impacts have been.

There can be no doubt that the population health impacts of these policies have been impressive. In a majority of European countries, and for a range of important causes of death, major declines have occurred that are largely or partly attributable to the implementation of health policies. These must also have contributed importantly to the increases in life expectancy that have occurred over the period 1970–2010. The total health impacts of these successes of health policy will be assessed in Chapter 14.

This chapter will first extend the area-by-area analysis by looking at the results for each country. The area-by-area analyses in Chapters 2 to 12 have covered most of the first three aims of this book. They have allowed an assessment of the extent to which different European countries vary in the implementation of effective health policies and the extent to which differences between European countries in implementation of these policies have impacted on trends and levels of corresponding health outcomes; they have also allowed the identification of some 'best practices' in health policy.

This chapter will go one step further by trying to identify which countries have generally been more successful than others in implementing effective health policies. This needs to be done before the fourth aim of this book, to identify the reasons for successes and failures of health policy in different countries, can be addressed. Subsequent chapters will use the results of the country-by-country analysis in this chapter to indicate opportunities for further health gains in Europe (another topic covered by

Chapter 14) and to analyse conditions for successful health policy-making (Chapter 15).

This comparative analysis can only be done with quantitative data and, therefore, some performance indicators derived from the analyses in the previous chapters will be developed. Both 'process' and 'outcome' indicators will be used, and the latter will make a further distinction between 'intermediate' and 'final' outcomes. Process indicators measure the degree of implementation of effective policies (e.g. by taking a country's score on the Tobacco Control Scale (TCS)). Intermediate outcome indicators measure the impact of these policies on the exposure of the population to health risks (e.g. by taking a country's prevalence of smoking). Final outcome indicators measure the impact on population health (e.g. by taking a country's lung cancer mortality rate).

This chapter is structured as follows. First, the results of the analyses reported in each of the 11 areas covered in the earlier chapters will be considered systematically to identify suitable performance indicators. This will be followed by an inter-country comparison for these performance indicators and the identification of countries that have generally been more successful than others in implementing effective health policies. The chapter will end by drawing a number of general conclusions.

Area-by-area summary

Tobacco

As Chapter 2 has shown, there is convincing evidence for the effectiveness of a range of tobacco control policies, including bans on smoking in public places; assistance to smokers to help them to quit; mass media campaigns and health warnings; bans on tobacco advertising, promotion and sponsorship; and raising tobacco taxes to discourage consumption.

The TCS was developed to measure a country's degree of implementation of these policies, and this shows that some European countries have much stricter tobacco control policies than others. In 2010, of the countries for which rankings are available, the United Kingdom, Ireland, Norway and Iceland had the highest scores, while Hungary, the Czech Republic, Luxembourg and Austria had the lowest scores.

There are large differences between countries in tobacco consumption, as measured by tobacco sales figures and survey-reported smoking. Currently, male smoking prevalence rates are particularly high in the former USSR (Roberts et al. 2012), while female smoking prevalence rates have become rather homogeneous across Europe, with the exception of some countries in the former USSR where female smoking rates have historically been low, although they are now rising (Perlman et al. 2007).

Differences in male smoking among countries partly reflect the impact of tobacco control policies. A country's score on the TCS correlates negatively with male smoking ($r = -0.39$), but not with female smoking ($r = 0.35$) (Fig. 13.1). This is because male smoking declined in many countries while tobacco control

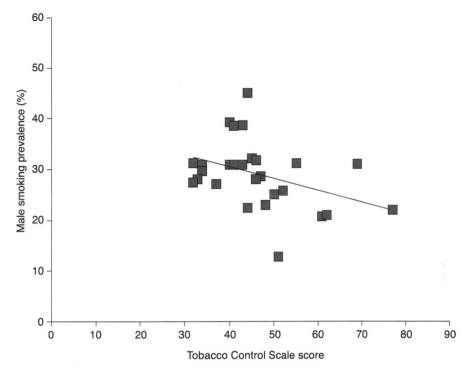

Figure 13.1 Association between a country's score on the Tobacco Control Scale and male smoking prevalence, ca. 2009

Sources: Joossens and Raw 2011; WHO Regional Office for Europe 2012

efforts were building up, and plausibly through these efforts, but female smoking was still on the rise.

There are large differences between countries in lung cancer mortality, the health indicator most closely related to smoking. Male lung cancer mortality rates are very high in some countries in central and eastern Europe and the former USSR, and relatively low in most Nordic countries and in the UK and Ireland. Female lung cancer mortality rates follow a different geographical pattern, with very low rates in southern Europe and many countries of the former USSR. Because of the dynamic nature of smoking trends and the long delay between exposure to tobacco smoke and lung cancer, one cannot expect current tobacco control efforts to be closely related to current lung cancer mortality rates. The latter, however, do reflect the accumulated exposure to smoking over several decades, and male lung cancer mortality rates may, therefore, partly reflect tobacco control efforts in the past (Shkolnikov et al. 1999).

The TCS score, male smoking prevalence rates and male lung cancer mortality rates are used as performance indicators for tobacco control policies. Table 13.1 presents the scores for each country on these indicators in the latest available year.

Table 13.1 Performance indicators by country for tobacco, alcohol and food policies

Country	Tobacco			Alcohol			Food		
	Tobacco Control Scale (0–100)[a]	Male smoking prevalence (%)	Male lung cancer mortality (deaths per 100,000 population)	Alcohol policy score (0–40)[b]	Alcohol consumption (litres per capita)[c]	Male cirrhosis mortality rate (deaths per 100,000 population)	Iodine deficiency (%)[d]	Fat intake (% of total energy intake)	Fruits and vegetable available per year (kg/capita)
Year	2010	2008	2007	2005	2009	2008	<2007	2007	2007
Nordic									
Finland	52	26	45	32	12	29	28	36	172
Sweden	51	13	28	36	9	8	30	36	205
Norway	62	21	45	35	8	5	47	35	220
Iceland	61	21	48		8	3	19	39	222
Denmark	46	28	63	17	13		48	36	209
Britain and Ireland									
United Kingdom	77	22	52	25	13	15	69	38	218
Ireland	69	31	53	26	13	9	56	35	219
Continental									
Netherlands	46	32	68	16	10	6	31	37	239
Belgium	50	25	79	12	12		67	40	201
Luxembourg	33	28	64	6	13	17	33	39	276
Germany	37		54	6	13		39	37	182
Switzerland	48	23	44	14	11	9	36	40	169
Austria	32	27	47	6	13	22	21	39	251

Mediterranean

France	55		62	14	13	16	33	42	214
Spain	46	32	65	8	13	13	35	42	243
Portugal	43	31	43	9	13	17	47	35	287
Italy	47	29	60	10	10	13	50	39	295
Malta	52	26	44	7	8	9		29	318
Greece	32		69	4	11	8	0	37	404
Cyprus	40	39	31	5	10	9	41	39	269
Western Balkans									
Slovenia	44	22	73	10	15	40	24	34	197
Croatia			85		13	39	22	33	193
Bosnia and Herzegovina							22		
Serbia		31	83			17	9	40	211
Montenegro		37	79		13		17	26	234
TFYR Macedonia					7		10	36	256
Albania							57	29	299
Central and eastern									
Poland	43		91	16	14	27	55	30	180
Czech Republic	34	30	71	5	17	25	13	36	144
Slovakia	41		69	9	15	40	15	34	154
Hungary	34		106	14	14	70	57	39	195
Romania	45	32	67	8	16	61	47	28	209
Bulgaria	40		62	7	11	32	11	31	132

(continued)

Table 13.1 (continued)

Country	Tobacco			Alcohol			Food		
	Tobacco Control Scale (0–100)[a]	Male smoking prevalence (%)	Male lung cancer mortality (deaths per 100,000 population)	Alcohol policy score (0–40)[b]	Alcohol consumption (litres per capita)[c]	Male cirrhosis mortality rate (deaths per 100,000 population)	Iodine deficiency (%)[d]	Fat intake (% of total energy intake)	Fruits and vegetable available per year (kg/capita)
Year	2010	2008	2007	2005	2009	2008	<2007	2007	2007
Former USSR									
Estonia	43	39	86	16	14	38	67	25	174
Latvia	44	45	76	14		25	77	36	168
Lithuania	41	39	79	13	13	56	60	27	187
Belarus		53	69				14	33	205
Ukraine		50	60				56	26	153
Republic of Moldova		51	50			106	27	21	108
Russian Federation			74				58	25	184
Georgia			32			29	4	21	102
Armenia		55	85				6	25	394
Azerbaijan		38	17				13	16	222
Average (SD)	46 (10)	32 (10)	62 (19)	14 (9)	12 (2)	26 (22)	35 (20)	33 (6)	217 (63)

Source: All data from WHO Regional Office for Europe (2012) unless specified in notes

Notes: TFYR Macedonia, the Former Yugoslav Republic of Macedonia; SD, standard deviation

[a]Tobacco Control Scale (Joossens and Raw 2011)

[b]Bridging the Gap Alcohol Policy score (Karlsson and Österberg 2007)

[c]Including unrecorded consumption (Anderson et al. 2012)

[d]Urinary iodine <100 µg/l (Andersson et al. 2007)

Alcohol

The harm attributable to alcohol is preventable and, as Chapter 3 has shown, there is a range of effective alcohol control policies. The three 'best buys' for alcohol control policy are price increase, limits on availability and bans on advertising (Edwards 1994). Various scales have been developed to measure the tightness and comprehensiveness of a country's alcohol control policies. These scales differ in their emphasis on different aspects of alcohol control but all show that northern European countries have stronger alcohol control policies than southern and central and eastern European, except that the last has relatively stringent drink driving controls.

There is a more than three-fold difference in recorded alcohol consumption between European countries. Estimates of unrecorded alcohol consumption are also available for many countries (but not for most of the former USSR, however), but if these are added to officially recorded alcohol consumption, the pattern of variation among countries remains largely the same. Alcohol consumption is relatively low in some northern and southern European countries (Rehm et al. 2006).

Differences between countries in alcohol consumption partly reflect the impact of alcohol policies. A country's score on one of the alcohol policy scales is negatively correlated with measures of alcohol consumption, as shown in Fig. 3.5 (p. 53).

There are also large differences between countries in cirrhosis mortality, the available health indicator most closely related to alcohol consumption. Male and female cirrhosis mortality rates are relatively high in the western Balkans, central and eastern Europe and the former USSR. These mortality rates are likely to reflect both the short- and the long-term health impacts of alcohol and may, therefore, partly reflect the impact of alcohol policies in the past.

The Bridging the Gap Alcohol Policy score, alcohol consumption in litres per capita (including unrecorded consumption) and male cirrhosis mortality are used as performance indicators for alcohol control policy. Table 13.1 shows the scores for each country on these indicators in the latest available year.

Food and nutrition

Although deficiency diseases have largely been eliminated, Chapter 4 has shown that iodine deficiency remains a problem in many European countries as a result of neglect of the most effective and sustainable countermeasure, iodization of salt.

There are large differences between countries in the percentage of the population with inadequate iodine intake. This varies between <20% in several countries in eastern Europe and >50% in the United Kingdom and Ireland, Belgium, Poland, Hungary, the Baltic states, Ukraine and the Russian Federation. These variations are likely to be partly caused by natural variations in iodine content of water and locally grown foods and partly to the use of iodized salt. There is a reasonably strong association between the penetration of iodized salt

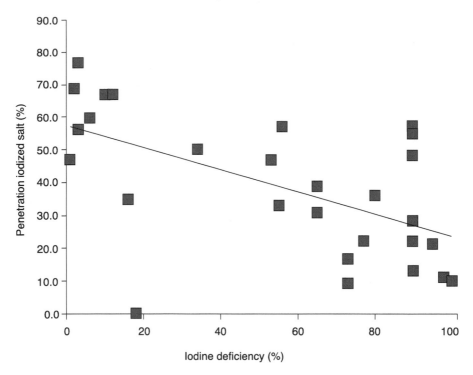

Figure 13.2   Association between penetration of iodized salt and prevalence of iodine deficiency, ca. 2008

Source: Calculated from Andersson et al. (2007)

in a country and the prevalence of iodine deficiency (Fig. 13.2). We will use the prevalence of iodine deficiency as a policy performance indicator.

Food policies that tackle nutrition-related risks of cardiovascular diseases were also reviewed in Chapter 4. Effective interventions to reduce fat and salt intake and to increase fruit and vegetable intake are available (Pomerleau et al. 2005), but evidence for population-level impacts could only be found in a few country-specific case studies, partly because national data on the implementation of these policies are not available. Nevertheless, some trends in food intake, for example intake of saturated fats, fruits and vegetables and salt, have been favourable in many European countries, probably partly as a result of health policies promoting better diets.

Currently, there are large differences between countries in food intake. Fat consumption (as a percentage of total energy intake) is relatively high in southern Europe, central and eastern Europe and the former USSR. The population average intake of salt is above recommended levels in all countries, but is particularly high in some central and eastern European countries. Fruit and vegetable consumption is traditionally highest in the Mediterranean region, and lowest in central and eastern Europe and the former USSR.

The available health indicator most closely related to these health policies is, of course, ischaemic heart disease mortality, but while this does correlate

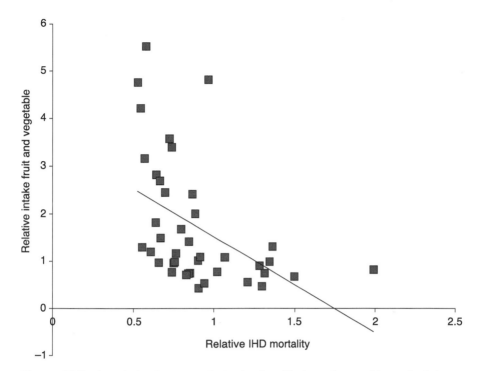

Figure 13.3 Association between relative intake of fruits and vegetables and relative mortality from ischaemic heart disease (IHD) (in both cases, value for European Union as a whole taken as 1), ca. 2008

Source: WHO Regional Office for Europe 2012

with fruit and vegetable consumption at the population level (Fig. 13.3), as it does at the individual level (Lock et al. 2005), ischaemic heart disease mortality is influenced by many other determinants, including smoking, risk factor detection and treatment, and medical care; therefore, this lack of association should not be interpreted literally.

For policies that tackle nutrition-related risks of cardiovascular diseases, fat intake and fruit and vegetable consumption will be used as performance indicators. Table 13.1 shows the scores for each country on these indicators in the latest available year.

Fertility, pregnancy and childbirth

Chapter 5 reviewed a wide range of policies regarding mother and child health and identified a number of effective policies, including access to contraception and safe abortion, prevention of multiple births in assisted reproduction, protection of pregnant women and children, smoking cessation during pregnancy, screening for congenital anomalies during pregnancy, access to safe delivery care and promotion of breastfeeding.

Information on national implementation of these policies was mostly limited to a narrow range of countries, but there were large differences in access to safe abortion, use of elective single embryo transfers, maternal and paternal leave arrangements, screening for congenital anomalies and delivery in breastfeeding-friendly hospitals.

There are also large differences between countries in a number of intermediate outcomes. Rates of induced abortion and teenage pregnancy are very high in many countries in the western Balkans, central and eastern Europe and the former USSR. Multiple birth rates vary between 2.5 and 4%, with high rates in the Czech Republic and Spain. Smoking during pregnancy varies between 5 and 25%, with high rates in Scotland and France. The prevalence of congenital anomalies at birth is high in Ireland and Malta. The percentage of babies breastfed at birth varies between 2% in France and 100% in Sweden.

Chapter 5 showed that some of these variations are likely to reflect variations in policy: multiple birth rates are lower in countries with a higher proportion of elective single embryo transfers; neonatal mortality from congenital anomalies is lower in countries with more extensive screening; and breastfeeding initiation rates are higher in countries with more deliveries in breastfeeding-friendly hospitals.

There are large differences between countries in health outcomes among children (as measured by perinatal mortality, fetal mortality, neonatal mortality and infant mortality for example) and mothers (as measured by maternal mortality). These indicators reflect the combined effect of between-country differences in background risk, in preventive activities and in medical care during pregnancy and childbirth, and should, therefore, be interpreted with caution. They are, however, also strongly related to intermediate outcomes of health policy, such as teenage pregnancies (Fig. 13.4).

It is necessary to limit performance indicators to those that are available for a reasonably large number of countries. Three indicators have been selected: one for health policies related to fertility (proportion of teenage pregnancies), one for health policies related to pregnancy (neonatal mortality) and one related to childbirth (maternal mortality). Table 13.2 presents these indicators for the latest available year.

Child health

Chapter 6 reviewed a wide range of child health policies: vaccination against diphtheria and measles, prevention of drowning and prevention of SIDS. It showed that effective health policies are available to reduce considerably the risk of morbidity or mortality from these causes.

Although there has been a gradual convergence of child vaccination programmes between European countries, there still are some important differences, for example in their organization (e.g. some countries have highly centralized systems and others decentralized). More importantly, however, there are large differences in intermediate outcomes as measured through actual immunization rates. As illustrated in Chapter 6, diphtheria immunization rates

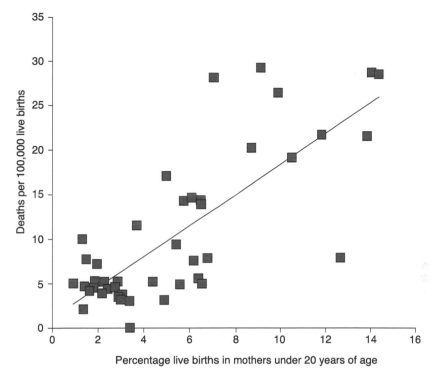

Figure 13.4 Association between teenage pregnancies and maternal mortality, ca. 2008

Source: WHO Regional Office for Europe 2012

plummeted in the 1990s in the former USSR as a result of system breakdown. Measles immunization decreased around the year 2000 in the United Kingdom and several other western European countries as a result of unfounded concerns among parents about the safety of vaccination. Currently, immunization rates are still suboptimal in many countries, with immunization rates below 95% for measles in Denmark, the United Kingdom, Ireland, Austria and Malta. In some other countries, such as Germany, the absence of a systematic immunization programme means that data are simply estimates and cannot be used in a timely manner to identify underserved groups. Incidence rates of diphtheria and measles also differ between countries, and during the 1990s, when immunization rates decreased in many countries in the European region, between-country differences in incidence clearly reflected the differences in immunization rates (Fig. 13.5).

A scoring system has been developed to summarize a country's degree of implementation of child safety policies. European countries appear to differ significantly in the implementation of these policies. Greece, Portugal and Spain have implemented relatively few policies, while Iceland, the Netherlands and Sweden have implemented many. Intermediate outcome data, in the form of safety behaviour, for example, are not available in this area, but countries

Table 13.2 Performance indicators by country for fertility/pregnancy/childbirth, child health and infectious disease control policies

Country	Fertility, pregnancy and childbirth			Child health			Infectious diseases		
	Percentage teenage pregnancies	Neonatal mortality (deaths per 1000 live births)	Maternal mortality (deaths per 100,000 live births)	Measles immunization rate (%)	Safety score[a]	Postneonatal mortality (deaths per 1000 live births)	AIDS incidence (new cases/100,000 population)	MRSA (% insensitive to methicillin)[b]	Influenza vaccination (%)[c]
Year	2008	2009	2007–9	2008	2009	2009	2009	2010	2008
Nordic									
Finland	2.2	2.0	3.9	99	39	0.6	0.5	0.4	47
Sweden	1.6	1.6	4.2	98	43	0.9	0.7	0.3	55
Norway	2.4	2.1	4.5	94		1.0	0.4	0.0	
Iceland	3.4	1.0	0.0	98	49	0.8	0.6	0.0	
Denmark	1.5	2.7	7.8	89		0.7	0.7	0.0	53
Britain and Ireland									
United Kingdom	6.2	3.2	7.6	92	40	1.5	1.2	5.7	73
Ireland	3.0	2.3	3.2	93	31	1.0	0.6	2.5	
Continental									
Netherlands	1.4	2.9	4.7	97	46	1.0	1.5	2.6	61
Belgium	2.8	2.6		99	30	1.4	1.1	2.1	
Luxembourg	1.8	1.4		99		0.7	1.4	18.2	82
Germany	2.3	2.6	5.2		39	1.3	0.6	0.2	63
Switzerland	0.9	3.1	5.0			0.9	1.9		51
Austria	3.3	2.5	3.0	83	41	1.3	0.8	1.7	65

(continued)

Mediterranean

France	2.0	2.4	7.2	98	40	1.1	1.6	0.2	
Spain	2.9	2.1	3.4	97	29	1.2	3.0	1.1	
Portugal	4.4	3.4	5.3	97	28	1.6	5.1	17.3	67
Italy	1.4	2.5	2.2	72	30	1.0	1.6	13.2	67
Malta	6.8	5.7	7.9			2.4	2.2	0.0	50
Greece	2.8	2.0		99	27	1.1	0.9	3.2	66
Cyprus	1.8	1.9		97	32	1.4	1.5	5.9	
Western Balkans									
Slovenia	1.3	1.6	10.0	97	41	0.8	0.5	2.2	
Croatia	3.7	4.3	11.6	96		1.0	0.3		
Bosnia and Herzegovina	10.5	10.5	19.2			4.1			28
Serbia	6.5	4.9	13.9	95		2.1	0.5	0.5	
Montenegro	5.7	4.1		95		1.7	0.5		
TFYR Macedonia	6.5	8.6		95		3.2	0.4		
Albania	5.0	2.5	17.1	99		5.3	0.8		
Central and eastern									
Poland	4.9	4.0	3.1	99		1.6	0.4	3.0	
Czech Republic	3.1	1.6	3.7		42	1.2	0.3	1.2	
Slovakia	6.6	3.1	5.0	99		2.6	0.0		9
Hungary	6.1	3.4	14.7	100	37	1.7	0.2	1.1	
Romania	11.8	5.5	21.7			4.3	1.0		29
Bulgaria	12.7	5.0	7.9	95		3.6	0.4	4.7	33

Table 13.2 (continued)

Country	Fertility, pregnancy and childbirth			Child health			Infectious diseases		
	Percentage teenage pregnancies	Neonatal mortality (deaths per 1000 live births)	Maternal mortality (deaths per 100,000 live births)	Measles immunization rate (%)	Safety score[a]	Postneonatal mortality (deaths per 1000 live births)	AIDS incidence (new cases/100,000 population)	MRSA (% insensitive to methicillin)[b]	Influenza vaccination (%)[c]
Year	2008	2009	2007–9	2008	2009	2009	2009	2010	2008
Former USSR									
Estonia	5.4	3.2		95	35	1.8	4.6	13.5	
Latvia	7.0	5.0	28.2	97	34	2.7	4.6	5.3	
Lithuania	5.6	2.8	4.9	96	33	2.1	1.6	12.5	
Belarus	6.4	3.1	5.6	97		3.8	4.0		
Ukraine	8.7	5.6	20.2	91		4.1	2.4		
Republic of Moldova	9.9	7.8	26.4	96		4.3	2.6		
Russian Federation	13.8	6.4	21.7	98		4.7			
Georgia	14.0	11.8	28.6	92		3.1	5.3		
Armenia	9.1	8.1	29.2	89		3.7	2.6		
Azerbaijan	14.3	6.0	28.5	95		3.8	0.7		
Average (SD)	**5.4 (3.8)**	**3.9 (2.4)**	**11.0 (8.9)**	**95 (5)**	**36 (6)**	**2.1 (1.3)**	**1.5 (1.4)**	**4.4 (5.4)**	**53 (18)**

Source: All data from WHO Regional Office for Europe (2012) unless specified in notes
Notes: MRSA, methicillin-resistant Staphylococcus aureus; TFYR Macedonia, the former Yugoslavian Republic of Macedonia; SD, standard deviation
[a]Child Safety Alliance safety grade (European Child Safety Alliance 2009)
[b]European Centre for Disease Control and Prevention 2012.
[c]Coverage among those 65 years and older (O'Flanagan et al. 2009)

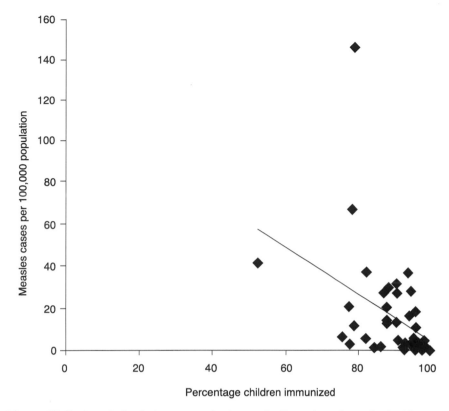

Figure 13.5 Association between measles immunization rate and measles incidence during the 1990s

Source: WHO Regional Office for Europe 2012

do differ in their final health outcomes, in the form of death rates from, for example, drowning. Some of these variations in health outcomes reflect variations in policy, as suggested by the negative correlation between a country's safety score and its rate of child mortality from drowning.

According to the case studies presented in Chapter 6, there have also been large differences between countries in the speed with which they have implemented policies to promote a supine sleeping position of infants, which helps to reduce the risk of sudden infant death. Although there are no internationally comparable data on the implementation of these policies or the associated behaviour change among parents, the fact that differences in timing of the policy change were reflected in time trends for mortality rates from SIDS (see Fig. 6.6) suggests that this can be used as a performance indicator. A preliminary review identified many inaccuracies in certification and coding of SIDS, and so the analyses here will use postneonatal mortality.

The following health policy performance indicators will be used for this area: measles immunization rate, child safety score and postneonatal mortality rate. Table 13.2 shows these indicators for the latest available year.

Infectious diseases

In addition to vaccination against childhood diseases, Chapter 7 reviewed infectious disease control policies in the field of HIV/AIDS, influenza, BSE, SARS and MRSA.

In the case of AIDS, the chapter identified several policies that are effective in reducing transmission, such as campaigns promoting safe sex, needle exchange programmes for intravenous drug users, and safe blood supply systems. In western Europe, some countries have responded rapidly and effectively, while other countries found it difficult to mount an effective response because of prevailing cultural attitudes to the major risk factors. Response was also delayed in central and eastern Europe and the former USSR. As a result, the course of the epidemic has differed significantly between countries. Currently, the incidence of HIV infection is very high in Ukraine, Estonia and the Republic of Moldova, and very low in Cyprus, Greece and the Netherlands. While some of this variation is likely to reflect other factors, such as the numbers of migrants (Del Amo et al. 2011), there is no doubt that it also partly indicates the success or lack of success of AIDS control policies.

For influenza, Chapter 7 identified vaccination as a (probably) effective strategy to reduce complications from influenza in vulnerable groups, such as the elderly. Although influenza vaccination of the elderly is recommended in most European countries, there are large differences in vaccination coverage. The percentage of elderly people immunized against influenza varies between 9% in Slovakia and 82% in Luxembourg. As Fig. 13.6 shows, there is a (weak) association between vaccination coverage and mortality from influenza in Europe.

While BSE and SARS were localized incidents and, therefore, do not lend themselves easily to systematic between-country comparisons, MRSA does. Effective policies to prevent drug resistance developing in *S. aureus* include restraint in the use of antibiotics, active surveillance and a 'search and destroy' strategy. Chapter 7 showed that European countries differ substantially in their implementation of these measures, and that between-country variations in the prevalence of MRSA in isolates of hospital patients reflect these policy variations.

Performance indicators for infectious disease control will be AIDS incidence, prevalence of MRSA isolates and influenza vaccination coverage. Table 13.2 shows these indicators for the latest available year.

Hypertension

Hypertension is a silent killer against which effective countermeasures are available, both in the field of primary prevention (including salt reduction and physical exercise) and in the field of secondary prevention (detection and treatment of hypertension in the asymptomatic phase). Chapter 8 has shown secondary prevention is effective in preventing the cardiovascular complications of hypertension, including stroke.

Compliance by health professionals with modern guidelines for the detection and treatment of hypertension has increased considerably in western Europe.

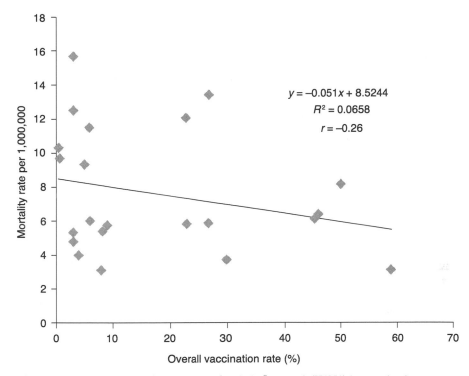

Figure 13.6 Association between pandemic influenza A (H1N1) immunization rate and cumulative mortality rate from pandemic influenza, 2009–2010

Sources: Kindly provided by Ralf Reintjes based on Mereckiene et al. (2012) and data from the European Centre for Disease Prevention and Control (http://www.ecdc.europa. eu, accessed 25 April 2012)

Simultaneously, awareness, treatment and control of hypertension in the population have increased. Comparative data on implementation of hypertension detection and control in different European countries are not available. What is known, however, is that implementation lags far behind in eastern Europe.

There are also large differences in prevalence of hypertension between European countries, and average systolic blood pressure tends to be lower in western Europe than in central and eastern Europe and the former USSR. While these variations may be caused by several factors, it is likely that, in part, differences in the implementation of hypertension detection and control are involved. The lower rates in western Europe result from a decline in blood pressure that has occurred over the past decades, and studies in some countries have shown that improved detection and control played at least some role in this decline.

There are also large differences between countries in mortality from cerebrovascular disease, the available health indicator most closely related to hypertension. Stroke mortality is much higher in central and eastern Europe than in western Europe, where rates have declined considerably from 1970 to 2010.

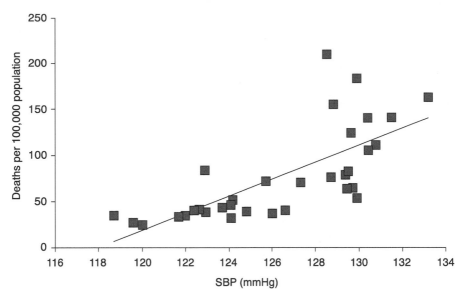

Figure 13.7 Association between average systolic blood pressure (SBP) and stroke mortality, women, ca. 2008

Sources: Danaei et al. 2011; WHO Regional Office for Europe 2012

Rates of stroke mortality are correlated with average blood pressure (Fig. 13.7), and the decline of stroke mortality has been stronger in countries with greater declines in blood pressure, supporting the idea that patterns of stroke mortality partly reflect progress in the management of hypertension.

Average systolic blood pressure among men and female mortality from cerebrovascular disease will be used as performance indicators. Table 13.3 presents these indicators for the latest available year.

Cancer screening

According to expert reviews and recommendations, three forms of cancer screening are effective in reducing mortality: cervical cancer, breast cancer and colon cancer screening. The last has not yet been implemented on a large enough scale to be analysed quantitatively, but the first two are, as shown in Chapter 9.

European countries differ in important ways in the implementation of effective cancer screening programmes. In order for cancer screening to have a population health impact, it is essential to reach a large proportion of the target group at risk: that is, to have a population-based national programme. Cervical cancer screening has been implemented on a national scale and using a population-based approach in all the Nordic countries, in the United Kingdom and in the Netherlands. Breast cancer screening has been implemented at a national level and using a population-based approach in most of the

Table 13.3 Performance indicators by country for hypertension, cancer screening, road traffic safety and air pollution policies

Countries	Hypertension		Cancer screening		Road traffic safety			Air pollution	
	Male average systolic blood pressure (mmHg)[a]	Female stroke mortality (deaths per 100,000)	Breast screening[b]	Cervical cancer mortality (deaths per 100,000)	Seat-belt use (%)[c]	Car occupant RTT deaths[d]	Pedestrian RTT deaths[e]	Annual SO₂ emission (tonnes/1000 persons)[f]	Urban ozone (μg/m³ per day)[g]
Year	2008	2008	<2000	2008	2007	2007	2007	2009	2009
Nordic									
Finland	135	40	2	1.5	89	0.9	0.2	11.1	1689
Sweden	132	39	2	2.3	96	0.7	0.1	3.2	2013
Norway	135	37	2	3.0	93	0.8	0.1	3.3	879
Iceland	130	35	2	0.0	88	1.2	0.1		
Denmark	130		1	3.1				2.7	2446
Britain and Ireland									
United Kingdom	131	45	2	2.6	91	0.6	0.2	6.5	1123
Ireland	135	39	1	4.7	86	1.2	0.4	7.4	1197
Continental									
Netherlands	131	34	2	2.4	94	0.5	0.1	2.3	1360
Belgium	129		1	3.5	79	1.2	0.2	7.1	2787
Luxembourg	131	40	2					6.3	
Germany	133		1	2.9	95	0.6	0.1	5.5	3130
Switzerland	131	27	1	1.2	86	0.5	0.2	1.7	4701
Austria	131	32	1	2.9	89	1.0	0.3	2.5	5097

(continued)

Table 13.3 (continued)

Countries	Hypertension		Cancer screening		Road traffic safety				Air pollution	
	Male average systolic blood pressure (mmHg)[a]	Female stroke mortality (deaths per 100,000)	Breast screening[b]	Cervical cancer mortality (deaths per 100,000)	Seat-belt use (%)[c]	Car occupant RTI deaths[d]	Pedestrian RTI deaths[e]	Annual SO_2 emission (tonnes/1000 persons)[f]	Urban ozone ($\mu g/m^3$ per day)[g]
Year	2008	2008	<2000	2008	2007	2007	2007	2009	2009
Mediterranean										
France	131	24	2	2.3	98	0.9	0.2	4.9	3859
Spain	130	34	2	2.6	89	1.2	0.3	9.4	5207
Portugal	135	70	1	4.8	90	1.1	0.3	7.2	3268
Italy	131	43	1	2.0	65	0.8	0.2	3.8	6196
Malta	132	51	0	2.4	96	0.2	0.2	18.0	
Greece	129	83	1	2.2	75	1.6	0.5	38.0	8084
Cyprus	131	41	2	1.7	81	1.1	0.4	21.5	
Western Balkans										
Slovenia	136	53	1	3.5	85	1.9	0.3	5.7	4959
Croatia	136	105	0	5.5		2.1	0.8		
Bosnia and Herzegovina			0	5.0		4.6	1.8		
Serbia	137	140		12.5	55	3.7	1.6		
Montenegro	135	78	0	8.5		5.2	1.4		
TFYR Macedonia	134		0	13.4		2.6	2.1		
Albania	134		0	4.2	30	8.5	7.5		

Central and eastern

Poland	135	64	1	7.8	74	2.1	1.4	22.6	3112
Czech Republic	134	71	2	5.2	90	1.8	0.6	16.6	4288
Slovakia	136	82	0	6.5		2.8	1.9	11.8	8051
Hungary	136	76	1	7.8	71	2.2	0.9	8.0	6809
Romania	133	154	0	16.2	80	5.5	0.8	21.4	4420
Bulgaria	133	163	0	9.1		3.3	1.3	86.5	3265
Former USSR									
Estonia	139	63	2	7.9	90	2.5	0.7	40.9	1675
Latvia	137	123	1	9.9	77	2.5	1.9	1.8	1260
Lithuania	137	110	1	11.5		2.6	1.5	10.8	2304
Belarus	137		0	6.6		3.1	2.6		
Ukraine	137	141	0	8.3					
Republic of Moldova	134	184	0	10.4		9.9	5.9		
Russian Federation	132	210	0	8.1	33	8.0	4.6		
Georgia			0	6.3			4.3		
Armenia			0	12.3		8.7	5.7		
Azerbaijan			0	7.0		10.8	6.9		
Average (SD)	**133 (3)**	**77 (49)**	**N/A**	**5.8 (3.8)**	**81 (17)**	**2.8 (2.8)**	**1.5 (2.0)**	**13.4 (17.0)**	**3584 (2058)**

Source: All data from WHO Regional Office for Europe (2012) unless specified otherwise in notes

Notes: TFYR Macedonia, the former Yugoslavian Republic of Macedonia; SD, standard deviation; N/A, not available

[a] Danaei et al. 2011

[b] Screening implementation: 0, no established programme; 1, regional programme or non-population-based national programme; 2, population-based national programme (von Karsa et al. 2008)

[c] Seat-belt wearing among front seat car occupants (WHO Regional Office for Europe 2009)

[d] Deaths from road traffic injury among car occupants, per 10,000 registered vehicles (calculated from data in WHO Regional Office for Europe, 2009)

[e] Deaths from road traffic injury among pedestrians, per 10,000 registered vehicles (calculated from data in WHO Regional Office for Europe 2009)

[f] Sulphur dioxide (Eurostat web site)

[g] Urban population exposure to air pollution by ozone (source: Eurostat web site add ref)

Nordic countries (with the exception of Denmark), the United Kingdom, the Netherlands, France, Spain, Cyprus, the Czech Republic and Estonia.

It has not been possible to study intermediate outcomes (i.e. screening participation rates), but final outcomes (i.e. mortality from cervical and breast cancer) could be examined. Cervical cancer mortality is higher in the eastern parts of Europe than in the western parts. Breast cancer mortality, however, has a different pattern of variation. It is lower in Mediterranean countries and in central and eastern Europe, and higher in the United Kingdom and Ireland, the continental region and the former USSR.

When European countries are stratified into three groups on the basis of their national income and geographical location, and cervical cancer mortality is compared within these groups between countries with and without a cervical cancer screening programme, those countries without a screening programme generally have higher mortality (Table 13.4). The same is true for breast cancer mortality; however, it is known from other sources that recent breast cancer mortality declines have also been determined by improvements in treatment.

The implementation of national population-based breast cancer screening and cervical cancer mortality rates will be used as performance indicators. Table 13.3 shows the performance of each country on these indicators.

Table 13.4 Differences in mortality from cervical and breast cancer between countries with and without systematic cancer screening

Europe area	Cervical cancer deaths per 100,000		Breast cancer deaths per 100,000	
	With screening	Without screening	With screening	Without screening
North	2.23	3.04	20.01	22.43
South	2.90	6.65	18.60	21.05
East	8.21	9.40	18.75	22.74

Source: Calculated from von Karsa et al. (2008) and WHO Regional Office for Europe (2012)

Mental health

Mental health policy is bedevilled by a lack of comparative data. The one exception is suicide deaths. Suicide rates have been falling across Europe until recently, although this trend has recently reversed, coinciding with the introduction of austerity policies (Stuckler et al. 2011). The reasons for the changes in suicide rates are not fully explained by existing research but seem likely to include broad welfare policies and reductions in access to the means of committing suicide, as well as other factors. It has not been possible to identify any reliable measure of mental health policies for use in European comparisons. In view of these uncertainties, no performance indicators will be used to compare countries for the area of mental health.

Road traffic safety

Road traffic safety policies are highly effective in reducing injury and, particularly, deaths. Substantial health gains have been achieved through improvements in road behaviour and in the design and safety of vehicles, equipment and road environments.

Reports by WHO, summarized in Chapter 11, suggest that European countries differ importantly in their road traffic safety policies. While differences in legislation have become rather small, there are important differences in law enforcement. There are also large differences in road infrastructure and vehicle safety. Unfortunately, no objective indicators of road traffic safety policies covering a large number of European countries are available. The analysis here will, therefore, focus on intermediate outcomes.

Despite the fact that seat-belt wearing (among car occupants) and helmet wearing (among motorcyclists) are both compulsory in all European countries, there are large variations in their use across Europe, probably as a result of differences in enforcement. Independently observed seat-belt wearing on front seats ranges from an extremely low 33% in the Russian Federation to an admirably high 96% in Sweden. Observed motorcycle helmet wearing is only 58% in Greece, but 100% in Switzerland and Norway.

The death rate from RTIs, as determined on the basis of police records, also varies substantially between countries, as do the death rates among different types of traffic participant. When death rates among car drivers and passengers are adjusted for the number of registered vehicles per country, they can be seen to be very high in the former USSR and the western Balkans. Some of these variations are likely to be caused by differences in enforcement of seat-belt and motorcycle helmet laws, as shown by Figures 11.1 and 11.2 (pp. 222 and 223).

Wearing seat-belts, the death rate among car drivers and passengers (adjusted for the number of registered vehicles) and the death rate among pedestrians (adjusted for the number of registered vehicles) will be used as performance indicators. Table 13.3 shows the performance of each country on these indicators.

Air pollution

Partly as a result of air pollution control measures, emission reductions have been achieved for sulphur dioxide, particulate matter and nitrogen oxides. As Chapter 12 has documented, air concentrations of sulphur dioxide and nitrogen oxides have declined, but it is unclear to what extent air concentrations of particulate matter (PM2.5) and ozone have declined as well.

We have not been able to find country-specific data on the implementation of air pollution control policies, but data on emissions and concentrations of various pollutants are available and suggest large differences in the success with which countries have reduced emissions. Several countries of southern and central and eastern Europe have been unable to reduce their sulphur dioxide emissions substantially, and currently the highest concentrations of sulphur dioxide in the air are mainly found in central and eastern Europe. Reductions in emissions of nitrogen oxides have also differed substantially among countries, partly because of differences in turnover of the vehicle fleet. High concentrations of nitrogen dioxide are found in urban centres across Europe.

Although it is quite likely that emission reductions and improvements in air quality have impacted on population health in Europe, there are no specific health outcomes that can be used as indicators. Air pollution has been linked to ischaemic heart disease and deaths from chronic obstructive pulmonary disease, but both are also strongly determined by other factors, such as smoking.

Sulphur dioxide emissions and urban ozone concentrations will be used as performance indicators. Table 13.3 shows the performance of each country on these indicators. Sulphur dioxide emissions (in tonnes per 1000 persons per year) are relatively high in Greece, Cyprus, Poland, Romania, Bulgaria and Estonia; for most of the former USSR, no comparable data are available. Exposure of urban populations to ozone is relatively high in Switzerland and Austria, and in many countries in Mediterranean and central and eastern Europe.

Country-by-country comparison

Overview of summary scores

The performance indicators for each policy area presented in Tables 13.1, 13.2 and 13.3 allowed us to calculate, for each country, a summary score indicating its relative success across all these areas. This summary score was constructed by determining, for each indicator, whether the country was in the upper, middle or lower tertile of the distribution, and by taking the difference between the percentage of scores in the upper tertile and the percentage of scores in the lower tertile. The results are shown in Table 13.5.

These summary scores can only be a crude indicator of a country's relative success. Each of the underlying performance indicators may have measurement problems and there are other factors that influence them, such as exposure to risk factors that are not targeted by health policies or the quality of a country's health care system. However, as long as the focus is on the big picture, this table provides an overall indication of the success of countries in implementing effective health policies.

First, this overall picture will be described briefly before discussing the performance of individual countries compared with others in the same region. The main reason for these region-wise comparisons is that it is probably less informative to compare countries with a high level of prosperity and a long tradition of public health policies, such as Norway, with countries that are much poorer and have only recently entered the EU, such as Bulgaria.

The overall picture that emerges from Table 13.5 is that there are important differences within Europe in health policy performance. The countries with overall best performance are Sweden (a difference of 89 percentage points between the percentage of indicators in the upper tertile and the percentage of indicators in the lower tertile), Norway (84 percentage points) and Iceland

Table 13.5 Summary scores for health policy performance

Country	Summary scores[a]			
	Observations	% in upper tertile	% in lower tertile	Difference (percentage points)
Nordic				
Finland	27	67	4	63
Sweden	27	89	0	89
Norway	25	84	0	84
Iceland	23	83	4	78
Denmark	21	48	5	43
Britain and Ireland				
United Kingdom	27	48	11	37
Ireland	26	46	8	38
Continental				
Netherlands	27	59	4	56
Belgium	23	35	17	17
Luxembourg	20	45	20	25
Germany	23	52	17	35
Switzerland	24	58	13	46
Austria	27	67	19	48
Mediterranean				
France	25	56	4	52
Spain	26	50	15	35
Portugal	27	33	15	19
Italy	26	54	23	31
Malta	24	54	13	42
Greece	25	40	24	16
Cyprus	24	54	21	33
Western Balkans				
Slovenia	26	35	19	15
Croatia	18	11	28	−17
Bosnia and Herzegovina	10	10	70	−60
Serbia	18	11	28	−17
Montenegro	17	18	35	−18
TFYR Macedonia	14	21	21	0
Albania	15	33	47	−13
Central and eastern				
Poland	24	17	21	−4
Czech Republic	25	32	20	12
Slovakia	23	17	35	−17

(continued)

Table 13.5 (*continued*)

Country	Summary scores[a]			
	Observations	% in upper tertile	% in lower tertile	Difference (percentage points)
Hungary	25	12	40	−28
Romania	24	8	50	−42
Bulgaria	24	8	42	−33
Former USSR				
Estonia	25	12	44	−32
Latvia	25	4	36	−32
Lithuania	25	12	40	−28
Belarus	16	13	38	−25
Ukraine	15	7	80	−73
Republic of Moldova	18	17	72	−56
Russian Federation	16	13	81	−69
Georgia	14	14	64	−50
Armenia	15	13	80	−67
Azerbaijan	15	20	53	−33
Average (SD)	**22 (5)**	**34 (23)**	**30 (23)**	**5 (43)**

Notes: TFYR Macedonia, the former Yugoslavian Republic of Macedonia; SD, standard deviation
[a]Summary scores were calculated from data in Tables 13.1 to 13.3. First, the total number of observations was determined. Then, for all available scores for each country, the percentage of scores falling in the upper tertile and the percentage falling in the lower tertile were calculated. Finally, a summary score was calculated for each country as the difference between the percentage of scores falling in the upper and the lower tertile

(78 percentage points). The countries with the worst overall performance are Ukraine (−73 percentage points), Russian Federation (−69 percentage points) and Armenia (−67 percentage points). These countries do better, or worse, than other countries for a wide range of policies.

These countries often combine better (or worse) 'process' indicators (such as scores for tobacco and alcohol control or the implementation of cancer screening) with better 'intermediate' and 'final' outcome indicators. As Tables 13.1, 13.2, and 13.3 show, Sweden, Norway and Iceland not only have good health outcomes but also have relatively high scores on the available 'process' indicators (the TCS, the Bridging the Gap Alcohol Policy score, the Child Safety score and breast cancer screening implementation).

Because countries are ordered in regional groups, it is easy to see that countries in the north on the whole do better than countries in the east: positive values for the summary score dominate the upper half of the table, while negative values dominate the lower half. There are, however, some interesting exceptions, which will be highlighted in the following sections.

One limitation of the performance indicators in Tables 13.1, 13.2, and 13.3 is that there are quite a few missing data, and that these do not occur completely at random: they tend to be more frequent in countries with lower scores on the available indicators. Therefore, a sensitivity analysis was carried out by imputing, for each country, all its missing data on the basis of the average value for the indicator in its region. For example, for a missing value in Denmark, the average of the other Nordic countries would be used, and for a missing value in Azerbaijan the average value for other countries of the former USSR would be used. This sensitivity analysis showed that country rankings were sufficiently robust (correlation coefficient between summary scores shown in Table 13.5 and summary scores partly based on imputed data is 0.98).

Nordic countries, the United Kingdom and Ireland, and continental Europe

As a group, the Nordic countries perform best, with usually good scores in all ten areas, but this group is not homogeneous. Denmark stands out as a country with a performance that is distinctly worse than that of other countries in this group (summary score of 43%). It has an average performance in many areas, including tobacco and alcohol, and its performance on measles immunization even falls in the lower tertile (see Tables 13.1, 13.2 and 13.3).

The performance of the United Kingdom is considerably below that of the Nordic countries, and similar to that of Ireland. The United Kingdom does not perform well on iodine deficiency, on fat consumption and on measles immunization (see Tables 13.1, 13.2 and 13.3). Ireland is not doing well on iodine deficiency and hypertension.

Among the continental European countries, the Netherlands does best, but it does dot not have a uniformly high level of performance and, therefore, scores lower (56%) than most of the Nordic countries, with the exception of Denmark. In this group, performance in the field of tobacco and alcohol control and indicators in the area of food are also often relatively low (see Tables 13.1, 13.2 and 13.3). Belgium (17%) performs worst in this group.

Mediterranean countries and western Balkans

As a group, the Mediterranean countries do only slightly less well than the continental European countries, which is remarkable given their shorter traditions of modern public health. They do less well on child safety. Again, this group is not homogeneous. France does best (52 percentage points) and Portugal has the worst performance (19 percentage points).

The countries in the western Balkans differ strongly in their performance. Bosnia and Herzegovina performs worst (–60 percentage points), while Slovenia performs best (15 percentage points). Albania scores better than expected on the basis of its low level of income, because of its favourable fat and fruit intake and high measles immunization rate, among other things.

Central and eastern Europe and the former USSR

The country in central and eastern Europe that scores best is the Czech Republic (12 percentage points). This is because of its good scores on a wide range of indicators: iodine deficiency, teenage pregnancy, postneonatal mortality, maternal mortality, child safety and AIDS incidence (see Tables 13.1, 13.2 and 13.3). Romania, by comparison, is among the worst performing countries in Europe and has low scores across the board, with the exception of iodine deficiency and fat consumption.

As a group, countries in the former USSR perform least well, and our evidence suggests that the Baltic states perform better than the rest, together with Belarus and Azerbaijan. Ukraine, the Russian Federation and Armenia perform worst, but do well on fat consumption.

Discussion and conclusions

The analysis reported in this chapter has shown that European countries differ significantly in the success they have achieved in implementing health policies. This is not only the case for each policy area individually but also across the board. The summary score that has been constructed shows that some countries have succeeded in implementing more effective health policies and in achieving overall better intermediate and final health outcomes than others. The question then becomes, what are the conditions which have allowed some countries to achieve so much better results than others? This question will be considered in Chapters 15 and 16, but the next chapter will first assess the overall health impact of these health policies.

References

Anderson, P., Møller, L. and Galea, G. (eds) (2012) *Alcohol in the European Union: Consumption, Harm and Policy Approaches.* Copenhagen: WHO Regional Office for Europe.

Andersson, M., de Benoist, B., Darnton-Hill, I. and Delange, F. (2007) *Iodine Deficiency in Europe: A Continuing Public Health Problem.* Geneva: Wold Health Organization and UNICEF.

Danaei, G., Finucane, M.M., Lin, J.K. et al. (2011) National, regional, and global trends in systolic blood pressure since 1980: systematic analysis of health examination surveys and epidemiological studies with 786 country-years and 5.4 million participants, *Lancet*, 377(9765):568–77.

Del Amo, J., Likatavicius, G., Perez-Cachafeiro, S. et al. (2011) The epidemiology of HIV and AIDS reports in migrants in the 27 European Union countries, Norway and Iceland: 1999–2006, *European Journal of Public Health*, 21(5):620–6.

Edwards, G. (1994) *Alcohol Policy and the Public Good.* Oxford: Oxford University Press.

European Centre for Disease Control and Prevention (2012) *Susceptibility of Staphylococcus aureus Isolates to Methicillin in Participating Countries in 2010.* Stockholm: European Centre for Disease Control and Prevention, http://ecdc.europa.eu/en/activities/surveillance/EARS-Net/database/Pages/table_reports.aspx (accessed 10 July 2012).

European Child Safety Alliance (2009) *Child Safety Report Card 2009. Europe Summary for 24 Countries*. Amsterdam: European Child Safety Alliance.

Joossens, L. and Raw, M. (2011) *The Tobacco Control Scale 2010 in Europe*. Brussels: Association of European Cancer Leagues.

Karlsson, K. and Österberg, E. (2007) *Scaling Alcohol Control Policies across Europe*. Brussels: Eurocare Bridging the Gap Project.

von Karsa, L., Anttila, A., Ronco, G. et al. (2008) *Cancer Screening in the European Union. Report on the implementation of the Council Recommendation on Cancer Screening*. Luxembourg: European Commission and International Agency for Research on Cancer.

Lock, K., Pomerleau, J., Causer, L., Altmann, D.R. and McKee, M. (2005) The global burden of disease attributable to low consumption of fruit and vegetables: implications for the global strategy on diet, *Bulletin of the World Health Organization*, 83(2):100–8.

Mereckiene, J., Cotter, S., Weber, J.T. et al for the VENICE Project Gatekeepers Group (2012) Influenza A(H1N1)pdm09 vaccination policies and coverage in Europe, *Eurosurveillance*, 17(4):18–27.

O 'Flanagan, D., Cotter, S. and Mereckiene, J. (2009) *National Seasonal Influenza Vaccination Survey in Europe, 2007/2008 Influenza Season*. Stockholm: European Centre for Disease Prevention and Control, Vaccine European New Integrated Collaboration Effort (VENICE).

Perlman, F., Bobak, M., Gilmore, A. and McKee, M. (2007) Trends in the prevalence of smoking in Russia during the transition to a market economy, *Tobacco Control*, 16(5):299–305.

Pomerleau, J., Lock, K., Knai, C. and McKee, M. (2005) Interventions designed to increase adult fruit and vegetable intake can be effective: a systematic review of the literature, *Journal of Nutrition*, 135(10):2486–95.

Rehm, J., Taylor, B. and Patra, J. (2006) Volume of alcohol consumption, patterns of drinking and burden of disease in the European region 2002, *Addiction*, 101(8):1086–95.

Roberts, B., Gilmore, A., Stickley, A. et al. (2012) Changes in smoking prevalence in seven countries of the former Soviet Union between 2001 and 2010, *American Journal of Public Health*, 102(7):1320–8.

Shkolnikov, V., McKee, M., Leon, D. and Chenet, L. (1999) Why is the death rate from lung cancer falling in the Russian Federation? *European Journal of Epidemiology*, 15(3):203–6.

Stuckler, D., Basu, S., Suhrcke, M., Coutts, A. and McKee, M. (2011) Effects of the 2008 recession on health: a first look at European data, *Lancet*, 378(9786):124–5.

WHO Regional Office for Europe (2009) *European Status Report on Road Safety*. Copenhagen: WHO Regional Office for Europe.

WHO Regional Office for Europe (2012) *European Health for All Database (HFA-DB)*. Copenhagen: WHO Regional Office for Europe, http://data.euro.who.int/hfadb/ (accessed 4 June 2012).

chapter fourteen

Past and future health gains

Johan Mackenbach, Marina Karanikolos and Martin McKee

Introduction

This chapter will make some quantitative estimates of the population health gains achieved through the past successes of health policy, and of what the future health gains might be if all European countries would adopt 'best practice' policies.

Because other data are not available, the analysis is limited to impacts of health policy on mortality. Mortality data by cause of death are available for most of the period 1970–2010 for most European countries and, therefore, lend themselves well to this kind of analysis. While we are aware of the limitations of mortality data, particularly of the fact that impacts of health policy on morbidity and quality of life will not be captured by them, we simply note that avoiding premature mortality is still, and will continue to be, an important goal of health policy.

Two outcome measures will be used: the number of deaths that have been or can be avoided and the number of PYLLs that have been or can be avoided. The second measure is added in because it gives more weight to deaths occurring at younger ages and, therefore, does justice to the idea that health policy should prioritize the avoidance of premature mortality.

The next section will briefly describe the methods used; this will be followed by the results outlining the health gains that have been achieved in the past and the health gains that can still be achieved in the future.

Methods

Our analysis intended to cover ten areas of health policy: all 11 areas covered by this book except for mental health, for which there was insufficient evidence for an impact of health policy on population health outcomes (see Chapter 10). For nine of these areas, one or more specific causes of death have been identified that can be (and often have been) influenced by health policy. The exception is control of air pollution, the health effects of which are likely to be spread across a range of causes of death (cardiovascular and respiratory causes, see Chapter 12). Table 14.1 presents the causes of death that have been selected for the analysis, with their ICD-10 code (World Health Organization 2010).

Initially, the number of deaths and PYLLs were determined for each of the selected causes in each country in 2009. The PYLLs were calculated as the number of years lost before the age of 85. This was done by multiplying the number of deaths occurring in each five-year age group with the difference between 85 and the mid-point of the age group (e.g. for each death occurring in the age group 20–25 the number of years of life lost was taken to be 85 − 22.5 = 62.5 years).

To estimate past health gains, the number of deaths or PYLLs that would have occurred in 2009 if the 1970 rates had still applied were calculated from the age-specific mortality rates for each of the selected causes in each country in 1970. This 'expected' number was compared with the 'observed' number to calculate the absolute and percentage reduction that had actually been achieved. This difference between 'expected' and 'observed' is labelled the 'saved' number of lives or PYLLs. By doing it in this way, instead of comparing age-standardized death rates between 1970 and 2009, the actual benefits accruing to each country's 2009 population could be estimated.

Mortality rates for 1970 could not be used for the countries of the former USSR and so 1981 was used as the comparator as this was the earliest available

Table 14.1 Causes of death selected for the analysis

Policy areas	Causes of death	ICD-10 code numbers[a]
Tobacco control	Lung cancer	C32–C34
Alcohol control	Liver cirrhosis[b]	K70–K74
	Other alcohol-related causes[c]	F10 Mental and behavioural disorders due to alcohol G31.2 Degeneration of the nervous system due to alcohol I42.6 Alcoholic cardiomyopathy K85.2 Alcohol-induced pancreatitis X45 Acute alcohol poisoning
Food	Ischaemic heart disease	I20–I25
Fertility, pregnancy and childbirth	Neonatal mortality[d]	Mortality from all causes in first month of life
	Maternal mortality[e]	O00–O99
Child health	All external causes (ages 1–19 years)	W00–X59
	Postneonatal mortality[d]	Mortality from all causes in months 2–11 of life

Policy areas	Causes of death	ICD-10 code numbers[a]
Infectious diseases	All infectious diseases[f]	A00–A99 and B00–B99
Hypertension	Cerebrovascular disease	I60–I69
Cancer screening	Cervical cancer	C53
	Breast cancer	C50
Mental health	None	
Road traffic safety	Road traffic accidents[g]	V01–V99
Air pollution	None	

Notes: The source of the mortality data is the WHO *European Mortality Database* (WHO Regional Office for Europe 2012), which is based on official data supplied by member countries. The baseline for all calculations is 2009 or the latest year for which data were available. Most countries had data for 2010, 2009 or 2008; exceptions were Azerbaijan, Georgia and Switzerland (2007), Denmark (2006), Belgium (2005), Albania (2004) and the former Yugoslavian Republic of Macedonia (2003). All calculations have been disaggregated by gender
[a]*International Classification of Diseases*, revision 10 (World Health Organization 2010)
[b]Not available for Armenia, Belarus, the Russian Federation, Ukraine, Switzerland
[c]Not available for Albania, Armenia, Azerbaijan, Belarus, Bulgaria, Greece, Montenegro, Russian Federation, Serbia, Slovakia, Slovenia, Switzerland, the former Yugoslavian Republic of Macedonia, Ukraine
[d]Because there is not a breakdown by age at death in weeks for infant mortality, these data are not available for Armenia, Belarus, Cyprus, Estonia, Portugal, Russian Federation, the former Yugoslavian Republic of Macedonia, and Ukraine; for these countries, infant mortality will be presented instead and included under postneonatal mortality
[e]Live births is used as denominator, not female population numbers by age
[f]Because of the predominance of secondary infections among the elderly, the analyses for this cause are restricted to those aged <75 years
[g]V01–V99 is all transport accidents, and also includes a small number of cases of non-road transport (water, air, etc.) and unspecified transport accidents

year for which comparable figures are available in the WHO mortality files. This is not expected to introduce serious bias in the calculations because no significant declines in all-cause mortality occurred in the USSR before 1981 (actually, mortality declines started much later, see Chapter 1). For Albania, 1987 was used as the comparator. Cyprus was excluded from the analysis of past health gains, because no data were available before 1999.

It is acknowledged that not all the declines in mortality between 1970 (or 1981) and 2009 can be attributed to health policy impacts. In many cases, other factors, such as improvements in medical care that led to increased survival from the conditions included in the analysis, will also have contributed to mortality declines. This issue will be considered in the discussion and conclusions of this chapter.

To estimate potential health gains that can still be obtained in the future a conceptually similar approach was followed. For this purpose, an 'expected' number was calculated and compared with the 'observed' number of deaths and PYLLs in 2009 (or latest available year). In this case, however, the 'expected' number of deaths or PYLLs was derived from a country with 'best practice' health policies in 2009: Sweden. Using each country's population numbers by age in 2009, the age-specific mortality rates in Sweden were used to calculate the number of deaths (and, subsequently, PYLLs) that could have been expected to occur in this country if the Swedish mortality rates had applied. As Chapter 13 has shown, Sweden has an exceptionally good record in most if not all of the areas of health policy covered by this book. Furthermore, as Chapter 16 will show, its performance is even better than might be expected given those of its characteristics that influence the ability to enact health policies. Consequently, the Swedish age-specific death rates for each cause of death in 2009 were used as the 'best practice' rates.

This 'expected' number of deaths or PYLLs in each country was then compared with the 'observed' number to calculate the absolute and percentage reduction that could potentially be achieved in the future if countries followed the Swedish example. This difference between 'expected' and 'observed' is referred to as the 'excess' deaths or PYLLs.

This approach worked well in a large majority of comparisons because Sweden indeed had lower mortality rates for most conditions than most other countries in 2009. However, in some cases, other countries had lower mortality rates. For example, women in the countries in the Caucasus have lower mortality rates from lung cancer than women in Sweden, not because of the superior tobacco control policies in these countries but because of a later start of the tobacco epidemic. The choice of Sweden as a benchmark country can, therefore, be well justified. Where countries had lower mortality than Sweden, their 'excess' deaths were arbitrarily set at zero.

Here again, it should be emphasized that not all the differences in mortality from the selected causes between a particular country and Sweden can be attributed to health policy – part of the differences may reflect other factors, such as differences in health care quality. This will be discussed further at the end of this chapter.

Results are presented by country as well as for Europe as a whole. As elsewhere in this book, Europe includes the European Region of the WHO, minus central Asia, Turkey and Israel. In the calculations, the mini-states of Andorra, Liechtenstein, Monaco, San Marino and Vatican City are also excluded.

In order to be able to present data for Europe as a whole, some values had to be imputed for countries where coding did not allow a detailed breakdown of causes of death. This mainly applied to alcohol-related causes, where precision to the level of the fourth digit in the ICD-10 codes was required. For cirrhosis, Georgia was used to impute values for Armenia; Lithuania for Belarus, the Russian Federation and Ukraine; and Germany for Switzerland. For other alcohol-related causes Lithuania was used to impute values for Belarus, the Russian Federation and Ukraine; Georgia for Armenia and Azerbaijan; Croatia for Serbia, Slovenia, Montenegro and the former Yugoslavian Republic of Macedonia; Italy for Greece; Germany for Switzerland; and the Czech Republic for Slovakia.

Results

Observed numbers of deaths and potential years of life lost in 2009

Detailed results on the observed number of deaths, by country, in 2009 or the latest available year are presented in Table 14.A1 in the Appendix to this chapter. Here only the total number of deaths and PYLLs in 2009 for Europe as a whole are presented (Table 14.2).

Table 14.2 shows how many deaths are still attributable to these causes of death, despite the progress that has been made in the past decades. The total number of deaths in Europe as a whole in 2009 was 8.2 million. Two of the largest, ischaemic heart disease and cerebrovascular disease, are included in the table; together they account for 2.7 million deaths. The smallest numbers of death of any cause in the table is maternal mortality, for which the number of deaths in Europe as a whole was below 1000 in 2009.

Each of these deaths is associated with a number of life-years lost. In the calculations, somewhat arbitrarily, the difference between the age at death and

Table 14.2 Observed number of deaths and potential years of life lost in Europe as a whole, by cause of death and gender, 2009

	Deaths 2009		*PYLLs 2009*	
	Men	*Women*	*Men*	*Women*
Lung cancer	273,904	91,510	4,554,207	1,404,925
Liver cirrhosis[a]	110,286	55,594	2,981,790	1,285,919
Other alcohol-related causes[b]	24,401	6,348	688,585	169,688
Ischaemic heart disease	837,733	870,405	11,526,208	5,803,037
Neonatal mortality[c]	21,828	16,515	1,849,424	1,399,335
Postneonatal mortality[c]	4,878	3,956	412,191	334,282
Maternal mortality		950		51,983
External causes (1–19 years)	6,422	2,569	464,842	190,825
Infectious diseases	57,925	21,537	1,602,582	571,888
Cerebrovascular disease	412,152	608,558	4,836,430	3,995,677
Cervical cancer		20,703		509,448
Breast cancer		129,396		2,198,915
Road traffic injury	60,733	19,620	2,603,447	720,736

Notes: PYLL, potential years of life lost
[a]Data were imputed for Armenia, Belarus, the Russian Federation, Ukraine, Switzerland
[b]Data were imputed for Albania, Armenia, Azerbaijan, Belarus, Bulgaria, Greece, Montenegro, the Russian Federation, Serbia, Slovakia, Slovenia, Switzerland, the former Yugoslavian Republic of Macedonia and Ukraine
[c]Separate neonatal and postneonatal were unavailable for Armenia, Belarus, Cyprus, Estonia, Portugal, the Russian Federation, the former Yugoslavian Republic of Macedonia and Ukraine; the figures for neonatal deaths in this table include all infant deaths for these countries

age 85 is taken as the number of years lost. This is older than the age used in previous calculations, which was once 64 and more recently 75. However, life expectancy at birth among women in Spain and France has already exceeded 85 years, and that among men in Sweden has reached almost 80 but on current trends would exceed 85 by 2030. The number of PYLLs per death varies among causes and depends on the average age at which deaths occur. The largest number of PYLLs per death applies to neonatal mortality (by definition, 85 years). However, some of the other causes also occur at relatively young ages, for example maternal mortality (an average of 55 PYLLs per death) and RTIs (an average of 43 PYLLs per death among men, and 37 PYLLs per death among women).

As a result, these causes of death rank somewhat higher on the basis of their PYLLs than on the basis of their number of deaths (Table 14.2). For example, while RTIs and cervical cancer cause a similar number of deaths among women in Europe as a whole, the total number of PYLLs is considerably higher for the first than for the second.

Past health gains: 'savings' in lives and potential years of life lost compared with 1970

Detailed results in each country for the number of deaths that have been avoided in 2009 through the reductions in mortality that have occurred since 1970 are presented in Table 14.A2 in the Appendix to this chapter. Without these gains, the number of deaths today would be very much larger. For example, among men, 351,000 deaths from ischaemic heart disease and 355,000 deaths from cerebrovascular disease have been avoided. Among women, the gains have also been large; 372,000 fewer deaths from ischaemic heart disease and 508,000 fewer deaths from cerebrovascular disease.

For some causes of death in women, however, the 'saved' number of deaths is negative: if the mortality rates of 1970 would still apply in 2009, the number of deaths from lung cancer would have been 45,000 fewer and that from breast cancer 16,000 fewer. In many countries, mortality rates from these two causes of death have increased among women, through changes in risk factor exposure that have not been sufficiently countered by health policy measures (in this case, tobacco control and breast cancer screening).

Table 14.3 presents the percentage reduction in the number of PYLLs, by cause and country, for both genders combined.

For many causes and in many countries, mortality would have been more than 100% higher in 2009 if the mortality declines had not occurred. The exceptions are, again, lung cancer and breast cancer, where developments among women have not been favourable. The largest relative impact of mortality declines can be seen for PYLLs avoided in maternal mortality, infectious diseases, infant mortality and external causes among children.

Here again enormous differences can be seen between countries. Among the Nordic counties, Denmark has had relatively modest percentage reductions in PYLLs since 1970, as has Belgium within the continental group of countries, which confirms the impression that these countries have been less successful

Table 14.3 Number of 'saved' potential years of life lost in 2009 by cause of death and country compared with 1970, as a percentage of deaths in 2009 both genders combined

	Lung cancer	Liver cirrhosis	Ischaemic heart disease	Infant mortality	Maternal mortality	External (1–19 years)	Infectious diseases	Cerebrovascular disease	Cervical cancer	Breast cancer	Road traffic injuries	Average
Nordic												
Finland	126	–76	327	399	714	394	452	380	382	15	394	319
Sweden	–21	52	324	333	501	450	74	240	341	47	537	262
Norway	–40	–7	390	302	651	385	98	364	286	45	318	254
Iceland	–28	31	434	617	0	2027	688	301	617	136	805	512
Denmark	–23	–53	372	317	17	202	62	101	419	42	330	162
Britain and Ireland												
United Kingdom	88	–78	307	297	103	244	136	357	254	65	240	183
Ireland	29	–54	267	503	694	298	465	424	33	38	181	261
Continental												
Netherlands	22	–2	539	239	483	751	111	288	337	52	605	311
Belgium	8	–5	235	429	484	317	123	290	108	21	172	198
Luxembourg	56	198	410	661	0	664	81	204	362	74	206	265
Germany	15	66	190	521	667	531	122	338	271	24	444	290
Switzerland	17	12	182	283	1886	410	216	399	465	64	437	397
Austria	26	98	191	564	2115	662	236	541	170	40	474	465

(continued)

Table 14.3 (*continued*)

	Lung cancer	Liver cirrhosis	Ischaemic heart disease	Infant mortality	Maternal mortality	External (1–19 years)	Infectious diseases	Cerebrovascular disease	Cervical cancer	Breast cancer	Road traffic injuries	Average
Mediterranean												
France	-18	227	178	330	347	550	174	427	70	5	233	229
Spain	-32	161	46	563	880	457	311	381	-53	-9	177	262
Portugal	-83	242	200	1263	677	977	550	365	190	16	266	424
Malta	8	199	124	404	0	0	2888	394	1278	42	99	494
Italy	14	268	220	742	2395	421	345	372	162	19	185	468
Greece	-23	200	0	841	710	402	1143	145	-34	-18	-11	305
Cyprus	N/A	N/A	N/A	N/A	N/A	N/A	N/A	N/A	N/A	N/A	N/A	N/A
Western Balkans												
Slovenia	-27	-33	55	2276	1305	499	3636	172	139	-35	247	748
Croatia	-46	-28	-27	983	387	311	1380	38	177	-39	136	297
Serbia	-56	60	-25	716	577	233	1371	-3	-4	-54	205	275
Montenegro	-46	86	31	887	0	375	5234	100	120	-37	166	629
TFYR Macedonia	-34	145	-35	405	1359	65	573	-32	113	-43	395	265
Albania	27	3585	-38	297	1069	-26	546	8	-59	-33	2	489

Central and eastern

Poland	-42	-54	12	495	1456	392	562	-12	72	-11	40	265
Czech Republic	19	-17	136	668	840	297	91	233	77	35	-61	211
Slovakia	24	-50	46	292	140	217	88	104	19	21	-61	76
Hungary	-56	-74	20	599	135	12	642	94	42	-18	-55	122
Romania	-39	-52	-40	405	389	0	391	24	2	-27	0	96
Bulgaria	-30	-69	45	217	642	144	189	36	-45	-38	15	101
Former USSR												
Estonia	44	N/A	158	377	0	225	44	236	59	6	180	133
Latvia	16	N/A	65	105	28	162	27	86	41	-9	212	73
Lithuania	13	N/A	36	235	0	120	59	26	-10	-12	123	59
Belarus	-4	N/A	-22	255	2189	32	-1	0	4	-10	23	246
Republic of Moldova	-3	N/A	9	193	58	104	69	-7	22	-20	135	56
Ukraine	32	N/A	-10	74	56	48	-57	10	0	-29	46	17
Russian Federation	36	N/A	-1	165	197	26	-4	14	7	-30	23	43
Georgia	34	N/A	213	97	-73	70	292	40	100	12	138	92
Armenia	-27	N/A	4	130	-6	8	108	17	72	-36	69	34
Azerbaijan	168	N/A	181	244	150	870	882	11	137	72	1236	395
Average	**4**	**161**	**140**	**481**	**591**	**349**	**595**	**183**	**164**	**9**	**227**	**264**

Notes: TFYR Macedonia, the former Yugoslavian Republic of Macedonia; N/A, data not available to allow the calculation of health gains

in their health policies than their immediate neighbours. Most countries in the central and eastern European region have done well in reducing infant mortality and infectious diseases but have not been so successful for many other causes of death. As already seen, many countries of the former USSR have had relatively modest declines in cause-specific mortality; among them, Ukraine has done least well.

Potential for future health gains: 'excess' deaths and potential years of life lost compared with Sweden

Detailed results on the number of deaths that can potentially be avoided if all countries would have the age-specific mortality rates of Sweden are presented in Table 14.A3 in the Appendix to this chapter.

As those figures show, the potential gains, expressed in absolute numbers of deaths, are simply stupendous. For example, among men in the whole of Europe, the potential gains by reducing deaths from lung cancer amount to around 150,000 deaths per year, for cirrhosis to around 79,000 deaths per year, and for RTIs to around 44,000 deaths per year. For each of these cases, more than half of all deaths occurring in 2009 in Europe as a whole could be avoided if all countries had Sweden's mortality rates. The largest gains would be achieved for ischaemic heart disease and cerebrovascular disease mortality – in the Russian Federation alone, the yearly number of deaths among men from these two causes would be 225,000 and 125,000 fewer, respectively, if this country had the mortality rates of our 'best practice' country.

Among women the results are slightly different. Overall, the potential gains are also enormous, but the distribution across causes of death differs from that among men (Table 14.A3 of the Appendix to this chapter). For lung cancer, the potential gains are minimal, because female lung cancer mortality in most countries is lower than in Sweden, which is already further advanced in the smoking epidemic. Several other causes also show smaller potential gains for women; however, for ischaemic heart disease and cerebrovascular disease, the absolute numbers of deaths to be avoided in Europe as a whole are even larger among women than among men. For cervical and breast cancer mortality, the number of deaths that could be avoided in Europe as a whole if all countries had the Swedish mortality rates is almost 11,000 and 24,000, respectively, corresponding to more than 50% and around 20% of all deaths from these causes in Europe as a whole (Table 14.A3 of the Appendix to this chapter).

Table 14.4 shows in more detail the percentage reduction in PYLLs, for both genders combined, that could be achieved if each country had the mortality rates of Sweden.

As could be expected from the information in the previous chapters, there are enormous differences between countries in the 'excess' PYLLs compared with Sweden. Averaged across all the causes in the analysis, the percentage 'excess' ranged from 5% in Iceland to a full 78% in the Republic of Moldova. Many countries in eastern Europe have average values above 50%, but even in many countries in western Europe, 20% or more of PYLLs could be avoided if these countries had the Swedish mortality rates. This clearly indicates both the

Table 14.4 'Excess' potential years of life lost in 2009, by cause of death and country, using the 'expected' values the country would have had if Swedish rates had applied, both genders combined[a]

	Lung cancer	Liver cirrhosis	Other alcohol related	Ischaemic heart disease	Infant mortality	Maternal mortality	External (1–19 years)	Infectious diseases	Cerebro-vascular diseases	Cervical cancer	Breast cancer	Road traffic injuries	Average
Nordic													
Finland	0	77	62	37	4	0	47	0	35	0	5	50	26
Sweden	0	0	0	0	0	0	0	0	0	0	0	0	0
Norway	22	0	24	0	20	0	46	0	4	18	0	45	15
Iceland	25	0	0	0	0	0	0	0	8	0	0	20	4
Denmark	52	70	81	0	25	78	47	8	45	23	36	51	43
Britain and Ireland													
United Kingdom	31	62	0	23	45	82	40	18	21	17	26	33	33
Ireland	32	43	0	32	21	57	51	5	21	56	32	55	34
Continental													
Netherlands	45	0	0	0	32	27	0	0	3	0	31	19	13
Belgium	47	53	20	5	36	51	44	44	29	15	37	74	38
Luxembourg	42	54	0	0	5	0	33	27	29	20	14	69	25
Germany	27	62	56	9	26	70	10	28	7	22	19	36	31
Switzerland	21	63	57	0	35	0	50	1	0	0	12	40	23
Austria	27	66	38	18	35	0	24	10	0	21	7	54	25

(continued)

Table 14.4 (continued)

	Lung cancer	Liver cirrhosis	Other alcohol related	Ischaemic heart disease	Infant mortality	Maternal mortality	External (1–19 years)	Infectious diseases	Cerebro-vascular diseases	Cervical cancer	Breast cancer	Road traffic injuries	Average
Mediterranean													
France	40	56	52	0	28	74	48	38	0	3	25	60	35
Spain	35	46	0	0	18	48	34	54	10	13	0	50	26
Portugal	14	61	0	0	30	76	29	78	54	48	10	67	39
Italy	24	40	0	0	28	23	30	39	17	0	20	67	24
Malta	16	0	0	27	54	0	0	0	19	0	22	28	14
Greece	36	0	0	27	19	52	47	0	48	0	3	80	26
Cyprus	0	0	0	24	24	0	0	21	0	0	13	75	13
Western Balkans													
Slovenia	40	80	52	6	0	60	17	0	52	49	18	68	37
Croatia	53	78	51	56	52	86	41	11	75	41	21	78	54
Serbia	61	52	51	53	64	81	53	10	83	79	41	71	58
Montenegro	56	46	52	22	56		33	0	65	54	21	74	43
TFYR Macedonia	48	30	51	62	77	58	76	63	88	55	31	50	58
Albania	15	0	51	56	67	41	90	6	80	0	0	72	40

Central and eastern

Poland	58	76	56	41	54	13	58	42	68	73	11	76	52
Czech Republic	43	73	0	54	12	28	61	14	57	55	0	69	39
Slovakia	41	84	0	72	55	82	67	14	73	71	10	68	53
Hungary	70	90	67	71	50	91	51	0	73	69	36	70	62
Romania	50	90	0	67	74	93	85	73	84	85	18	75	66
Bulgaria	46	76	0	56	70	74	79	57	86	74	25	79	60
Former USSR													
Estonia	30	77	86	66	28	0	75	77	63	67	18	66	54
Latvia	37	79	88	79	67	94	84	81	82	67	31	74	72
Lithuania	37	88	62	78	48	0	86	76	78	80	27	77	62
Belarus	37	89	63	88	46	0	88	83	87	66	10	82	61
Ukraine	29	88	62	89	73	94	87	94	86	78	35	80	74
Republic of Moldova	43	96	87	87	78	97	88	90	89	82	27	77	78
Russian Federation	41	89	63	86	69	93	92	92	90	75	30	86	75
Georgia	0	78	0	51	83	97	75	67	86	52	14	61	55
Armenia	51	80	0	79	75	94	85	79	75	49	42	45	63
Azerbaijan	0	88	0	61	74	92	32	66	87	12	0	0	43
Average	**34**	**57**	**32**	**38**	**42**	**49**	**50**	**35**	**49**	**38**	**19**	**59**	**42**

Notes: TYR Macedonia, the former Yugoslavian Republic of Macedonia
[a]Values of 0 indicate that a country has equal or lower mortality rates compared with Sweden

potential for further health gain in the future and the missed opportunities of the past and the present.

If different causes of death are examined, the average percentage 'excess' PYLLs varies between a low 19% for breast cancer and a staggering 57% for cirrhosis, 57% for maternal mortality, and 59% for RTIs (Table 14.4). The last values are very high indeed, but hide even larger country-specific values. For example, many countries of the former USSR could potentially lower their numbers of PYLL from many of these causes by more than 80 or even 90%. The relatively low average percentage 'excess' PYLLs for breast cancer (Table 14.4) perhaps indicates that even Sweden could do better on this cause: several countries, including countries in the rich western part of the region, have lower breast cancer mortality rates than Sweden.

Discussion and conclusions

Gains in health since 1970 for the causes analysed in this chapter have clearly been enormous. While not all of these declines can be attributed to health policies, part of the decline in all these causes can be, as shown in the previous chapters. For example, some of the declines in lung cancer and ischaemic heart disease can be attributed to tobacco control; some of the declines in external cause mortality among children to injury prevention, and some of the declines in death rate from RTIs to road safety measures, and so on. It is impossible to estimate the specific contribution of preventive health policies to these declines, but even if these accounted for only half or a quarter of the cause-specific declines, the successes would be immense.

At the same time, not all countries have been equally successful in bringing down mortality from these preventable causes, as shown again by the calculations in this chapter. The relative reductions in PYLLs since 1970 confirm what has been illustrated in the earlier chapters: many countries in the eastern part of Europe have done less well than countries in western Europe, and that some countries in western Europe have done less well than their neighbours. These differences clearly highlight some of the main failures of health policy in Europe.

The calculations of the 'excess' deaths and PYLLs compared with the benchmark country, Sweden, show how large the potential is for further health gains. Some of the differences between Sweden and other European countries may reflect other factors, but, again, part of the differences is likely to be a result of Sweden's superior health policies, for example in the fields of tobacco and alcohol control, injury prevention and cancer screening.

We hope that the enormous reductions in deaths and PYLL that can theoretically be achieved will inspire policy-makers around Europe to redouble their efforts in implementing the best practices observed elsewhere.

Appendix

Table 14.A1 Observed deaths in 2009

	Lung cancer	Liver cirrhosis	Other alcohol related	Ischaemic heart disease	Neonatal	Postneonatal	Maternal	External (1–19 years)	Infectious diseases	Cerebrovascular disease	Cervical cancer	Breast cancer	Road traffic injuries
Men													
Albania	507	2	118	1,593	61	119		98	45	1,521			278
Armenia	1,080	448	6	4,150	258			67	199	1,300			145
Austria	2,481	1,098	360	7,185	125	50		20	194	1,869			434
Azerbaijan	485	1,437	14	3,380	575	314		38	305	3,959			61
Belarus	3,141	2,237	415	25,519	301			173	893	7,411			1,215
Belgium	5,250	803	242	6,380	168	96		32	465	3,072			855
Bulgaria	3,285	1,475	102	8,065	221	144		70	324	10,352			854
Croatia	2,363	966	254	4,885	96	23		13	133	3,268			471
Cyprus	175	34	4	462	22			1	17	159			78
Czech Republic	4,191	1,434	135	12,101	109	76		52	304	4,820			757
Denmark	2,160	632	630	3,257	98	27		21	160	1,969			231
Estonia	510	179	172	1,881	34			12	85	534			88
Finland	1,468	912	354	6,024	66	12		21	87	1,756			276
France	23,247	5,659	2,526	21,525	1,027	519		241	2,258	13,497			3,353
Georgia	767	665	9	3,053	437	109		48	207	3,743			270
Germany	30,642	9,832	4,534	67,403	858	436		143	3,249	23,576			2,882
Greece	5,656	614	48	7,461	123	81		39	208	6,654			1,333

(continued)

Table 14.A1 (continued)

	Lung cancer	Liver cirrhosis	Other alcohol related	Ischaemic heart disease	Neonatal	Postneonatal	Maternal	External (1–19 years)	Infectious diseases	Cerebrovascular disease	Cervical cancer	Breast cancer	Road traffic injuries
Hungary	6,185	3,537	662	15,588	180	83		43	183	6,246			847
Iceland	64	5	2	204	4	1		1	1	75			12
Ireland	1,121	209	7	2,919	96	44		23	75	872			203
Italy	26,924	5,408	256	38,176	789	319		143	2,326	25,318			4,260
Latvia	920	280	311	4,027	60	28		29	180	1,721			187
Lithuania	1,288	770	143	6,416	65	44		59	269	2,102			356
Luxembourg	168	40	0	189	3	3		0	22	147			34
Malta	126	17	3	319	11	2		0	1	103			11
Montenegro	240	40	31	256	20	9		1	3	203			54
Netherlands	6,709	557	148	6,004	283	95		23	408	3,462			508
Norway	1,259	139	145	2,843	83	35		20	112	1,376			208
Poland	17,819	5,061	1,706	25,407	947	351		195	1,236	15,913			3,856
Portugal	3,076	1,168	147	3,950	211			30	914	6,127			838
Republic of Moldova	884	1,813	378	7,506	187	104		69	541	2,824			373
Romania	8,617	7,530	262	27,021	690	503		250	1,553	22,490			2,170
Russian Federation	47,110	32,279	5,980	278,933	8,182			3,227	25,417	143,803			22,053
Serbia	4,133	756	437	6,759	202	77		35	189	7,232			635
Slovakia	1,749	1,090	65	7,717	111	98		36	118	2,660			419
Slovenia	778	449	119	1,059	19	6		3	19	867			166
Spain	18,685	3,878	282	20,320	585	307		23	228	13,216			2,234

Sweden	1,958	473	260	8,204	96	64	115	1,999	3,111			223
Switzerland	2,076	803	379	4,637	117	35	31	166	1,585			325
TFYR Macedonia	624	104	92	1,280	181		22	75	1,725			108
Ukraine	13,572	10,673	1,978	136,369	2,724		745	11,394	40,343			5,051
United Kingdom	20,411	4,780	686	47,306	1,403	664	210	1,363	19,171			2,021
Europe	**273,904**	**110,286**	**24,401**	**837,733**	**21,828**	**4,878**	**6,422**	**57,925**	**412,152**			**60,733**
Women												
Albania	150	0	15	1,065	47	108	45	21	1,661	18	138	75
Armenia	242	129	4	3,875	196	0	17	53	1,864	63	497	34
Austria	1,288	395	82	7,756	89	43	9	97	3,274	161	1,502	143
Azerbaijan	133	1,244	7	2,695	338	266	19	104	5,130	67	251	26
Belarus	365	1,082	118	25,236	210		51	220	10,172	315	1,194	373
Belgium	1,410	442	101	5,110	140	66	18	359	4,720	169	2,268	296
Bulgaria	623	382	25	6,360	168	135	25	148	12,088	346	1,313	239
Croatia	635	311	46	5,657	95	21	7	58	4,656	114	898	145
Cyprus	49	10	43	215	10		1	7	218	6	102	14
Czech Republic	1,505	663	171	13,664	85	71	18	190	7,372	311	1,607	269
Denmark	1,732	306	49	2,979	76	20	8	101	2,663	106	1,246	93
Estonia	136	87	64	2,451	22		3	30	851	59	236	31
Finland	601	337	654	5,510	56	26	9	56	2,624	54	819	80
France	6,968	2,388	8	16,219	877	381	103	1,191	18,780	741	11,634	1,020
Georgia	146	233	1,224	2,835	312	87	12	61	4,466	86	500	67

(continued)

Table 14.A1 (continued)

	Lung cancer	Liver cirrhosis	Other alcohol related	Ischaemic heart disease	Neonatal	Postneonatal	Maternal	External (1–19 years)	Infectious diseases	Cerebrovascular disease	Cervical cancer	Breast cancer	Road traffic injuries
Germany	13,815	5,034	9	65,723	683	345	37	65	1,857	37,974	1,524	17,466	1,060
Greece	1,136	207	108	4,461	115	52	4	11	120	8,839	134	1,914	314
Hungary	2,824	1,391	1	17,598	147	85	18	13	113	7,899	396	2,169	270
Iceland	69	1	1	146	1	3	0	0	0	84	2	36	1
Ireland	698	108	54	2,209	73	27	3	5	46	1,242	93	676	63
Italy	7,897	3,807	69	37,338	620	269	13	56	1,209	38,299	378	12,195	1,082
Latvia	184	181	40	4,566	49	31	7	11	80	2,915	98	438	72
Lithuania	242	377	0	8,001	39	33	0	17	97	3,671	198	594	101
Luxembourg	72	26	0	116	6	3	0	2	8	191	7	85	13
Malta	38	4	0	327	7	2	0	0	0	161	2	79	5
Montenegro	75	13	5	161	15	6	0	2	2	317	12	73	23
Netherlands	3,714	314	60	4,378	226	91	4	12	266	5,377	205	3,213	202
Norway	834	96	40	2,535	49	29	1	8	78	1,954	73	671	53
Poland	6,114	2,185	221	22,368	729	300	8	75	619	20,451	1,748	5,242	1,173
Portugal	757	381	16	3,608	152		7	6	388	8,158	271	1,620	226
Republic of Moldova	186	1,746	128	9,060	112	73	18	29	118	3,348	192	457	98
Romania	2,004	4,399	64	26,276	470	415	51	103	468	26,815	1,739	3,153	674
Russian Federation	8,945	16,127	1,760	306,244	6,089		388	1,362	7,474	228,731	6,187	23,517	8,054
Serbia	1,332	219	74	6,115	143	70	6	6	84	9,492	471	1,614	162
Slovakia	478	454	22	9,295	77	60	6	13	95	3,321	213	746	116

Spain	3,213	1,529	43	15,294	467	250	17	44	944	17,941	643	6,129	619
Sweden	1,664	203	53	6,808	87	47	3	6	164	4,491	139	1,395	81
Switzerland	1,008	411	102	4,398	112	29	1	11	93	2,540	91	1,268	90
TFYR Macedonia	96	28	13	786	124		1	9	40	1,864	44	240	21
Ukraine	2,404	5,375	573	174,613	2,077		129	256	3,450	60,139	2,218	8,089	1,513
United Kingdom	15,426	2,793	260	35,425	1,110	500	74	99	1,015	30,511	959	11,678	586
Europe	**91,510**	**55,594**	**6,348**	**870,405**	**16,515**	**3,956**	**950**	**2,569**	**21,537**	**608,558**	**20,703**	**129,396**	**19,620**

Note: TFYR Macedonia, the former Yugoslavian Republic of Macedonia

Table 14.A2 Saved lives in 2009 compared with 1970

	Lung cancer	Liver cirrhosis	Ischaemic heart disease	Infant	Maternal Mortality	External (1–19 years)	Infectious disease	Cerebrovascular disease	Cervical cancer	Breast cancer	Road traffic injuries
Men											
Albania	138	203	-574	552		-27	119	-17			-29
Armenia	-397	N/A	-369	340		-24	45	128			108
Austria	1,564	1,327	7,604	1,005		137	660	9,359			2,208
Azerbaijan	938	N/A	6,714	2,053		270	1,514	214			877
Belarus	-547	N/A	-5,595	796		45	-144	-1,016			306
Belgium	301	118	8,734	1,195		101	243	8,249			1,696
Bulgaria	-880	-1,029	4,008	883		96	525	659			195
Croatia	-1,148	-341	-2,270	1,187		40	895	-64			820
Cyprus	N/A	N/A	N/A	N/A		N/A	N/A	N/A			N/A
Czech Republic	1,391	-6	9,981	1,317		130	439	7,003			-378
Denmark	-180	-311	9,572	449		37	2	1,777			841
Estonia	105	N/A	2,396	116		20	31	1,105			171
Finland	1,958	-690	10,007	373		82	408	4,899			1,103
France	-2,903	11,919	19,084	5,390		1,306	2,586	52,828			8,173
Georgia	174	N/A	6,911	514		17	268	2,178			380
Germany	11,604	8,480	78,672	7,163		759	2,518	74,487			13,417
Greece	-1,763	1,210	242	1,770		142	1,164	3,914			-117
Hungary	-2,690	-2,533	1,334	1,727		-1	1,308	4,787			-393
Iceland	-41	-1	414	31		13	2	185			77
Ireland	101	-111	4,707	668		43	243	2,592			433

Italy	−3,803	13,144	44,326	8,409	605	3,838	51,278	9,827
Latvia	−47	N/A	2,363	120	49	23	1,226	471
Lithuania	−28	N/A	1,477	244	54	39	−218	451
Luxembourg	105	69	401	60	9	0	161	85
Malta	5	30	150	51	4	22	215	14
Montenegro	−95	36	54	233	9	137	171	120
Netherlands	2,982	−12	23,782	980	182	35	8,534	2,911
Norway	−469	7	7,067	359	77	44	3,487	655
Poland	−7,485	−2,357	−2,840	6,711	668	8,625	−5,231	1,892
Portugal	−2,614	2,370	4,903	2,589	242	2,314	15,453	2,238
Republic of Moldova	−116		896	524	53	−115	22	449
Romania	−3,554	−3,832	−12,564	4,715		3,117	−495	
Russian Federation	10,258	N/A	381	14,065	619	−4,770	14,048	7,367
Serbia	−2,017	318	−2,074	1,801	53	1,538	−1,419	1,536
Slovakia	566	−465	1,373	576	67	207	2,105	−231
Slovenia	−223	−157	135	615	19	468	578	450
Spain	−7,946	5,179	1,199	5,298	521	3,900	31,756	3,946
Sweden	−60	104	18,707	587	79	125	3,868	1,135
Switzerland	780	481	3,007	501	112	355	4,730	1,453
TFYR Macedonia	−203	123	−418	612	11	348	−710	435
Ukraine	2,735	N/A	−9,373	2,197	234	−6,010	1,260	2,736
United Kingdom	20,725	−3,571	106,881	6,396	509	1,141	50,717	5,315
Europe	**17,223**	**29,702**	**351,406**	**85,172**	**7,361**	**28,207**	**354,806**	**73,144**

(continued)

Table 14.A2 (continued)

	Lung cancer	Liver cirrhosis	Ischaemic heart disease	Infant	Maternal Mortality	External (1–19 years)	Infectious disease	Cerebrovascular disease	Cervical cancer	Breast cancer	Road traffic injuries
Women											
Albania	-45	147	-614	442	13	-16	100	-302	-7	-43	4
Armenia	-126	N/A	561	250	0	17	62	-97	44	-250	52
Austria	-684	441	8,128	725	19	40	196	12,690	207	189	696
Azerbaijan	94	N/A	4,961	1,588	46	186	918	-470	117	166	243
Belarus	30	N/A	4,143	506	23	7	68	311	62	-339	40
Belgium	-854	163	5,624	824	20	48	-30	11,111	214	251	673
Bulgaria	-60	-79	8,821	569	30	24	270	4,846	-144	-599	110
Croatia	-374	-9	-3,110	1,123	20	16	505	72	150	-485	266
Cyprus	N/A	N/A	N/A	N/A	N/A	N/A	N/A	N/A	N/A	N/A	N/A
Czech Republic	-828	30	8,469	960	23	56	69	9,467	187	40	-181
Denmark	-1,249	39	8,319	253	1	13	21	2,728	280	156	358
Estonia	-27	N/A	3,475	95	N/A	9	21	2,358	44	-35	67
Finland	-341	-184	5,377	267	7	17	148	7,426	186	-63	330
France	-4,298	4,846	13,615	3,856	173	492	1,103	61,347	649	-565	3,303
Georgia	112	N/A	8,771	402	-22	15	158	3,314	130	-4	136
Germany	-8,813	3,167	50,004	4,945	246	264	424	101,186	3,747	276	5,102
Greece	-321	680	634	1,349	29	44	535	5,700	-51	-855	80
Hungary	-1,887	-762	3,356	1,237	23	2	538	10,156	221	-404	-144

Country											
Iceland	-44	7	185	25	N/A	3	8	173	13	15	13
Ireland	-354	-43	3,286	539	20	30	173	3,402	34	6	146
Italy	-4,379	3,620	49,470	6,416	298	148	1,659	56,157	553	-831	2,641
Latvia	-27	N/A	4,113	57	1	8	9	2,991	45	-105	119
Lithuania	-51	N/A	4,395	181	N/A	22	33	99	19	-186	144
Luxembourg	-55	18	178	39	N/A	3	3	214	22	10	16
Malta	-30	2	-38	38	N/A	3	13	280	16	25	1
Montenegro	-46	21	82	210	N/A	2	78	136	19	-27	26
Netherlands	-3,031	144	16,499	681	21	61	77	12,373	578	1,175	932
Norway	-672	2	4,879	232	6	17	26	4,921	161	104	126
Poland	-4,224	141	-5,948	4,810	116	263	2,794	-3,268	992	-1,299	556
Portugal	-684	1,464	3,747	1,996	48	86	1,096	19,071	534	-97	507
Republic of Moldova	9		2,214	394	11	32	127	732	52	-149	138
Romania	-811	-1,974	-10,540	3,697	196	N/A	1,749	6,583	-156	-1,313	N/A
Russian Federation	808	N/A	59,886	9,486	763	139	-359	43,668	2,128	-9,691	995
Serbia	-908	273	-2,192	1,719	34	32	838	-2,191	-41	-949	499
Slovakia	-172	-141	146	434	7	27	26	3,891	25	17	-74
Slovenia	-188	-43	242	568	11	7	242	866	68	-247	140
Spain	-1,159	3,381	2,324	3,757	152	157	1,556	42,525	-308	-1,938	1,169
Sweden	-1,135	136	18,060	392	9	34	33	5,237	299	496	459
Switzerland	-713	-69	1,063	327	18	41	155	6,731	332	624	518
TFYR Macedonia	-18	66	-200	624	14	5	196	-768	44	-113	122

(continued)

Table 14.A2 *(continued)*

	Lung cancer	Liver cirrhosis	Ischaemic heart disease	Infant	Maternal Mortality	External (1–19 years)	Infectious disease	Cerebrovascular disease	Cervical cancer	Breast cancer	Road traffic injuries
Ukraine	863	N/A	17,551	1,333	81	142	−1,755	8,257	641	−3,070	751
United Kingdom	−7,820	−1,857	72,073	4,533	69	143	353	63,700	2,288	3,751	2,315
Europe	**−44,514**	**13,625**	**372,010**	**61,881**	**2,523**	**2,641**	**14,235**	**507,621**	**14,394**	**−16,355**	**23,394**

Note: TFYR Macedonia, the former Yugoslavian Republic of Macedonia

Table 14.A3 Excess deaths in 2009 compared with Sweden

	Lung cancer	Liver cirrhosis	Other alcohol related	Ischaemic heart disease	Infant	Maternal	External (1–19 years)	Infectious diseases	Cerebrovascular disease	Cervical cancer	Breast cancer	Road traffic injuries
Men												
Albania	193	0	63	586	118		86	0	1,170			212
Armenia	733	346	0	3,060	194		57	146	915			72
Austria	921	702	137	1,141	66		2	0	0			238
Azerbaijan	0	1,238	0	1,358	668		5	188	3,246			0
Belarus	1,963	1,895	215	21,535	149		150	718	5,989			1,000
Belgium	3,339	325	0	0	101		8	231	428			617
Bulgaria	1,869	1,115	0	2,962	257		54	149	8,479			676
Croatia	1,593	762	139	2,269	57		3	32	2,325			370
Cyprus	50	1	0	0	9		0	0	0			59
Czech Republic	2,471	963	0	5,998	22		29	73	2,631			513
Denmark	1,195	380	488	0	35		9	36	594			108
Estonia	314	127	142	1,194	12		9	59	284			59
Finland	463	649	207	2,283	0		9	0	387			153
France	11,950	2,888	993	0	450		92	943	0			1,961
Georgia	153	503	0	940	459		36	123	2,970			173
Germany	12,843	5,481	2,110	0	358		0	1,096	0			920
Greece	3,236	50	0	0	40		17	0	2,952			1,066
Hungary	4,586	3,111	420	9,638	129		21	0	4,070			622
Iceland	17	0	0	12	0		0	0	3			5

(continued)

Table 14.A3 (continued)

	Lung cancer	Liver cirrhosis	Other alcohol related	Ischaemic heart disease	Infant	Maternal	External (1–19 years)	Infectious diseases	Cerebrovascular disease	Cervical cancer	Breast cancer	Road traffic injuries
Ireland	524	46	0	676	37		12	0	51			104
Italy	14,197	2,390	0	0	320		30	882	5,981			2,873
Latvia	596	192	261	2,917	58		24	135	1,320			137
Lithuania	822	645	71	4,771	58		50	206	1,502			282
Luxembourg	92	20	0	0	0		0	12	47			23
Malta	53	0	0	50	7		0	0	6			1
Montenegro	150	15	17	0	17		0	0	93			40
Netherlands	3,709	0	0	0	123		0	20	0			125
Norway	421	0	25	0	32		8	8	71			97
Poland	12,380	3,533	834	5,872	719		104	489	8,873			2,979
Portugal	1,052	675	0	0	74		9	675	3,162			595
Republic of Moldova	503	1,697	310	6,186	235		59	482	2,358			292
Romania	5,178	6,634	0	14,532	899		205	1,106	17,900			1,676
Russian Federation	30,884	27,407	3,121	225,327	5,743		2,907	22,885	124,893			18,940
Serbia	2,752	403	240	1,860	181		19	18	5,442			465
Slovakia	1,056	886	0	5,237	124		23	17	1,775			295
Slovenia	432	355	65	0	0		0	0	433			118
Spain	10,310	1,854	0	0	169		28	1,027	242			1,171
Sweden	0	0	0	0	0		0	0	0			0
Switzerland	706	454	183	0	49		14	0	0			150

TFYR Macedonia	376	32	49	492		144	16	36	1,450			62
Ukraine	7,332	8,945	979	115,406		2,010	641	10,489	32,791			4,038
United Kingdom	8,848	1,943	0	44		976	61	0	1,318			593
Europe	**150,262**	**78,660**	**11,069**	**436,348**		**15,103**	**4,795**	**42,279**	**246,151**			**43,882**
Women												
Albania	0	0	5	458	0	107	42	0	1,271	0	0	53
Armenia	0	79	0	3,058	11	147	14	5	1,335	27	178	8
Austria	0	211	33	1,834	0	41	4	0	0	33	233	70
Azerbaijan	0	1,155	0	1,281	26	437	10	6	4,225	0	0	0
Belarus	0	876	62	20,433	0	84	45	41	7,020	171	0	285
Belgium	0	221	42	0	1	69	11	178	502	13	768	205
Bulgaria	0	206	0	2,508	3	213	21	0	9,581	228	193	170
Croatia	0	210	19	3,267	5	64	4	0	3,096	46	242	105
Cyprus	0	0	0	0	0	0	0	0	8	0	11	8
Czech Republic	0	441	0	8,230	0	18	12	5	3,814	159	161	179
Denmark	481	197	142	0	3	21	5	11	542	29	508	48
Estonia	0	55	40	1,588	0	4	2	3	284	37	22	18
Finland	0	216	32	1,934	0	11	6	0	266	0	9	32
France	0	1,074	307	0	31	331	63	163	0	0	2,489	473
Georgia	0	146	0	821	30	325	9	0	3,149	26	0	29
Germany	0	3,041	699	3,556	19	240	22	226	0	162	3,927	321
Greece	0	0	0	0	1	31	5	0	4,782	0	258	215
Hungary	154	1,159	46	11,649	16	120	7	0	4,003	240	654	179

(continued)

Table 14.A3 (continued)

	Lung cancer	Liver cirrhosis	Other alcohol related	Ischaemic heart disease	Infant	Maternal	External (1–19 years)	Infectious diseases	Cerebrovascular disease	Cervical cancer	Breast cancer	Road traffic injuries
Iceland	14	0	0	10	0	0	0	0	0	0	2	0
Ireland	0	41	0	463	14	1	2	0	96	44	226	30
Italy	0	2,383	0	0	229	0	26	92	7,574	0	2,367	540
Latvia	0	126	54	3,161	55	6	10	34	1,994	61	79	50
Lithuania	0	302	20	6,137	29	0	15	33	2,449	147	100	70
Luxembourg	0	17	0	0	3	0	2	1	26	1	24	9
Malta	0	0	0	121	4	0	0	0	27	0	23	1
Montenegro	0	2	2	0	11	0	2	0	184	4	3	18
Netherlands	0	0	0	0	102	0	1	0	0	0	948	63
Norway	0	4	16	0	7	0	5	4	0	8	32	14
Poland	0	1,417	14	3,789	546	0	50	0	8,252	1,217	213	843
Portugal	0	145	0	0	36	4	0	194	3,887	107	45	132
Republic of Moldova	0	1,687	112	7,939	138	17	26	64	2,621	151	79	69
Romania	0	3,962	0	16,643	639	45	91	87	20,540	1,438	346	490
Russian Federation	0	13,130	952	242,119	4,049	342	1,278	4,803	186,804	4,115	4,195	6,792
Serbia	0	54	29	2,631	132	4	2	0	7,230	361	568	97
Slovakia	0	353	0	7,019	66	4	9	8	1,835	143	88	71
Slovenia	0	133	9	0	2	0	2	0	502	19	137	25
Spain	0	603	0	0	118	4	21	200	0	0	0	236

Sweden	0	0	0	0	0	0	0	0	0	0	0	0
Switzerland	0	254	60	0	55	0	6	0	0	0	184	25
TFYR Macedonia	0	0	5	351	93	0	7	10	1,590	23	54	6
Ukraine	0	4,312	290	150,770	1,487	116	228	2,497	44,570	1,498	1,261	1,093
United Kingdom	612	1,537	0	0	693	53	59	0	4,383	79	3,071	61
Total	**1,261**	**39,750**	**2,992**	**501,772**	**10,772**	**746**	**2,123**	**8,664**	**338,440**	**10,588**	**23,699**	**13,136**

Note: TFYR Macedonia, the former Yugoslavian Republic of Macedonia

References

WHO Regional Office for Europe (2012) *European Mortality Database.* Copenhagen: WHO Regional Office for Europe, http://data.euro.who.int/hfamdb/ (accessed 10 July 2012).

World Health Organization (2010) *International Classification of Diseases*, revision 10 (updated 23 November 2010). Geneva: World Health Organization, http://www.who.int/classifications/icd/en/ (accessed 24 June 2012).

chapter fifteen

The will and the means to implement health policies

Martin McKee and Johan Mackenbach

Introduction

The previous chapters in this book offer many examples of success in health policy, but also reveal many missed opportunities. As Chapter 14 has shown, Europe is undoubtedly much healthier as a result of the successes, but much more can be gained if the performance of all countries is improved to the level of the best. And even in the best-performing countries, there is more that could be done. Consequently, while this book cannot claim to be comprehensive, these findings offer the beginning of an agenda for better health in Europe in the 21st century. Yet the findings also beg an important question. Why is it that some countries have been able to enact effective policies while others have not? This chapter and the next one will seek to answer this question.

To examine this question, this chapter will first present a general framework for analysis and then look back at Chapters 2–12 to identify what conditions for successful policy-making can be identified in each of these area-specific analyses. Chapter 16 will complement the qualitative analysis of Chapter 15 with a quantitative analysis of the conditions for successful health policies.

General framework

The different nature of health policies

The health policies reviewed here are very different in nature, and it is, therefore, likely that the conditions for their success are partly different too. One aspect in which these areas differ is their relative dependence on three different 'implementation modes' for prevention: service provision, health promotion and health protection. Table 15.1 illustrates this for each of our policy areas (as defined and specified in Chapters 2–12).

Table 15.1 Relative dependence of 11 health policies on service provision, behaviour change and intersectoral policies[a]

Policy area	Service provision	Health promotion	Health protection
Tobacco	+	++	++
Alcohol	−	+++	++
Food and nutrition	−	+++	++
Fertility, pregnancy, childbirth	+++	+	+
Child health	++	++	+
Infectious disease control	++	++	+
Hypertension detection and treatment	++++	+	−
Cancer screening	++++	+	−
Mental health	+++	+	+
Road safety	−	+	++++
Air pollution	−	−	+++++

Note: [a]For each policy area, a total of 5+ is allocated across the different modes

For example, while the success of tobacco control policies is partly dependent on service provision (in the form of counselling and nicotine replacement therapy for those who want to stop smoking), it predominantly depends on health promotion (such as mass media campaigns on the dangers of smoking, graphic pictorial warning labels on packs, etc.) and health protection measures (such as restrictions on sales to young people and bans on smoking in public places).

As Table 15.1 shows, the relative dependence of the 11 areas on each of these three modes of implementation is profoundly different: hypertension detection and treatment and cancer screening are almost entirely dependent on service provision, while air pollution control is entirely dependent on health protection. Most of the other areas present a mix.

Successful alcohol and food and nutrition policies do not require substantial service provision but are mainly dependent on health promotion and health protection. Policies in the areas of fertility/pregnancy/childbirth, child health, infectious disease control and mental health are relatively more dependent on service provision (e.g. in the form of contraception and safe abortion, screening for congenital anomalies, immunizations, prudent use of antibiotics, and antidepressant therapy) but also require some health promotion (e.g. in the form of education of parents to prevent cot death) and health protection (e.g. in the form of fences around swimming pools to prevent drowning and the removal of the means of committing suicide). Policies in the areas of road safety are mostly dependent on health protection measures but also require some health promotion (e.g. to reduce drunk driving and increase seat-belt wearing).

Clearly, conditions for successful health policy must be different for these 11 areas. While service provision requires that the health sector assume a lead role and engage in continuous active involvement, health protection is often led by other sectors. All involve costs, but in different ways. For example, service provision may incur financial costs while health protection may be politically costly where it challenges powerful vested interests, as may be health promotion if it challenges behaviours that are subject to different preferences.

A simple model

Chapters 2 to 12 have shown that countries differ in the degree to which they have chosen to, and/or have been able to, implement effective strategies to improve population health. Some have not even tried to initiate a policy; some have developed one but have failed to implement it; some have implemented a policy but have been unable to maintain or adapt it when circumstances change; and some have succeeded in developing small-scale or local programmes but have been unable to scale them up to cover the whole population. Even among those that have implemented wide-ranging policies, few have established monitoring systems to enable them to be evaluated. Yet, a few have developed, implemented and evaluated their policies, adapted them in the light of these evaluations, and achieved real improvements in population health. What can explain these differences?

Generally speaking, the implementation of health policies is dependent on there being both the 'will' and the 'means' to do something about a problem. Figure 15.1 summarizes a simple conceptual framework linking these elements.

Will

The first step in achieving a will to do something is to get it on the policy agenda. Kingdon (1984) identified three independent processes that are involved in achieving this: problems, proposals and politics. For an issue to arrive on the agenda, at least two must coincide at a critical time, a so-called policy window.

Problems

Problems refer to how decision-makers are persuaded to pay attention to one issue rather than another. Here, many different actors can play a role. One set includes the various media outlets, which have tremendous discretion on what they choose to cover. If an editor of a major newspaper decides to focus on an issue over a period of time, it may be difficult, at least in a democracy, for politicians to resist doing something. Indeed, it may be that democracy as such is important to make politicians responsive to emerging concerns among the public, although this may depend on the electoral system and the perceived electoral threat to the incumbent government.

Television programmes that shock can also have a major impact by bringing the scale and nature of an otherwise hidden problem to public attention.

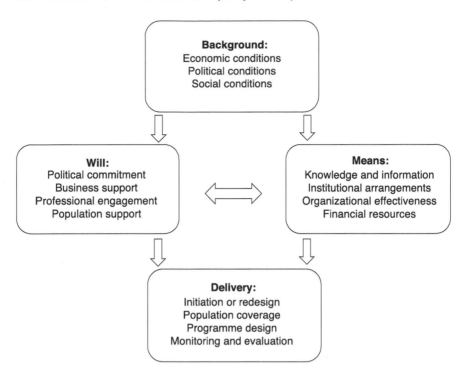

Figure 15.1 A simple conceptual framework outlining the conditions for effective health policy-making

This need not be a documentary. The 1966 television play *Cathy come home*, broadcast in the United Kingdom, is credited with raising awareness of the problems of homelessness and stimulating the creation of a non-governmental organization, Crisis, to tackle it (Franklin 1999).

The media also respond to evidence that a problem exists. This evidence can be produced by statutory bodies, such as national statistics authorities, drawing attention to a newly developing trend, or entities such as public health observatories and academic researchers analysing data in innovative ways to reveal the existence of a previously unnoticed problem. Such focus need not be limited to problems that have already arisen; there are several examples of Foresight programmes, such as those in the United Kingdom (Georghiou 1996) and the Netherlands (van der Meulen 1999), that scan the horizon to identify issues that have not yet emerged but can be predicted with reasonable certainty, although these have tended to focus on technology rather than health. An exception is the United Kingdom Government's Foresight report *Tackling Obesities: Future Choices* (Kopelman et al. 2007). Such evidence can also be generated by civil society organizations, compiling accounts from those affected by a problem and releasing it to the media or conducting polling to show that an issue overlooked by politicians is a matter of concern to the public.

Problems may also become visible through the actions of individuals, particularly where they have a high degree of public visibility, for example as politicians or media celebrities. This may be inadvertent; when Kylie Minogue was diagnosed with breast cancer, bookings for mammography in the target age group doubled in two weeks, and six weeks later it was still a third higher than previously (Chapman et al. 2005).

However, there are also powerful forces that work to keep problems off the agenda, by presenting evidence that deflects attention away from the issue concerned. Examples include the food industry seeking to attribute the obesity epidemic to inadequate physical activity, and, therefore, a matter of individual responsibility, and the tobacco industry seeking to discredit the overwhelming evidence on the dangers of second-hand smoke (McKee and Diethelm 2010).

Proposals

Proposals refer to what might be done to address a problem that has been identified. It is more likely that something will be done if there is consensus on what will work; if the proposed solution is consistent with prevailing norms, such as those that relate to the respective roles of the individual and the state; if there is no powerful opposition; and if it is inexpensive in monetary and political terms.

Success will depend on someone assembling the evidence that a policy will be effective and ideally cost-effective. This requires functioning institutions, such as university research units or national public health bodies. It also requires dedicated streams of research functioning to undertake and evaluate small-scale evaluations, to synthesize evidence from elsewhere and to model its likely impacts. The proposal should be coherent with the national context, and so it should take account of the performance of the institutions that already exist, including law enforcement agencies and trading standards offices.

Those engaged in the development of proposals can make it more likely that they will be adopted by finding ways to reduce the costs and practical obstacles to implementation and by increasing public and political support for them, through advocacy. For example, a major factor in the expansion of bans on smoking in public places was the demonstration that they worked, in that people did comply with the bans, although this was greatly encouraged by making the owner of the property responsible for enforcement through fines and withdrawal of licences, rather than depending on penalties against smokers (Bauer et al. 2007). Again, it is necessary to counter the powerful vested interests that sow confusion about effective policies, such as the efforts by the tobacco industry and its front organizations to convince politicians, misleadingly, that bans on smoking in public places would lead to falls in revenue in bars and restaurants (Scollo et al. 2003).

Politics

Politics comprises those factors that influence agendas, such as changes in government. It also includes political norms, such as those on the role of the state and the individual. In general, left-wing governments tend to favour greater state intervention and right wing governments less, but there are many exceptions. One element that has, so far, received less attention than it merits is the extent to which a country is ethnically or linguistically heterogeneous. Research among American states and worldwide has shown that political entities that are more fragmented are less willing to invest in public goods that benefit everyone (Alesina et al. 2001).

Politics also relates to the access that those seeking to influence health policy have to politicians. For example, the tobacco industry uses its claims to corporate social responsibility to obtain access to politicians (Fooks et al. 2011). Another aspect falling within this definition of politics is the pattern of prevailing values in society, including norms about the relationship between the individual and the state and willingness to bear short-term costs for long-term gains.

Window of opportunity

The combination of problems, policies and politics is more likely to be effective if they come together in a window of opportunity. This may be a scandal, a disaster or an individual tragedy that creates popular demands for action, causing politicians to search for some way that they can be seen to respond. It may also arise when someone known to be sympathetic to addressing an issue is appointed to a position of influence, or when it becomes apparent that it is possible to link one policy to another that is being implemented, for example by attaching a health policy measure to legislation on a related issue, perhaps on the basis of evidence from a health impact assessment.

Later in this analysis it will be seen that some of the differences between countries in implementation of health policies can indeed be traced back to differences in political will – sometimes based on long-standing differences in political orientations, sometimes based on single events that spurred political commitment. Professional engagement has also often played an important role; in some countries, organizations of health professionals have been very active in promoting policies to prevent the problems that they see in their clinics and offices. Whether the population supports the policy, or even takes the initiative in asking for the policy, also is an important factor, particularly when awareness and compliance are important for the success of the policy.

Means

Creating the will to enact an identifiable health policy is only the first step. It is then necessary to find the means to implement it. This requires several things. First, there must be adequate financial resources. Although health policies vary greatly in cost, and some, such as increased tobacco taxation, can be income generating, it will inevitably be easier for wealthy countries than poor ones to introduce many policies, particularly those based on service provision.

Second, there must be functioning institutions. Some relate to the overall effectiveness of the functions of government, such as the ability to draft and enact legislation in legislatures and the ability of the courts to enforce the law.

These vary considerably within Europe, and not only because of differences in resources. The situation is complicated in federal states, illustrated by the challenges in implementing a nationwide ban on smoking in public places in Germany (Stafford 2010). Other conditions will vary depending on the policy in question but may include organizational and managerial capacity to engage those responsible for implementing it, including those in sectors as diverse as education, transport, housing, police and regional development, among others. Consequently, it is always going to be easier to implement policies that enhance health in countries with effective governments.

Conditions for successful health policy: insights from the different areas

Chapters 2 to 13 have identified many aspects of health policy that are important for its success. For areas that partly or wholly depend on service provision, such as hypertension detection and control and cancer screening, a population-based approach that ensures wide coverage is important. For areas that partly depend on health promotion, such as tobacco and alcohol control, a comprehensive approach that tackles several determinants of unhealthy behaviour simultaneously is important in achieving success. For areas that depend on health protection, the involvement of other sectors than the health sector is crucial. In all cases, it is self-evident that a programmatic, evidence-based approach is desirable. The question that concerns us here is how does one create the conditions for successful policy delivery? Table 15.2 summarizes some of the insights that can be gleaned from chapters 2–12.

Will

The earlier chapters have given us several examples of how the will arose to address certain problems. In a few rare cases this happened rapidly. For example, as described in Chapter 7, the threat of a SARS epidemic was first noted when the Global Public Health Intelligence Network, a Canadian web-crawling system, was able to identify and publicize extremely rapidly the emergence of a previously unknown and potentially fatal viral infection in southern China (Mykhalovskiy and Weir 2006). Speed of response has characterized many infectious disease outbreaks throughout history, but in many of the other policy areas it has taken many years for an issue to be seen as a problem requiring concerted action. This was frequently the case with those issues involving a degree of personal choice, such as smoking and drinking. Many governments were all too willing to abdicate their responsibilities to their citizens.

In such cases, civil society organizations played an important role, using graphic means to demonstrate the scale of the disease burden involved. The statement that half of all smokers will die from their habit and of these half will die before reaching retirement age, is a simple message that is easy to convey. Media campaigns showing the victims of drunk drivers starkly convey the human consequences that lie behind the statistics. The organization

Table 15.2 Conditions for successful health policy mentioned in Chapters 2 to 12

Policy area	Will	Means
Tobacco	Advocacy by civil society (+) Clarity of message (+) Framework Convention on Tobacco Control (+) Tobacco industry influence (–)	International exchange of evidence (+) Tobacco industry influence (–) Corruption (–)
Alcohol	Cognitive dissonance (–) Alcohol industry influence (–)	Availability of evidence (+) Economic collapse (–) European integration (–) Lack of industry regulation (–)
Food	Lack of awareness (iodine) (–) Advocacy groups (+) Collaboration with industry (+)	Availability of evidence (+) European integration (±) Working across government (+)
Fertility, pregnancy and childbirth	Pronatalist policies (–) Rejection of abortion (–)	Availability of registrations (+) Lack of evidence (–) International collaboration (+)
Child health	Professional engagement (+) Advocacy groups (+) Immunization scares (–) United Nations Convention on the Rights of the Child (+)	Disruption of health system (–) International collaboration (+) Genuine communication (+) Professionals in media (±)
Infectious diseases	Reluctance to regulate (–) Civil society involvement (+) Stigma of deviant behaviour (–)	Surveillance systems (+) Centralized systems (+) International collaboration (+) Forward-looking institutions (+)
Hypertension	Professional compliance (+) Evidence of amount of hidden salt in food (+)	Availability of evidence (+) Drug availability (+)
Cancer screening	Professional advocacy (+) Professional inertia (–)	Availability of evidence (+) Screening register (+) Effective organization (+)
Mental health	Evidence on hidden burden of disease (+) Professional awareness (+) Stigma (–)	Lack of outcome data (–)
Road traffic safety	Aversion of 'nanny state' (–) High political support (+)	Availability of evidence (+) Innovation in industry (+) International collaboration (+) European integration (+)
Air pollution	Engagement with environmental movement (+)	Availability of evidence (+) Innovation in industry (+) European integration (+) Low vehicle turnover (–)

Consensus Action on Salt and Health has made visible the large quantities of salt hidden in many processed foods (MacGregor and Sever 1996). Air pollution became recognized as a political problem requiring concerted action not as a consequence of concerns about health (at least not after some of the major pollutants from burning coal had been tackled in the 1950s, for example as a response to high death rates in London smogs (Davis et al. 2002)) but rather because of the damage being done to trees by acid rain. In this case it was the environmental movement that was key.

In several cases, individuals have played a critical role in raising awareness of certain health issues, and in advocating policy action. The British television chef Jamie Oliver placed the problem of junk food being served to children in schools firmly on the policy agenda, shocking the public by revealing just how some of the food being given to their children was produced, such as the now infamous 'Turkey Twizzlers', in which reconstituted turkey meat was combined with a soup of chemicals to produce a product containing over 20% fat (Morgan 2006). In the 1980s the French and Italian oncologists Maurice Tubiana and Umberto Veronesi exploited their connections with, respectively, Francois Mitterrand and Bettino Craxi to drive forward the first ever EU programme in health, Europe against Cancer (Mele and Compagni 2010). Again in the United Kingdom, a television presenter, Ann Diamond, placed the issue of SIDS in the public eye after she lost a baby (McKee et al. 1996a).

Professional bodies have also played a role, such as the paediatricians in the Netherlands who identified the rising rate of postneonatal death in the 1980s and initiated a campaign to reduce it, based on emerging evidence on the role of sleeping position (McKee et al. 1996a; Mackenbach 2011). In the United Kingdom, the Royal College of Physicians played a major role in highlighting the damage caused by smoking (Berridge 2007).

The media too have contributed to agenda setting. The high levels of antibiotic-resistant infections in British hospitals were the subject of a campaign by a major newspaper and, although the reporting was often inaccurate and misleading (Goldacre 2008), it made the issue a major political concern, acting as a symbol of the failings of the government at the time (Boyce et al. 2009).

Elsewhere, inaction has persisted because an issue is not recognized as a matter for policy action. The scale of iodine deficiency in Europe described in Chapter 4 is remarkable and extremely easy to rectify, but it has yet to come anywhere close to the political agenda in most countries. Chapter 8 describes how far there is still to go to reduce the toll of death and disability caused by stroke in Europe (Kim and Johnston 2011), something that should be easily achievable given existing knowledge about how to control hypertension. What progress has been made is largely a result of the gradual increase in awareness among health professionals, which has occurred largely by passive diffusion. The evidence set out in Chapter 9 on the effectiveness of organized, as opposed to opportunistic, cancer screening programmes is another example of where the problem seems clear but has yet to reach the policy agenda in many countries.

In some cases, however, inaction, or more often delayed action, results partly from the efforts of powerful vested interests to suggest that there is no problem. The most notorious example is second-hand smoking, where the tobacco industry conducted a major campaign to generate misleading research and to pursue alternative, spurious explanations, with the central aim of creating sufficient confusion about whether exposure was harmful. This even included efforts to redefine the standards used in epidemiology (Ong and Glantz 2001). Another example was the failure to respond in a timely manner to the emergence of BSE in the United Kingdom, where the interests of the agricultural industry were prioritized over human health (Chapter 7) (McKee et al. 1996b).

Similar factors can be discerned in the development of proposals for policy, Kingdon's (1984) second process facilitating policy action. Politicians may accept the problem exists but they may not know what to do about it. Academic research to demonstrate the effectiveness of policies is essential, but its findings must be translated into information that can be understood by policymakers and which is seen as salient to their concerns (Innvaer et al. 2002). Understanding of how best to translate evidence into policy has increased greatly in recent years and is summarized in the material produced in the SUPPORT project (Lavis et al. 2009).

Civil society organizations have sometimes played an important role in the dissemination of evidence about what works. One of the most effective has been Globalink, a coalition of organizations dedicated to counteracting the activities of the international tobacco industry (Wipfli et al. 2010). A more recent example is the emergence of a coalition of women's organizations campaigning against misinformation about immunization to prevent human papilloma virus infection (Laurent-Ledru et al. 2011). However, there are many other European organizations, often joining together under the umbrella of the European Public Health Alliance, who exchange knowledge on what has been found to work in different settings.

Once again, opposition by vested interests can play a role in blocking policy. The tobacco industry has promoted the views that bans on smoking in public places are unenforceable, that they will reduce revenues in the hospitality industry and that tax increases will increase smuggling (Howell 2011). In these, and in other areas, their goal is to persuade policy-makers that any measures they may be contemplating are too difficult. Their arguments are, of course, based on gross distortions of the evidence. Similar tactics can be discerned by parts of the food industry in their opposition to simple, clear and easily understood 'traffic light' labelling of foodstuffs (Lobstein and Davies 2009), and the alcohol industry in its efforts to persuade policy-makers that the, obvious to most people, link between alcohol and violence is far more complicated than people simply getting drunk and picking fights (McKee 2006). However, there are also some examples of industry playing a positive role, as in the reformulation of some foods to remove TFAs in the Netherlands and measures by the car industry to improve vehicle safety.

The final element of Kingdon's (1984) framework for agenda setting is the political dimension. The opportunity to introduce an EU restriction on tobacco advertising following the election of a Labour Government in the United Kingdom in 1977 has already been mentioned. However, individual politicians may also play a role. For example, David Byrne, then Irish Attorney General and later European Commissioner for Health, recognized the scope to implement a ban on smoking in public places, building on experience in New York.

Turning to national values, religious matters play a limited role in health policy except in relation to reproductive health. As was noted in Chapter 5, Ireland and Malta, both of which prohibit termination of pregnancy on grounds of fetal abnormality, have the highest proportions of neonatal deaths from these causes. This may also be a factor in the high rate of teenage pregnancy in Malta, where the Catholic Church has long opposed sex education in schools and the use of contraception (Massa 2009).

Health policy may also be influenced by political views about the appropriate role of the state. In the Nordic countries, Sweden and Finland have traditionally seen the state playing a greater role in the lives of their citizens (Bambra 2011), for example through their imposition, at least until they were compelled to abandon some of them by European law, of stringent controls on alcohol sales. In contrast, Denmark has, at least since the 1960s, taken a much more libertarian approach. As a consequence, death rates from tobacco- and alcohol-related diseases rose rapidly in Denmark during the 1970s and 1980s, opening up a substantial gap in life expectancy with Sweden (Chenet et al. 1996).

Domestic health policy may also be influenced by international factors. In some cases, as in the EU, some policies relevant to health are made at the European level anyway (McKee et al. 2002). However, the Framework Convention on Tobacco Control has provided a means for civil society to hold governments to account for their actions. The same is true of the Convention on the Rights of the Child (United Nations General Assembly 1989). However, supranational policies may also impede policy-making, as was the case with Denmark's efforts to implement a ban on TFAs or Finland's challenges in maintaining an effective policy on alcohol within the European single market (Chapter 4) (Chenet et al. 1997).

Any consideration of political factors cannot ignore the role of certain industries, in particular the tobacco industry and also, to some extent, the food and alcohol industries. In some countries, links with politicians have been very close. Germany and Austria, for example, are considered by the tobacco industry to be especially supportive of their activities. It is now known that a number of senior scientists in Germany advising on tobacco policy were being paid by the industry (Gruning et al. 2006). There have been persistent concerns about alleged involvement by senior politicians in Montenegro in tobacco smuggling into Italy (Sisti 2009).

Means

The will to implement health policies is not enough. Countries must have the means to do so. Most obviously, they must have the necessary resources. This obviously requires money, although as noted above, some policies such as taxation of harmful substances can be income generating. Therefore, a country with a higher gross national product is likely, all else being equal, to find it easier to implement policies. Countries faced with economic crises, such as those in the former USSR in the early 1990s and countries in southern Europe in the economic crisis that arose in 2008, face major problems in maintaining policies previously put in place.

Yet resources are more than simply money. Money is a means to buy labour and goods, and if these are not available in a country then money by itself will be of little use. Many health policies require actions by skilled workers, both in the health sector and beyond. Consequently, the effective implementation of many health policies will only be possible if they can build on the presence of a trained workforce. That workforce also needs the tools to do the job. One reason for the poor control of hypertension in the countries of the former USSR is the affordability of medicines (Chapter 8) (Roberts et al. 2012). Resources are also required for physical infrastructure. One of the reasons for the high death rate from RTIs in countries in the former USSR is the poor state of the road network. Low turnover of a country's vehicle fleet, because of economic constraints, will reduce the speed with which emissions of air pollutants can be reduced (Chapter 12).

Health policies also require functioning information systems. These are necessary to identify those at greatest need. For example, surveys on smoking behaviour, on knowledge of the health effects of smoking and of how people are influenced by tobacco marketing are essential to develop effective tobacco policies. Similar information is required to counter hazardous alcohol consumption. Information systems are also essential to monitor the performance of a health policy in order to identify when and where to intervene if problems arise. In the absence of an effective information system, containing socio-demographic data, it will not be possible to identify groups with low levels of uptake of immunization or cancer screening. Information is also necessary to monitor the environment. For example, policies to reduce air pollution have been based on data on the levels of noxious substances that were previously unavailable (Chapter 13).

However, some areas have proven resistant to the creation of effective information systems. One example is mental health, where suicide rates are recognized to be a very limited indicator of the effectiveness of policies but remain in widespread use because of the absence of detailed and consistent data on the prevalence of mental illness. The seminal Global Burden of Disease study, led by Chris Murray and Alan Lopez, made visible the scale of human misery caused by mental illness by incorporating not only mortality but also disability (Murray 2001). In similar ways, other academic studies have helped to raise awareness of other health problems. The American physician Ancel Keys led the Seven Country study, which included a number of European countries, to establish the association between dietary cholesterol and heart disease and led to the term 'Mediterranean diet' being coined (Menotti et al. 1996), while the French physician Michel de Lorgeril, working in Lyon, showed that shifting to such a diet lowered the risk of heart disease (de Lorgeril and Salen 2006). Tobacco control efforts would have been impossible without research demonstrating the link between smoking and lung cancer, such as that by Richard Doll and Austin Bradford Hill (Doll and Hill 1954).

Perhaps the most important factor in determining whether a health policy can be implemented is the effectiveness of the government. Governments vary greatly in their ability to carry out core functions. These range from the ability to collect taxes to the ability to organize collective health care or education systems. The World Bank has characterized government effectiveness as having three major components: the quality of the civil service and its independence from political pressures, the quality of policy formulation and implementation, and the credibility of the government's commitment to such policies (Kaufmann et al. 2002). It has operationalized each of these using data from a range of sources, such as the degree of public satisfaction with different types of infrastructure, the time spent by private sector management in dealing with government officials and the speed with which decisions are made. Clearly, a government that is unable to collect taxes, as in Greece and many countries in the former USSR, will be unable to implement many complex health policies.

There are many reasons why governments are ineffective. One is the calibre of the civil servants, a problem in those countries that pay such low wages that the most skilled individuals emigrate, move full-time into the private sector or devote much of their time to second jobs. Another is rapid turnover within bureaucracies so that institutional memory is lost. However, it is equally important to avoid the rigidity that prevents bureaucracies from incorporating new knowledge. Few countries succeed in getting the balance right. Yet another problem is corruption. Indeed, corruption at all levels may be the most important reason why many public health policies are not implemented effectively. Corruption may be low level, for example where police take bribes rather than enforce road safety legislation, or high level, where politicians and senior officials are complicit in tobacco smuggling. Unfortunately, public health professionals have, until recently, been unwilling to confront the impact of organized crime on health (Reynolds and McKee 2010).

A related issue is trust in government. It will be more difficult to persuade the public to act on messages set out by governments if they distrust them. In the United Kingdom, trust in government was seriously eroded by the BSE affair (McKee and Coker 2009), which made it more difficult to counteract the misleading media coverage of the safety of the MMR vaccine some years later (Chapter 6) (Gardner et al. 2010).

An institutional infrastructure to develop policies that are appropriate to the national context is essential. This may involve sophisticated marketing campaigns to disseminate health promotion messages, as is done in a number of western European countries in relation to tobacco. Another example is the creation of organized cancer screening programmes, such as those in Finland and the United Kingdom, comprising call and recall systems, integrated management follow-up of those identified as positive and systems of quality assurance. The same considerations apply to immunization programmes. As was seen in Chapters 7 and 9, it seems easier to put such programmes in place in countries with integrated health care delivery systems, often associated with funding from taxation, than in more fragmented ones, which tend to be associated with payment from social insurance.

Conclusions

This chapter has argued that governments must have both the will and the means to implement effective health policies and has given a large number of examples of how differences between countries in the implementation of effective health policies can arise. In countries where there is a lack of means, intentions remain just that. In such cases, policy intentions are no more than dreams set out in reports that gather dust on bookshelves, because countries lack the resources, the infrastructure or the organizational capacity to make things happen. Yet other countries have the means to implement effective policies but lack the will to do so. They may not realize they have a problem; they may not be aware that there is a solution, or they may be unwilling to let health policy interfere with other interests. To better understand the role of these different contexts it is necessary to take a more quantitative approach. This will be done in Chapter 16.

References

Alesina, A., Glaeser, E.L. and Sacerdote, B. (2001) *Why Doesn't the US have a European-style Welfare System?* Cambridge, MA: National Bureau of Economic Research.

Bambra, C. (2011) Health inequalities and welfare state regimes: theoretical insights on a public health 'puzzle', *Journal of Epidemiology and Community Health*, 65(9): 740–5.

Bauer, U., Juster, H., Hyland, A. et al. (2007) Reduced secondhand smoke exposure after implementation of a comprehensive statewide smoking ban: New York, June 26, 2003 – June 30, 2004, *MMWR Morbidity and Mortality Weekly Report*, 56(28):705–8.

Berridge, V. (2007) Medicine and the public: the 1962 report of the Royal College of Physicians and the new public health, *Bulletin of the History of Medicine*, 81(1):286–311.

Boyce, T., Murray, E. and Holmes, A. (2009) What are the drivers of the UK media coverage of meticillin-resistant *Staphylococcus aureus*, the inter-relationships and relative influences? *Journal of Hospital Infection*, 73(4):400–7.

Chapman, S., McLeod, K., Wakefield, M. and Holding, S. (2005) Impact of news of celebrity illness on breast cancer screening: Kylie Minogue's breast cancer diagnosis, *Medical Journal of Australia*, 183(5):247–50.

Chenet, L., Osler, M., McKee, M. and Krasnik, A. (1996) Changing life expectancy in the 1980s: why was Denmark different from Sweden? *Journal of Epidemiology and Community Health*, 50(4):404–7.

Chenet, L., McKee, M., Osler, M. and Krasnik, A. (1997) Alcohol policy in the Nordic countries, *British Medical Journal*, 314(7088):1142–3.

Davis, D.L., Bell, M.L. and Fletcher, T. (2002) A look back at the London smog of 1952 and the half century since, *Environmental Health Perspectives*, 110(12):A734–735.

Doll, R. and Hill, A.B. (1954) The mortality of doctors in relation to their smoking habits; a preliminary report, *British Medical Journal*, 1(4877):1451–5.

Fooks, G.J., Gilmore, A.B., Smith, K.E. et al. (2011) Corporate social responsibility and access to policy elites: an analysis of tobacco industry documents, *PLoS Medicine*, 8(8):e1001076.

Franklin, B. (1999) *Social Policy, the Media and Misrepresentation*. London: Routledge.

Gardner, B., Davies, A., McAteer, J. and Michie, S. (2010) Beliefs underlying UK parents' views towards MMR promotion interventions: a qualitative study, *Psychology and Health Medicine*, 15(2):220–30.

Georghiou, L. (1996) The UK technology foresight programme, *Futures*, 28:359–77.

Goldacre, B. (2008) *Bad Science*. London: Fourth Estate.

Gruning, T., Gilmore, A.B. and McKee, M. (2006) Tobacco industry influence on science and scientists in Germany, *American Journal of Public Health*, 96(1):20–32.

Howell, F. (2011) The Irish tobacco industry position on price increases on tobacco products, *Tobacco Control*, Epub ahead of print (PMID: 22170338).

Innvaer, S., Vist, G., Trommald, M. and Oxman, A. (2002) Health policy-makers' perceptions of their use of evidence: a systematic review, *Journal of Health Service Research Policy*, 7(4):239–44.

Kaufmann, D., Kraay, A. and Zoido-Lobaton, P. (2002) *Governance Matters II*. Washington DC: World Bank.

Kim, A.S. and Johnston, S.C. (2011) Global variation in the relative burden of stroke and ischemic heart disease, *Circulation*, 124(3):314–23.

Kingdon, J. (1984) *Agendas, Alternatives and Public Policies*. Boston, MA: Little Brown.

Kopelman, P., Jebb, S.A. and Butland, B. (2007) Executive summary: Foresight 'Tackling Obesities: Future Choices' project, *Obesity Reviews*, 8(suppl 1):vi–ix.

Laurent-Ledru, V., Thomson, A. and Monsonego, J. (2011) Civil society: a critical new advocate for vaccination in Europe, *Vaccine*, 29(4):624–8.

Lavis, J.N., Oxman, A.D., Lewin, S. and Fretheim, A. (2009) SUPPORT tools for evidence-informed health policymaking (STP), *Health Research and Policy Systems*, 7(suppl 1):I1.

Lobstein, T. and Davies, S. (2009) Defining and labelling 'healthy' and 'unhealthy' food, *Public Health Nutrition*, 12(3):331–40.

de Lorgeril, M. and Salen, P. (2006) The Mediterranean-style diet for the prevention of cardiovascular diseases, *Public Health Nutrition*, 9(1A):118–23.

MacGregor, G.A. and Sever, P.S. (1996) Salt: overwhelming evidence but still no action – can a consensus be reached with the food industry? CASH (Consensus Action on Salt and Hypertension), *British Medical Journal*, 312:1287–9.

Mackenbach, J.P. (ed.) (2011) *Successen van preventie 1970–2010 [Successes of Prevention 1970–2010]*. Rotterdam: Erasmus Publishing/Erasmus MC, Department of Public Health.

Massa, A. (2009) Malta 'burying head in sand' on sexual health, *Sunday Times*, 29 November, http://www.timesofmalta.com/articles/view/20091129/local/malta-burying-head-in-sand-on-sexual-health.283759 (accessed 11 July 2012).

McKee, M. (2006) A European alcohol strategy, *British Medical Journal*, 333(7574): 871–2.

McKee, M. and Coker, R. (2009) Trust, terrorism and public health, *Journal of Public Health*, 31(4):462–5.

McKee, M. and Diethelm, P. (2010) How the growth of denialism undermines public health, *British Medical Journal*, 341:c6950.

McKee, M., Fulop, N., Bouvier, P. et al. (1996a) Preventing sudden infant deaths: the slow diffusion of an idea, *Health Policy (Oxf)*, 37:117–35.

McKee, M., Lang, T. and Roberts, J.A. (1996b) Deregulating health: policy lessons from the BSE affair, *Journal of the Royal Society of Medicine*, 89(8):424–6.

McKee, M., Mossialos, E. and Baeten, R. (eds) (2002) *The Impact of EU Law on Health Care Systems*. Brussels: PIE Peter Lang.

Mele, V. and Compagni, A. (2010) Explaining the unexpected success of the smoking ban in Italy: political strategy and transition to practice, 2000–2005, *Public Administration*, 88:819–35.

Menotti, A., Keys, A., Blackburn, H. et al. (1996) Comparison of multivariate predictive power of major risk factors for coronary heart diseases in different countries: results from eight nations of the Seven Countries Study, 25-year follow-up, *Journal of Cardiovascular Risk*, 3(1):69–75.

van der Meulen, B. (1999) The impact of foresight on environmental science and technology policy in the Netherlands, *Futures*, 31:7–23.

Morgan, K. (2006) School food and the public domain: the politics of the public plate, *Political Quarterly*, 77:379–87.

Murray, C.J.L. (2001) *The Global Burden of Disease 2000 project: aims, methods and data sources*. Cambridge, MA: Harvard Burden of Disease Unit, Center for Population and Development Studies.

Mykhalovskiy, E. and Weir, L. (2006) The Global Public Health Intelligence Network and early warning outbreak detection: a Canadian contribution to global public health, *Canadian Journal of Public Health*, 97(1):42–4.

Ong, E.K. and Glantz, S.A. (2001) Constructing sound science and good epidemiology: tobacco, lawyers, and public relations firms, *American Journal of Public Health*, 91(11):1749–57.

Roberts, B., Stickley, A., Balabanova, D., Haerpfer, C. and McKee, M. (2012) The persistence of irregular treatment of hypertension in the former Soviet Union, *Journal of Epidemiology and Community Health*, 66:1079–82.

Reynolds, L. and McKee, M. (2010) Organised crime and the efforts to combat it: a concern for public health. *Globalisation and Health*, 6:21.

Scollo, M., Lal, A., Hyland, A. and Glantz, S. (2003) Review of the quality of studies on the economic effects of smoke-free policies on the hospitality industry, *Tobacco Control*, 12(1):13–20.

Sisti, L. (2009) *The Montenegro Connection*. Washington DC, Center for Public Integrity.

Stafford, N. (2010) Campaigners hope a vote for a complete smoking ban in Bavaria will spread to other German states, *British Medical Journal*, 341:c3631.

United Nations General Assembly (1989) *Convention on the Rights of the Child*. New York: United Nations.

Wipfli, H.L., Fujimoto, K. and Valente, T.W. (2010) Global tobacco control diffusion: the case of the framework convention on tobacco control, *American Journal of Public Health*, 100(7):1260–6.

chapter sixteen

Conditions for successful health policies

Martin McKee and Johan Mackenbach

Introduction

Chapter 13 provided a series of indicators by which it was possible to assess the achievements of different countries on key areas of health policy identified in Chapters 2–12. This chapter will ask whether we can quantitatively explain the observed differences in performance on the basis of the factors identified in Chapter 15. To do so, the indicators that capture relevant aspects of these factors must be identified. After this, the chapter will report on a number of exploratory analyses: determinants of a country's overall score on health policy performance, determinants of a country's performance on individual indicators, and characteristics of outliers.

Indicators of 'will' and 'means'

Financial resources

The first factor to be considered is financial resources. These are likely to be important in the development and implementation of health policy. Within Europe, variations in national income are well known (Table 16.1). The richest countries in the year 2000 were Luxembourg, Norway and Switzerland. The poorest countries were the Republic of Moldova, Albania and Azerbaijan. Although there is a clear distinction in average income level, measured as GDP per capita in American dollars in 2000, between the different parts of Europe, with the north and west of Europe being considerably richer than the east, there is also considerable heterogeneity within regions, for example within the western Balkans (with Slovenia being more than six times richer than Albania) and within the former USSR (with Belarus being almost five times richer than

Table 16.1 Economic, cultural and political background factors, ca. 2000[a]

Countries	Gross domestic product	Survival values	Democracy	Government effectiveness	Left-wing party	Ethnic fraction-alization
Year	2000	2000–2006	2000	2002	1990–2009	2001
Nordic						
Finland	26,402	0.94	10.0	2.21	34.40	0.1315
Sweden	27,174	2.09	10.0	2.07	68.77	0.0600
Norway	41,777	2.17	10.0	2.02	59.34	0.0586
Iceland	31,489	1.63	10.0	2.07	21.35	0.0798
Denmark	30,468	1.87	10.0	2.17	32.96	0.0819
Britain and Ireland						
United Kingdom	27,032	1.31	10.0	1.93	63.33	0.4737
Ireland	31,389	1.18	10.0	1.68	11.45	0.1206
Continental						
Netherlands	31,927	1.94	10.0	2.09	31.86	0.1054
Belgium	29,692	1.13	10.0	1.99	49.86	0.5554
Luxembourg	63,392	1.13	10.0	2.17	32.57	0.5302
Germany	29,051	0.44	10.0	1.81	45.19	0.1682
Switzerland	34,414	1.90	10.0	2.25	28.57	0.5314
Austria	31,574	1.43	10.0	1.98	31.78	0.1068
Mediterranean						
France	27,311	0.94	9.0	1.61	37.42	0.1032
Spain	24,945	0.51	10.0	1.82	60.23	0.4165
Portugal	19,606	0.49	10.0	1.20	37.48	0.0468
Italy	27,142	0.85	10.0	0.93	28.84	0.1145
Malta	19,442			1.10	9.32	0.0414
Greece	20,707	0.55	10.0	0.84	53.06	0.1576
Cyprus	20,274	0.13	10.0	1.17	17.68	0.0939
Western Balkans						
Slovenia	19,043	0.38	10.0	0.88	49.36	0.2216
Croatia	9,775	0.31	8.0	0.34		0.369
Bosnia and Herzegovina	5,798			−0.97		0.6300
Serbia	7,244	−1.03	7.0	−0.21		0.5736

Countries	Gross domestic product	Survival values	Democracy	Government effectiveness	Left-wing party	Ethnic fraction-alization
Year	2000	2000–2006	2000	2002	1990–2009	2001
Montenegro	4,877	–1.24	7.0	–0.29		0.5736
TFYR Macedonia	6,358	–0.72	6.0	–0.46		0.5023
Albania	3,177	–1.14	5.0	–0.59		0.2204
Central and eastern						
Poland	10,834	–0.60	9.0	0.56	32.54	0.1183
Czech Republic	16,044	0.38	10.0	0.93	37.98	0.3222
Slovakia	11,844	–0.43	9.0	0.47	28.10	0.2539
Hungary	13,025	–1.22	10.0	1.01	51.47	0.1522
Romania	6,151	–1.60	8.0	–0.14	59.05	0.3069
Bulgaria	6,374	–1.52	8.0	0.09	24.67	0.4021
Former USSR						
Estonia	10,405	–1.19	9.0	0.81	26.11	0.5062
Latvia	8,119	–1.27	8.0	0.59	18.10	0.5867
Lithuania	8,566	–1.00	10.0	0.61	46.91	0.3223
Belarus	12,188	–1.23	–7.0	–1.06		0.3222
Ukraine	5,644	–1.72	6.0	–0.71		0.4737
Republic of Moldova	2,420	–1.69	7.0	–0.63		0.5535
Russian Federation	8,305	–1.88	–5.0	–0.32		0.2452
Georgia	4,310		5.0	–0.76		0.4923
Armenia	4,333		5.0	–0.22		0.1272
Azerbaijan	3,722		–7.0	–0.87		0.2047

Notes: TFYR Macedonia, the former Yugoslavian Republic of Macedonia
[a]For sources and definitions, see text

the Republic of Moldova). On average, richer countries are expected to have implemented more health policies than poorer countries.

Values

European countries differ not only in their economic situation but also in their cultural, political and institutional conditions. The World Values Survey has identified two dimensions that explain a large amount of variation in a wide range of national indicators (Inglehart 2000; World Values Survey 2012). One is a traditional/secular–rational scale, reflecting the contrast between societies in which religion is very important and those in which it is not. Societies near the traditional pole emphasize the importance of parent–child ties and deference to authority, along with traditional family values, while rejecting divorce, abortion, euthanasia and suicide. Such societies have high levels of national pride and a nationalistic outlook. Societies with secular–rational values have the opposite preferences on all of these topics. The second relates to the transition from industrial society to postindustrial societies. This is the survival/ self-expression scale. Increasing prosperity means that more people in advanced industrialized countries take basic survival for granted. As a consequence, their priorities have shifted from basic economic and physical security towards subjective well-being, self-expression and quality of life.

It is the second that is of potentially most relevance to health policy as it is plausible that those societies that have moved beyond a focus on basic survival towards self-expression will be more likely to invest in their future well-being by enacting health-enhancing measures. Populations of richer countries tend to have different value orientations compared with populations of poorer countries: as the World Values Survey consistently shows, people in the latter are more likely to exhibit survival values, reflecting the challenges they face on a day-to-day basis, whereas those in the former, who have overall fewer immediate concerns about survival, are oriented towards self-expression values.

Although the association between average income and position on the World Values Survey scale of survival/self-expression is quite strong, there are important deviations from this general pattern (Table 16.1). For example, Finland is as rich as the other Nordic countries but the value orientation of its population on this scale is more traditional, perhaps because Finland has only relatively recently exited from the Russian sphere of influence. A population that adheres more closely to values of self-expression might be expected to look more to the future and to invest in measures that will enhance future health. In contrast, a country where values are dominated by survival may view such investments as a luxury. This is consistent with what is known about how messages about individual behaviour are presented. Therefore, it is often argued that smokers living in severely deprived environments may feel that there is little point in quitting, seeing it as one of their few pleasures in a life that they expect will be short given what they have observed among their friends and families (a view borne out by research measuring time preferences of smokers at different levels of income; Scharff and Viscusi 2011). Given how widespread this view is, it is plausible that it will be echoed among policy-makers.

Democracy

As noted above, health policies are forms of purposeful collective behaviour and often require initiation, or at least approval, by political institutions. Most countries in northern and western Europe have long democratic traditions, but during the 20th century many countries in the south and east have had shorter or longer periods of autocratic government. In the year 2000, all European countries had forms of parliamentary democracy, but in the western Balkans and in the former USSR not all countries had fully functional democracies. The quality of democracy has been assessed by independent researchers with the so-called Polity IV index (Table 16.1). This scores a country's democratic system from −10 (least democratic) to +10 (most democratic) based on the competitiveness of political participation, constraints on the chief executive and competitiveness of executive recruitment (Marshall et al. 2010). Although there is a positive correlation between average income and the democratic nature of political systems (Marshall et al. 2010), the correlation is far from perfect, as is evident from the fact that within the countries of the former USSR Belarus has a relatively high level of economic development but a partly autocratic political system, whereas the much poorer Republic of Moldova has a better functioning democracy. Democratically elected governments would be expected to be more responsive to the needs of populations and, therefore, to be more active in implementing health policies.

Government effectiveness

Whether governments are able to implement health policies is also likely to depend on their overall effectiveness, as determined by, for example, the professionalism of the civil service, the functioning of government departments and agencies and the absence of corruption. The summary index of government effectiveness developed by the World Bank indicates large variation within Europe (Table 16.1). Poorer countries tend to have less-effective governments ((Marshall et al. 2010), but within the same category of prosperity there are some notable variations. For example, Italy has a much lower effectiveness score than Spain, and richer Belarus has a much lower effectiveness score for its government than poorer Lithuania. Countries with a higher score on government effectiveness would be expected not only to have implemented more health policies but also to have achieved better intermediate and final outcomes.

Political composition of governments

What health policies governments pursue is ultimately a matter of political choice or, in some cases, ideology. Within Europe, the main political parties (under varying names) have traditionally been the social-democrats on the left, the Christian-democrats in the centre and the 'liberals' or conservatives on the right. Since the 1980s, there have been large differences between countries in the share that each of these parties have had in government. The average share of the total number of cabinet posts held by social democratic parties varied between 9% in Malta and 69% in Sweden. There is no association with average income. Social democratic governments have tended to pursue more egalitarian policies than governments dominated by other political parties, for example by implementing universal health insurance or social security. As noted in Chapter 1, some studies have reported better health outcomes in countries with longer periods of social democratic rule. One might expect these countries also to have implemented more health policies.

Ethnic fractionalization

Collective behaviour requires that countries view themselves collectively, in other words that each person sees their fellow citizen as their neighbour. This may be less likely in countries that are more heterogeneous, on linguistic, religious or ethnic grounds (Kvist et al. 2012). Events during and immediately after the Second World War led to states that were largely homogeneous; those that were not, such as Switzerland and Belgium, had addressed the issue by means of a high degree of devolution to the cantons and communities. In south-eastern Europe, the multiethnic state of Yugoslavia spilt into ethnically homogeneous states in the 1990s, with the exception of Bosnia and Herzegovina, which remains politically fragmented along ethnic lines, and Macedonia, with its large Albanian population (Glenny 1996). The situation is quite different in eastern Europe and the former USSR, with Slovakia and Romania having large Hungarian populations and Bulgaria having a large Turkish population. Ukraine is divided between ethnic Ukrainians and Russians (McKee 2009). The Russian Federation is a complex multiethnic state but has addressed this by a degree of decentralization to regions and *oblasts* (Danishevski et al. 2006). On the basis of evidence from elsewhere, it would seem likely that some of these countries provide less-fertile ground for public health policies. Data on fractionalization on ethnic, linguistic and religious grounds were assembled for all countries of the world from a range of sources, particularly censuses, around 2001 (Norwegian Social Science Data Services 2011). Data for Europe are shown in Table 16.1.

Correlations between variables

Clearly, it is to be expected that many of these variables are correlated with one another, which they indeed are (Table 16.2). Wealthier countries are more likely to have populations that place a greater emphasis on self-expression rather than the immediate problems of survival. Democracy is also associated with economic development, with the relationship likely to be bidirectional. The same is true for the association between wealth and government effectiveness; richer countries can afford bureaucracies that employ people with higher skills and with greater access to information. Somewhat similar arguments apply to the associations with survival/ self-expression values. Those living in a democracy may need to worry less about their immediate survival, while the threat of electoral defeat provides a stimulus for investment and effective government. The reasons for the associations between self-expression and electoral success by left-wing parties and ethnic fractionalization are less clear. Nor is it immediately clear why there should be an association between ethnic fractionalization and government effectiveness – although it may be easier to build up effective government in more homogeneous nations.

Table 16.2 Correlations between potential explanatory variables

	GDP (2000)	Survival values	Democracy	Government effectiveness	Left-wing parties	Ethnic fractionalization
GDP	1.00	**0.84**	**0.47**	**0.86**	0.06	0.32
Survival/ self-expression values		1.00	**0.51**	**0.89**	**0.50**	**0.50**
Democracy			1.00	0.07	0.07	0.13
Government effectiveness				1.00	0.31	**0.44**
Left-wing parties in cabinet					1.00	0.04
Ethnic fractionalization						1.00

Notes: GDP, gross domestic product; bold indicates $p < 0.10$

As noted in Chapter 15, several of these variables relate to both the will and the means to implement health policy. However, some are more closely related to one than the other. For example, GDP per capita and government effectiveness relate mainly to the means of implementation, while survival/self-expression values, democracy (providing a means for public concerns to be brought to the attention of policy-makers), low levels of ethnic fractionalization (increasing willingness to invest in public goods) and left-leaning parties (with their greater emphasis on collective provision) are more closely related to the will to take action.

Determinants of overall health policy performance

Indicators of 'will' and 'means' versus the health policy performance summary score

Chapter 13 described the calculation of a summary score for health policy performance, indicating a country's relative success across all 11 areas considered. This summary score was constructed by determining, for each indicator, whether the country was in the upper, middle or lower tertile of the distribution, and by taking the difference between the country's percentage of scores in the upper tertile and its percentage of scores in the lower tertile. Values of the score ranged between –73% in Ukraine to 89% in Sweden (Table 13.5, p. 279). Factors that might contribute to differences in these scores are now considered. As several of the factors introduced in the previous section are correlated with the summary score (Table 16.3), as well as with each other (Table 16.2), a multivariate regression analysis was carried out. As can be seen in the univariate analyses in Table 16.3, all except left-wing parties are significantly associated with the health policy performance summary score, with survival/self-expression values coming out strongest.

Table 16.3 Correlations of possible explanatory factors with health policy performance score

Variable	Correlation coefficient
Log gross domestic product	**0.85**
Survival/self-realization values	**0.94**
Democracy	**0.53**
Government effectiveness	**0.86**
Left-wing parties in cabinet	0.08
Ethnic fractionalization	**–0.55**

Note: Bold indicates $p < 0.10$

There was no theoretical basis for assuming that one factor would be more important than the others; consequently, the multivariate regression used a forward selection procedure, in which each variable was entered sequentially on the basis of the strength of its correlation. Given the non-linear distribution of GDP/capita, its log value was used.

In the multivariate analysis, two variables were significantly associated with the summary score: survival/self-realization values and ethnic fractionalization. The more a country's population is oriented towards self-realization values, the higher is its score; the more a country is ethnically fragmented, the lower is its score. On their own, survival/self-realization values explained almost 87% of the variation in the summary score ($r^2 = 0.869$) while the addition of ethnic fractionalization increased this to almost 90% ($r^2 = 0.899$). These findings indicate that performance on health policy is driven substantially by the dominant values in the population, for example because a popular demand to do something is communicated to politicians. However, the will to take action seems to be reduced in more fragmented societies, where there may be less willingness to invest in policies that benefit everyone. The results of the multivariate regression yield the following equation:

Health Policy Performance Score = 18.207 + 27.384 (survival values)
– 40.064 (ethnic fractionalization)

This can be used to estimate predicted scores for each country and calculate the difference from what would be expected on the basis of their dominant values and ethnic composition. The results are shown in Fig. 16.1 for those countries with more than 20 data points to generate the health policy performance summary score. These results indicate that Malta, Finland, Spain, Iceland and Sweden performed better than expected on the basis of these indicators of 'will', while Denmark, Slovakia, the United Kingdom and the Netherlands performed worse than expected.

The preceding analyses relate primarily to the extent to which countries have the will to implement health policies. The analysis will now turn to their performance in relation to the means to do so. The wealth of each country,

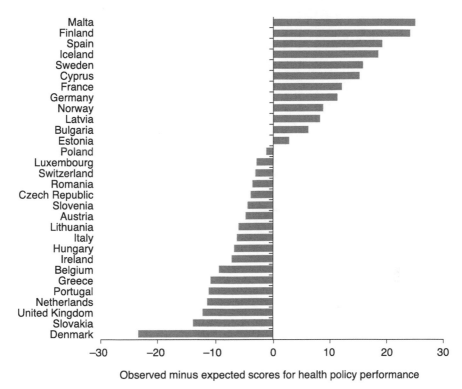

Figure 16.1 Observed minus expected scores for health policy performance, based on a country's survival/self-expression vales and ethnic fractionalization

Note: This was calculated by estimating the expected score for each country by inserting its values on the survival/self-expression and ethnic fractionalization scores into the regression-based formula given in the text and subtracting the expected score from the observed score. For example, Denmark scored 43 on the health policy performance summary score while its expected value was 66, giving a difference of –23

captured by GDP per capita, is used as an indicator of their means. The results are shown in Fig. 16.2. A polynomial trend line has been added to show which countries are performing better or worse than expected. There is one clear outlier, Sweden, which performs much better than would be expected given its level of economic development, although Norway and Iceland are not far behind.

Conditions for successful health policy: insights by country

The discussion will now move to considering how these findings compare with previous assessments of health policy and public health capacity and performance. Three studied have been identified that attempted to compare the performance of the countries studied here in developing and implementing health policy: a comparison of Finland, Sweden, Denmark, the Netherlands,

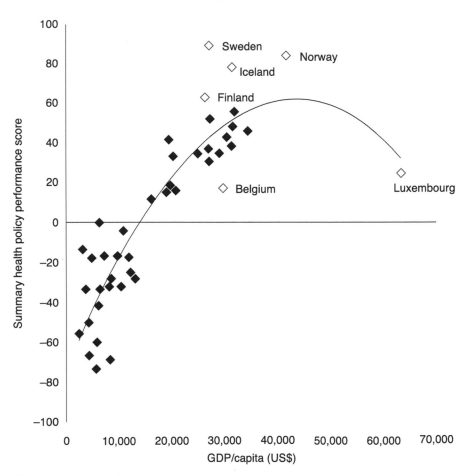

Figure 16.2   Association between national income (as gross domestic product (GDP)) and health policy performance summary score

Germany and France (Allin et al. 2004); a comparison of Finland, Ireland, France, Greece, Albania, Hungary and Lithuania (Ritsatakis and Makara 2009); and a comparison of all the EU-27 Member States (Brand and Aluttis 2011). These provide some insights into why some countries do better or worse than their immediate neighbours, or than what could be expected on the basis of the determinants of health policy performance analysed in the previous section.

Among the Nordic countries, Denmark performs less well than the other countries, including its immediate neighbour Sweden, and less well than could be expected based on its country's value orientation and lack of ethnic fractionalization (Fig. 16.1). Denmark's poor summary score reflects its relatively low scores in almost all areas of health policy: tobacco control, alcohol control, iodine deficiency, neonatal and maternal mortality, measles immunization, breast cancer screening and road traffic safety. Yet in comparative studies of processes and conditions of health policy, Denmark is consistently described as a country with well-developed and well-resourced policies that are supported by strong legal frameworks and a well-functioning public health infrastructure (Allin et al. 2004), and a country with an excellent data infrastructure and a well-trained workforce (Brand and Aluttis 2011) without any apparent differences from Sweden. It is unlikely, therefore, that Danish Governments have lacked the means to achieve better performance; rather it seems that they lack the will to intervene strongly to counter health risks related to modern lifestyles. An in-depth comparison of health policy documents from the four Nordic countries shows that while the health problems are the same, Finnish, Swedish and Norwegian documents have a strong emphasis on social relations, living conditions and participation, while Danish health policy documents focus on individual behaviour, responsibility and autonomy (Vallgårda 2007, 2011).

In continental Europe, Belgium stands out as an underperformer, both in comparison with its immediate neighbours, the Netherlands and France, and in comparison with all other countries at a similar level of income. It has a relatively low score on survival/self-expression values and a relatively high score on ethnic fractionalization (Table 16.1), which may partly explain its low performance. Descriptions of the Belgian public health infrastructure indeed highlight the problems inherent in its federal structure, many elements of which are divided between the Flemish and Walloon communities. However, it performs worse than expected even after survival/self-realization values and ethnic fractionalization is taken into account (Fig. 16.1). One possible explanation is that it lacks the means to implement policies: other reports suggest that Belgium may have suffered historically from a shortage of skilled public health professionals (Ritsatakis and Makara 2009). More recently, however, Belgium has developed an extensive public health infrastructure, including a number of well-resourced agencies and well-developed information resources (Brand and Aluttis 2011) so it may perhaps be expected to score more highly in the future.

Among the Mediterranean countries, Portugal and Greece have the lowest levels of performance but these are, of course, also relatively poor countries, and they lie very close to the trend line when their scores are plotted against log GDP per capita (Fig. 16.2). By comparison, Malta and Cyprus do better at the same level of national income. In cross-national comparisons of health policy, Greece is described as a country with a weakly developed public health tradition. Systematic health policy-making in Greece is hampered by a chaotic financing system, frequent changes of government, lack of law enforcement, a medicalized public health system and a deficient data infrastructure (Ritsatakis and Makara 2009). Both Greece and Portugal have a weak public health infrastructure, with gaps in information and in training and organizational problems (Brand and Aluttis 2011). The same applies to Cyprus, but it has a highly centralized public administration system, which may make health policy development and implementation easier. Malta has a much better developed public health infrastructure, which has been attributed, in part, to the legacy of British colonial rule and the strong persisting professional and educational links between public health in Malta and that in the United Kingdom (Brand and Aluttis 2011).

Within the western Balkans, Slovenia is doing better than its neighbours, which is perhaps not surprising in view of its historical heritage, its greater wealth and early accession to the EU. It lies just above the trend line when scores are plotted against GDP per capita (Fig. 16.2). More surprising is the better than expected position of Albania, which although it is among the poorest countries in Europe does not do worse than most countries that have emerged from the former Yugoslavia, and actually does better than countries such as Romania and Bulgaria. In international comparative studies of health policy, Albania is often seen as a country with a poor public health infrastructure that is unprepared to deal with non-communicable diseases (Ritsatakis and Makara 2009). Epidemiological studies have shown, however, that because of effective infectious disease control and continuing low income Albania has managed to reduce infant and infectious disease mortality effectively over the past half century without a rapid rise in non-communicable diseases, reflecting its almost complete isolation from the rest of Europe during communist rule (Gjonca and Bobak 1997; Gjonca et al. 1997). This advantage may be temporary, as Albania may now be threatened by the advent of western lifestyles (Shapo et al. 2004). It still has a high measles immunization rate, a low fat intake and a high fruit and vegetable intake, and relatively low rates of neonatal, post-neonatal and cerebrovascular disease mortality, but it must begin to build up a public health infrastructure geared towards dealing with non-communicable diseases.

In central and eastern Europe, the best-performing country is the Czech Republic, like Slovenia a country with a history of attachment to the central European traditions of the Austro-Hungarian empire and richer than other countries in its group. It has a relatively well-developed public health infrastructure (Brand and Aluttis 2011). In contrast to some other countries in the region, Romania's public health infrastructure is not only poor resourced but also still very much oriented towards the management of infectious diseases (Brand and Aluttis 2011), despite the fact that non-communicable disease rates are very high in this country. Romania and Bulgaria both perform close to what would be expected, after adjustment for survival/self-expression values and ethnic fractionalization, although this may reflect their high scores on the latter, with large numbers of ethnic Hungarians in Romania and Turks in Bulgaria, and of Roma in both.

Among the countries of the former USSR, the Baltic states together with Belarus do somewhat better than the rest, which is perhaps not surprising in view of the higher national income of the former, although their scores are below the trend line with GDP per capita, indicating less good performance than expected given their resources. More surprising is the fact that, compared with the two other Baltic states Lithuania is not performing better. In international comparisons of health policy, Lithuania is often seen as an exemplary country, with a long tradition of epidemiological studies of non-communicable diseases, high-level political commitment to health promotion and a series of high-profile national programmes to improve population health (Ritsatakis and Makara 2009). This has, however, not enabled Lithuania to perform better than its neighbours in tobacco control, alcohol control, prevention of iodine deficiency, hypertension management, cervical cancer screening or road safety.

There must have been a large gap between intentions and implementation. Recently, life expectancy trends have diverged between Estonia (where sustained progress has been observed since 2000) and Latvia (where life expectancy has stagnated) and Lithuania (where life expectancy has even declined somewhat, partly because of a striking increase in deaths from alcohol-related diseases) (Jasilionis et al. 2011).

Determinants of performance on individual indicators

Indicators of 'will' and 'means' versus individual health policy performance indicators

Although values for the survival/self-realization and ethnic fractionalization scores explained most of the variation in health policy performance summary scores, a more detailed analysis of the performance on individual measures of health policy reveals that, in many cases, there is a strong association with

Table 16.4 Results of regression analyses of performance in health policies on possible explanatory factors

	Variable	Beta value	Significance	Correlation coefficient
Tobacco control score	Survival	0.419	0.024	0.176
Male smoking	Survival	−0.715	<0.001	0.545
	Left-wing parties	−0.432	0.001	0.752
Male lung cancer	Survival	−0.606	<0.001	0.368
Alcohol policy score	Government effectiveness	0.435	0.21	0.189
Alcohol consumption	Survival	−0.571	0.002	0.326
Male cirrhosis	Survival	−0.819	<0.001	0.617
	Left-wing parties	0.276	0.027	0.692
Iodine deficiency	None			
Fat as percentage of total energy intake	Log GDP	0.695	<0.001	0.482
Fruit and vegetable consumption	Log GDP	1.420	<0.001	0.159
	Government effectiveness	−1.130	0.004	0.393
Teenage pregnancy rate	Log GDP	−1.685	<0.001	0.649
	Democracy	−0.411	0.012	0.737
Neonatal mortality	Democracy	−0.803	<0.001	0.645

(continued)

Table 16.4 *(continued)*

	Variable	Beta value	Significance	Correlation coefficient
Maternal mortality	Democracy	−0.662	<0.001	0.438
Measles immunization rate	None			
Child safety score	Government effectiveness	0.438	0.047	0.192
Postneonatal mortality	Log GDP	−0.496	0.001	0.714
	Democracy	−0.468	0.001	0.811
AIDS incidence	None			
MRSA rate	None			
Influenza vaccination rate	Log GDP	0.758	0.001	0.575
Male systolic blood pressure	Survival	−0.607	<0.001	0.369
Female stroke mortality	Log GDP	−1.770	<0.001	0.867
Cervical cancer mortality	Log GDP	−1.989	<0.001	0.796
Seat-belt wearing	Government effectiveness	0.575	0.003	0.331
Occupant mortality	Log GDP	−1.720	<0.001	0.797
Pedestrian mortality	Log GDP	−0.837	<0.001	0.7
Sulphur dioxide emissions	Government effectiveness	−0.569	0.002	0.324
Ozone	None			

Notes: GDP, gross domestic product; MRSA, methicillin-resistant *Staphylococcus aureus*

other potential explanatory variables. This section describes the results of a multivariate analysis to identify which of these variables has the greatest ability to explain performance on each aspect of health policy. Once again, multivariate regressions were undertaken, entering each variable sequentially on the basis of its correlation with the policy in question. This was undertaken for all of the areas of health policy with the exception of the existence of a breast cancer screening programme, as it could only take values of 0, 1 or 2. The results are summarized in Table 16.4. Only those variables retained in the equation are shown.

GDP was the main predictor of performance in nine of the health policy areas, survival/self-expression values in six, government effectiveness in five, democracy in three, involvement of left-wing parties in two and ethnic fractionalization in none. Clearly, given the intercorrelation of the variables, performance is likely to be determined by some variables acting through their impact on others, such as higher GDP per capita encouraging a move away from an emphasis on survival values and towards self-expression. Unfortunately, the limited number of countries and the amount of missing data preclude undertaking the structural equation modelling that would be necessary to tease out these relationships. None of the potential explanatory factors offered any significant explanation of performance in relation to iodine deficiency, AIDS incidence, ozone levels or measles immunization (in the last, virtually all countries reported levels in excess of 90% except for Austria and Malta).

Performance in a number of areas was clearly associated with greater availability of resources. For example, wealthier countries have higher levels of fruit and vegetable consumption but they also have a higher proportion of fat in their diets. Wealthier countries also had lower teenage pregnancy rates, lower postneonatal mortality rates, higher rates of influenza immunization, lower death rates from stroke and from cervical cancer, and lower death rates from RTIs, among both vehicle occupants and pedestrians. All of these associations are intuitive: wealthier people can afford more fruit and vegetables, but they also live in countries where there is a high degree of penetration of energy-dense high-fat products. Greater resources can be spent on health care, such as cervical screening, detection and treatment of blood pressure, and immunization. They also make it possible to maintain roads and enable people to buy more modern and, therefore, safer cars.

A higher score on the survival/self-expression scale was associated with stronger tobacco control, lower male smoking, lower lung cancer mortality among men, lower levels of alcohol consumption and cirrhosis among men and lower systolic blood pressure. This is consistent with the idea that the adoption of self-expression values encourages individuals and their political leaders to invest in the future, specifically in policies that will prolong life and health.

Government effectiveness emerges as significantly associated with alcohol policy, where the ability to enforce restrictions on access and sanctions against drunk driving and related matters are important. Similarly, the ability to develop, implement and enforce measures to increase the safety of children's environments is clearly linked to the effectiveness of government. The association between government effectiveness and seat-belt wearing is also unsurprising, given the importance of law enforcement in this area. The association with sulphur dioxide emissions may reflect the effectiveness of environmental protection agencies.

The observed associations between democracy and the three measures of maternal and child mortality are perhaps more surprising, although they may signify that governments that are more responsive to their citizens invest more in health and welfare services. In a secondary analysis, it was shown that the percentage of GDP spent on health was significantly associated with both maternal and postneonatal mortality, but not neonatal mortality itself. However, in a subsequent analysis when both democracy and expenditure on health were included in the equation, only democracy was significant.

The involvement of left-wing parties in government seemed to contribute relatively little explanatory power. The exceptions were with cirrhosis, where greater left-wing participation in government was associated with higher levels of mortality, after adjustment for survival/self-realization values, and male smoking, where it was associated with lower rates. However, neither association was particularly strong, and it is possible that they were the result of confounding by some unmeasured variable.

The strengths of the associations observed must be interpreted with some caution, given the limitations of the data on both performance measures and potential explanatory variables, the fact that some data were missing, particularly in the former USSR, and the relatively small number of countries included in the analysis. Nonetheless, it is striking that the explanatory variables chosen can explain over 60% of the variation in male smoking, mortality from cirrhosis, teenage pregnancy, neonatal mortality, postneonatal mortality, mortality from cervical cancer and stroke among women, deaths from RTIs, and sulphur dioxide emissions.

In exploratory analyses, a variety of other measures were looked at, including density of physicians (as an indicator of the skills level in the workforce), health expenditure as a percentage of GDP (as an indicator of the priority placed by governments on health), total government expenditure (as an indicator of the perceived role of the state) and linguistic fractionalization. Although each correlated with some of the performance measures, none added significantly to those presented above.

These findings indicate that a substantial amount of the variation among countries in their performance in a majority of the areas of health policy studied can be attributed to the availability of resources, the values held by their citizens, the quality of democracy and the effectiveness of the governments. The next question, discussed below, is whether it is possible to explain the performance of those countries that do better or worse than would be expected given their situation with respect to these variables.

Outliers

This section examines those countries that differ for a specific health policy performance indicator from what would be expected on the basis of the associations identified above. In some cases, these could be explained readily by factors other than health policy.

Looking first at smoking control, as assessed by the TCS (Fig. 16.3), several countries stand out as scoring much higher than would be expected based on the prevailing values of their citizens, suggesting that governments have led public opinion in the quest for better health rather than followed it. The country furthest from the trend line is the United Kingdom, where successive governments have made a clear commitment to reduce smoking rates. The decentralized nature of health policy in the United Kingdom may have made this easier. For example, the decision by Scotland to ban smoking in public places placed substantial pressure on the English health minister at the time, who was known to be reluctant to do so.

The good performance of the United Kingdom may also be linked to the existence of very effective non-governmental organizations, in particular the campaigning group Action on Smoking and Health (ASH) and professional body, the Royal College of Physicians. Some of the Royal Colleges in the United Kingdom have recognized the important role that a respected professional

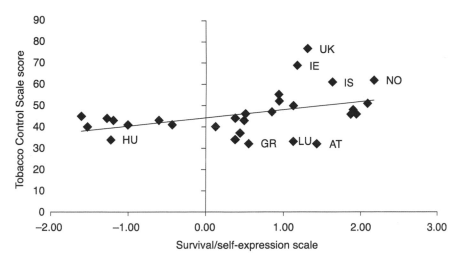

Figure 16.3 Association between survival/self-expression values and score on the Tobacco Control Scale

Notes: AT, Austria; IE, Ireland; IS, Iceland; GR, Greece; HU, Hungary; LU, Luxembourg; NO, Norway; UK, the United Kingdom

voice can play in promoting health policy. This is different from the situation in many other parts of Europe, where professional bodies have focused more on employment issues. Ireland too has been the lead in action against tobacco, with ASH Ireland playing a very effective role, benefiting from a strong evidence base assembled by the TobaccoFree Research Institute Ireland, a company established by a previous government. Norway and Iceland have also been ahead of the curve in taking action against tobacco.

In contrast, Luxembourg, Austria, Greece and Hungary seem to have lagged behind public opinion. Luxembourg has a weak public health infrastructure and scores less well than would be expected on many of the measures evaluated in this book. The company Austria Tabac, owned by Gallaher's since privatization in 2001, has benefited from long-standing political connections, as well as the absence of an effective anti-tobacco voice in Austria. The tobacco industry in Hungary has benefited from close links with successive governments, particularly the Ministry of Agriculture (Szilagyi and Chapman 2003).

A more detailed study looked recently at the political factors related to differing responses to the tobacco epidemic and to smoking rates (Bogdanovica et al. 2011). It found smoking prevalence to be significantly higher in countries with higher scores for corruption, material deprivation and gender inequality, but lower in wealthier countries, those with higher social spending, life satisfaction and human development scores. In the multivariate analysis, however, only the corruption perception index was independently related to smoking prevalence. Exposure to tobacco smoke in the workplace was also correlated with corruption, independently of smoking prevalence, but not with measures for the implementation of national smoke-free policies.

Turning to policies on alcohol control, three Nordic countries, Norway Sweden and Finland, stand out as having policies that are more advanced than would be expected even allowing for the high level of effectiveness of their governments (Fig. 16.4). All three have experienced major problems with alcohol in the past, with the development of strong temperance movements in the 20th century (Bengtsson 1938). Measures have included retail monopolies with limits on times when alcohol can be purchased, coupled with high taxes. However, as noted in Chapter 3, Finland and Sweden have been compelled to weaken their policies as a consequence of EU accession (Chenet et al. 1997). In contrast, policies on alcohol in Germany, Austria, and Denmark lag behind what might be expected. This is a strong indication that these countries lack the political will to tackle this issue, even though all three have high levels of alcohol-related problems.

Teenage pregnancy rates are also closely associated with national income (Fig. 16.5). Malta and the United Kingdom have much higher rates than would be expected. The high rates in Malta have, as noted in Chapter 15, been attributed to inadequate sex education in schools, reflecting the strong opposition by the church. The situation in the United Kingdom has long been a matter of concern and seems to reflect a more general problem of adolescent health, illustrated by high rates of teenage smoking, illicit drug use and teenage drinking (McKee 1999).

Turning to indicators of policy related to fertility and maternal health, there is a relatively strong association between scores on the democracy index and neonatal and maternal mortality. Countries doing worse than expected include Romania and Bulgaria (results not shown), both of which have health systems

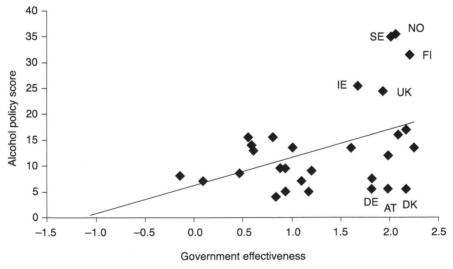

Figure 16.4 Association between government effectiveness and alcohol policy score (using Bridging the Gap score)

Notes: AT, Austria; DE, Germany; DK, Denmark; FI, Finland; IE, Ireland; NO, Norway; SE, Sweden; UK, the United Kingdom

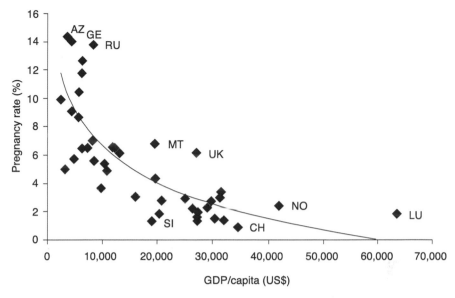

Figure 16.5 Association between national income (as gross domestic product (GDP)) and teenage pregnancy rate

Notes: AZ, Azerbaijan; CH, Switzerland; GE, Georgia; LU, Luxembourg; MT, Malta; NO, Norway; RU, the Russian Federation; SI, Slovenia; UK, the United Kingdom

facing severe problems of underfunding, weak delivery systems and loss of skilled workforce through migration (McKee et al. 2007).

There is an association between government effectiveness and child safety scores albeit weak (Fig. 16.6). Countries scoring higher than expected, suggesting that their governments have placed a higher priority on child safety, include Iceland, the Netherlands and the Czech Republic. Countries scoring lower than expected include Belgium, Spain, Portugal and Greece.

There is a close association between postneonatal mortality and national income. However, Albania, the Russian Federation, Belarus and Malta all do rather worse than would be expected, whereas Finland and Croatia do rather better (results not shown).

There are few obvious outliers in the association between national income and influenza immunization rate, although the United Kingdom does rather better than might be expected (results not shown).

The death rate from cervical cancer is correlated with national income, which may partly reflect the capacity to implement a screening system (Fig. 16.7). For example, high rates are seen in many of Europe's poorest countries. However, among these, the very high rate in Romania stands out. Among high-income countries, the rate in Ireland is somewhat higher than expected, reflecting the late introduction of an organized screening programme, which was only implemented in 2008. The death rate in Finland is substantially lower than expected, consistent with its exemplary organized screening programme, which has been in place for many years.

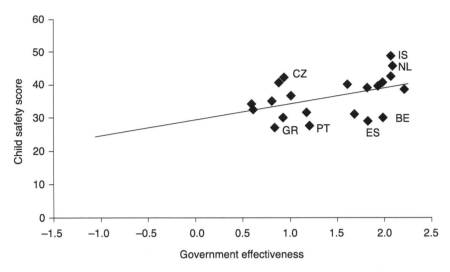

Figure 16.6 Association between government effectiveness and child safety score

Notes: BE, Belgium; CZ, Czech Republic; ES, Spain; GR, Greece; IS, Iceland; NL, Netherlands; PT, Portugal

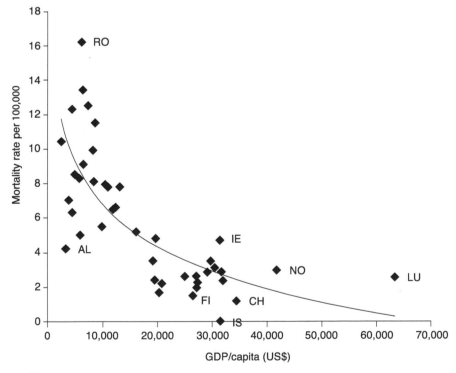

Figure 16.7 Association between national income (as gross domestic product (GDP)) and deaths from cervical cancer

Notes: AL, Albania; CH, Switzerland; FI, Finland; IE, Ireland; IS, Iceland; LU, Luxembourg; NO, Norway; RO, Romania

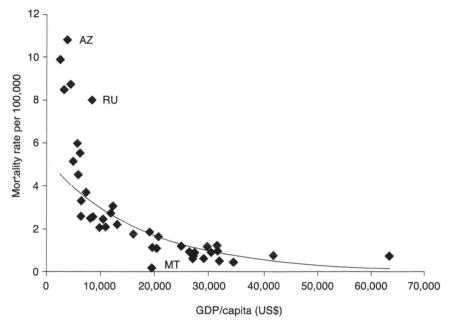

Figure 16.8   Association between national income (as gross domestic product (GDP)) and mortality among vehicle occupants

Notes: AZ, Azerbaijan; MT, Malta; RU, the Russian Federation

There are no obvious outliers in the association between government effectiveness and seat-belt wearing except for the Republic of Moldova and the Russian Federation, where rates are even lower than would be expected given the very low scores on this measure (results not shown).

Deaths among occupants of motor vehicles and pedestrians are highly correlated with each other, and with national income (Fig. 16.8). As previously noted, less wealthy countries are unable to construct and maintain safer roads, while those living in them are unable to purchase safer vehicles. Death rates are, however, particularly high in the Russian Federation and Azerbaijan, as well as in some other former Soviet countries. Looking at Europe as a whole obscures the quite large relative differences among some of the wealthier countries (Fig. 16.9). The extremely low rates in Malta are likely to reflect the high traffic density and thus the limited opportunities for speeding. However, there is no obvious reason, in terms of resources and infrastructure, why Ireland, Belgium and Iceland should perform so much worse than the Netherlands and Switzerland. Some of these differences are consistent with different intensities of enforcement of traffic rules (Fitzpatrick and Nicholson 2010; Aalsma et al. 2012), as set out in Chapter 11.

There is considerable scatter around the trend line for government effectiveness and sulphur dioxide emissions, although one country, Bulgaria, stands out as having exceptionally high values, even allowing for its low score on this measure (results not shown).

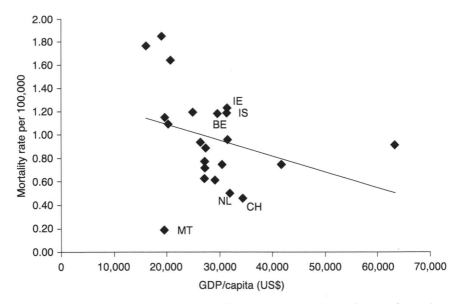

Figure 16.9 Association between national income in countries with gross domestic product (GDP) per capita greater than US$ 15,000 and mortality among vehicle occupants

Notes: BE, Belgium; CH, Switzerland; IE, Ireland; IS, Iceland; MT, Malta; NL, Netherlands

Discussion and conclusions

The analyses presented in this chapter have several limitations. The first is that the data are incomplete: there are particularly serious gaps in our ability to assess health policy in many countries in the former USSR and western Balkans. While the sensitivity analysis showed a high correlation between the health policy performance summary score as used in these analyses and a score based on imputation for all missing values (see Chapter 13), the possibility cannot be excluded that some of the results are biased through the non-randomness of missing values for specific indicators (e.g. because non-availability of data stems from a lack of interest in a particular health policy). Also, the health policy performance summary score, although evidence based, needs further validation. An attempt to undertake a principal components analysis was unsuccessful, as the data did not meet the statistical preconditions for such an analysis; consequently, it was appropriate to look at each area individually. Other limitations relate to the inherent problems of using routinely collected data (e.g. cross-country differences in cause-of-death registration) and to the small number of countries on which the multivariate analysis was based.

More fundamentally, an analysis using only national data fails to capture inequalities within countries. European countries are far from homogeneous, as studies of health inequalities within countries have shown time and again (Mackenbach et al. 1997, 2008). Over the past decades, trends in mortality have been more favourable among those with higher socioeconomic positions

(Mackenbach et al. 2003), particularly in countries in the eastern part of Europe (Leinsalu et al. 2009). It is likely that some of the contrasts that this book has highlighted between countries are even larger on a subnational scale, partly as a result of differential impacts of health policies (Schaap et al. 2008; Stirbu et al. 2010).

Despite these limitations, the results provide important new insights into the determinants of health policy in Europe. They suggest that national health policies reflect, to a considerable extent, the priorities of the populations. Where citizens are preoccupied with survival on a daily basis, governments are less likely to look to the future and to develop policies that will improve the length and quality of the lives of their citizens in the years to come. It could be argued, however, that it is the responsibility of governments to lead public opinion rather than just following it. There are several examples in the preceding chapters of where this appears to be the case, and where substantial health gains have been achieved as a result.

The results also suggest that national health policies reflect the availability of the means to implement them. Wealthier countries are in a better position than poorer countries because they have the resources necessary to develop policies and put them into practice. However, there are important exceptions: some countries do much better than their national income would predict (suggesting that they have put more priority on health policy, resulting in important health gains) while other countries do worse than their national income would predict.

Overall, Sweden stands out as a high performer. To a considerable extent, this is what would be expected: it is a wealthy country, it has at least until recently been ethnically homogeneous and its population places a high priority on values conducive to prevention of health problems. Nonetheless, its overall score is even higher than would be predicted taking these factors into account. The analyses here could not provide an explanation for this high level of performance, but it is noted that Sweden has been described in international comparative studies as a country with a long public health tradition and a strong public health infrastructure (Allin et al. 2004). In contrast, its neighbour Denmark has many of the same advantages but performs significantly worse, probably because of its more libertarian cultural traditions.

In many cases, the results of the quantitative analysis could be interpreted on the basis of the qualitative insights obtained in Chapter 15. Where policies differ, it is often a matter of political will, with a combination of factors involved. These include individuals, institutions and context. For example, the role of civil society organizations, as well as the energy of those individuals working with them, helps to explain the relative success of the United Kingdom and Ireland in tobacco policy. In contrast, the closeness of the tobacco industry with successive governments in countries such as Denmark, Germany and Austria provides a plausible explanation for their relatively poor performance. The long history of alcohol problems, and strong responses to them, in the Nordic countries go some way to explaining the good performance of those countries in this area. The achievements of Finland's renowned cervical screening programme are apparent in its low death rate from cervical cancer. In some cases, countries may be outliers for different reasons. For example, the high teenage pregnancy rate in Malta has been attributed to the role of the church in opposing sex education in schools, while similarly poor performance in the United Kingdom seems to relate to a more general problem of alienation of adolescents.

The next and final chapter of this book will turn to the policy recommendations following from this analysis.

References

Aalsma, M.C., Carpentier, M.Y., Azzouz, F. and Fortenberry, J.D. (2012) Longitudinal effects of health-harming and health-protective behaviors within adolescent romantic dyads, *Social Science and Medicine*, 74(9):1444–51.

Allin, S., Mossialos, E., McKee, M. and Holland, W. (2004) *Making Decisions on Public Health: A Review of Eight Countries*. Brussels: European Observatory of Health Systems.

Bengtsson, H. (1938) The temperance movement and temperance legislation in Sweden, *Annals of the American Academy of Political and Social Science*, 197:134–53.

Bogdanovica, I., McNeill, A., Murray, R. and Britton, J. (2011) What factors influence smoking prevalence and smoke free policy enactment across the European Union Member States, *PLoS One*, 6(8):e23889.

Brand, H. and Aluttis, C. (2011) *Reviewing public health capacity in the EU. Final report*. Maastricht: Maastricht University Press.

Chenet, L., McKee, M., Osler, M. and Krasnik, A. (1997) Alcohol policy in the Nordic countries, *British Medical Journal*, 314(7088):1142–3.

Danishevski, K., Balabanova, D., McKee, M. and Atkinson, S. (2006) The fragmentary federation: experiences with the decentralized health system in Russia, *Health Policy Planning*, 21(3):183–94.

Fitzpatrick, P. and Nicholson, A.J. (2010) Road safety in Ireland: enforcement is the key, *Irish Medical Journal*, 103:69.

Gjonca, A. and Bobak, M. (1997) Albanian paradox, another example of protective effect of Mediterranean lifestyle? *Lancet*, 350(9094):1815–17.

Gjonca, A., Wilson, C. and Falkingham, J. (1997) Paradoxes of health transition in Europe's poorest country: Albania 1950–90, *Population and Development Review*, 23(3):585–609.

Glenny, M. (1996) *The Fall of Yugoslavia: The Third Balkan War*. London: Penguin.

Inglehart, R. (2000) Globalization and postmodern values, *Washington Quarterly*, 23:215–28.

Jasilionis, D., Meslé, F., Shkolnikov, V. and Vallin, J. (2011) Recent life expectancy divergence in Baltic countries, *European Journal of Population*, 27(4):403–31.

Kvist, J., Fritzell, J., Hvinden, B. and Kangas, O. (2012) *Changing Social Equality: The Nordic Welfare Model in the 21st Century*. Bristol: Policy Press.

Leinsalu, M., Stirbu, I., Vågerö, D. et al. (2009) Educational inequalities in mortality in four Eastern European countries: divergence in trends during the post-communist transition from 1990 to 2000, *International Journal of Epidemiology*, 38(2):512–25.

Mackenbach, J.P., Kunst, A.E., Cavelaars, A.E. et al. (1997) Socioeconomic inequalities in morbidity and mortality in western Europe. The EU Working Group on Socioeconomic Inequalities in Health, *Lancet*, 349(9066):1655–9.

Mackenbach, J.P., Bos, V., Andersen, O. et al. (2003) Widening socioeconomic inequalities in mortality in six Western European countries, *International Journal of Epidemiology*, 32(5):830–7.

Mackenbach, J.P., Stirbu, I., Roskam, A.J. et al. (2008) Socioeconomic inequalities in health in 22 European countries, *New England Journal of Medicine*, 358(23):2468–81.

Marshall, M.G., Jaggers, K. and Gurr, T.R. (2010) *Polity IV Project: Political Regime Characteristics and Transitions, 1800–2009*. Denver, CO: Center for Systemic Peace.

McKee, M. (1999) Sex and drugs and rock and roll. Britain can learn lessons from Europe on the health of adolescents, *British Medical Journal*, 318(7194):1300–1.

McKee, M. (2009) The poisoning of Victor Yushchenko, *Lancet*, 374(9696):1131–2.

McKee, M., Balabanova, D. and Steriu, A. (2007) A new year, a new era: Romania and Bulgaria join the European Union, *European Journal of Public Health*, 17(2):119–20.

Norwegian Social Science Data Services (2011) *Fractionalization Data*. Oslo: Norwegian Social Science Data Services, http://www.nsd.uib.no/macrodataguide/set.html?id=16& sub=1 (accessed 18 June 2012).

Ritsatakis, A. and Makara, P. (2009) *Gaining Health. Analysis of Policy Development in European Countries for Tackling Noncommunicable Diseases*. Copenhagen: WHO Regional Office for Europe.

Schaap, M.M., Kunst, A.E., Leinsalu, M. et al. (2008) Effect of nationwide tobacco control policies on smoking cessation in high and low educated groups in 18 European countries, *Tobacco Control*, 17(4):248–55.

Scharff, R.L. and Viscusi, W.K. (2011) Heterogeneous rates of time preference and the decision to smoke, *Economic Inquiry*, 49(4):959–72.

Shapo, L., McKee, M., Coker, R. and Ylli, A. (2004) Type 2 diabetes in Tirana City, Albania: a rapid increase in a country in transition, *Diabetes Medicine*, 21(1):77–83.

Stirbu, I., Kunst, A.E., Bopp, M. et al. (2010) Educational inequalities in avoidable mortality in Europe, *Journal of Epidemiology and Community Health*, 64(10):913–20.

Szilagyi, T. and Chapman, S. (2003) Hungry for Hungary: examples of tobacco industry's expansionism, *Cent European Journal of Public Health*, 11(1):38–43.

Vallgårda, S. (2007) Public health policies: a Scandinavian model? *Scandinavian Journal of Public Health*, 35(2):205–11.

Vallgårda, S. (2011) Addressing individual behaviours and living conditions: four Nordic public health policies, *Scandinavian Journal of Public Health*, 39(6 suppl):6–10.

World Values Survey (2012) [website]. Stockholm: Institute for Futures Studies, http://www.worldvaluessurvey.org/index_surveys (accessed 24 June 2012).

chapter seventeen

Conclusions

Martin McKee and Johan Mackenbach

This book began with a description of the remarkable opportunity offered
to anyone seeking to understand the impacts of health policy by the natural
laboratory that is formed by the diverse countries of Europe. Over the 40 years
that were surveyed for the book, the populations of European countries have
followed very different trends in health. The scale and nature of these diverse
trends are most easily visible when presented as mortality and life expectancy.
Life expectancy has increased almost continuously in the Nordic countries,
in the United Kingdom and Ireland, and in continental and Mediterranean
Europe. Yet in central and eastern Europe and parts of the former USSR,
life expectancy was already stagnating in 1970 and only began to improve in
the 1990s – in some cases, particularly the former USSR, even later. As a result,
life expectancy at birth (for both sexes combined) now varies from 69 years in
the Russian Federation to 82 years in Switzerland, an astonishing 13 years. In
1970, the gap between the best (Sweden) and worst (Romania) of the countries
we have been examining was only seven years.

This divergence in life expectancy can be traced back to diverging trends in
mortality from a wide range of causes of death, many of which have become
amenable to various health policies. Among these, we have studied some of the
most important, including from some infectious diseases; lung, cervical and
breast cancer; ischaemic heart disease and cerebrovascular disease; cirrhosis;
maternal and infant mortality; suicide; and road traffic and other injuries.
While some European countries have experienced rapid and/or early declines
in mortality from these causes, others could be shown to have made no progress
at all or are only doing so, and to a limited extent, in the last few years.

There are few magic bullets in public health. Changes in the number of deaths
from a particular cause almost always reflect the interplay of a wide range of
factors, some within the control of individuals and governments and others
not. Yet the series of detailed analyses in this book have shown that, at least
in part, the explanation for these declines in mortality from some causes has
been the implementation of effective health policies. The analyses covered 11

important areas of health policy: tobacco; alcohol; food and nutrition; fertility, pregnancy and childbirth; child health; infectious disease; hypertension; cancer screening; mental health; RTIs; and air pollution. For ten of these areas, there is good evidence that preventive interventions are effective in reducing death rates among populations and that differences in how and when countries implemented these policies partly explain the health trends observed. The one exception is mental health; this does not necessarily mean that health policy has had no effect but rather that the burden of disease from mental illness is dominated by disability, about which there are few data, and those that are available, on suicides, are problematic because of factors such as cultural differences in the stigma attached to such deaths.

We have been able to document a long list of successes in health policy in the years between 1970 and 2010. Tobacco killed over 100 million people worldwide in the 20th century, comparable with the number of casualties in wars. However, tobacco control policies implemented since the 1960s have contributed to declines in mortality from many causes, including lung cancer (although in many countries not yet among women) and ischaemic heart disease. Policies to reduce hazardous drinking have contributed to declines in mortality from cirrhosis and RTIs. Policies to reduce fat and salt intake and to increase consumption of fruit and vegetables have almost certainly contributed to declines in mortality from ischaemic heart disease and cerebrovascular disease. Policies related to fertility, pregnancy and childbirth have helped to reduce maternal and neonatal mortality. Child health policies have helped to reduce postneonatal mortality and deaths from injury among children. Immunization and other measures to prevent and control infections have reduced incidence and mortality from a range of infectious diseases. Detection and treatment of hypertension has contributed to declines in mortality from ischaemic heart disease and cerebrovascular disease. Cancer screening has helped to reduce mortality from cervical cancer and breast cancer. Measures to make driving safer have contributed to declines in RTIs. Reductions in air pollution have almost certainly reduced mortality from a range of causes, including ischaemic heart disease and chronic obstructive pulmonary disease.

The exact contribution that these health policies have made to better population health is likely to be substantial, even if it cannot be ascertained with precision. Except in cases such as immunization, there is rarely a direct link between a policy and a health outcome. For example, the remarkable reductions in deaths from ischaemic heart disease that have been observed in many countries result from a combination of reduced smoking rates, better diets, improved management of hypertension and a range of other factors, including advances in health care. The precise contribution that each has made to a decline in mortality in a particular country at a particular time will vary. Finally, to make the exercise of assessing the effects of health policies manageable, we have been selective in the indicators we have chosen to capture the results of health policy. For example, smoking is implicated in many diseases beyond lung cancer and ischaemic heart disease, including cancers at a range of sites such as larynx, kidney and bladder; peripheral vascular disease; and chronic airways disease. It also exacerbates many other disorders and harms those exposed to second-hand smoke.

This means that calculations of the gains that have already been achieved, and those that might be achieved in the future, are of necessity imprecise. While noting this caveat, it can be shown that there would have been many more deaths in Europe as a whole if the age-specific mortality rates in 1970 from the causes selected had still applied in 2009: around 850,000 more each year from cerebrovascular disease, 700,000 more from ischaemic heart disease, 150,000 more from neonatal and postneonatal mortality and 100,000 more from RTIs. These figures are enormous. To take only the last of these, the achievements are the equivalent of preventing a jumbo jet crash every single day. In relative terms, the health gains have been greatest for mortality from maternal causes (a seven-fold reduction), infectious diseases (six-fold reduction) and infant mortality (five-fold reduction). In terms of the number of PYLLs, the gains have also been very great.

These successes have, however, not been shared equally between countries. Using a set of 18 quantitative performance indicators covering all of the ten areas where successful health policies could be identified, a summary health policy performance score was constructed that allowed a comparison of countries. As a group, the Nordic countries have been most successful: most of these countries have implemented a large number of the health policies known to be effective and they have achieved correspondingly good population health outcomes. Most of the other western European countries have also performed quite well, but with large variations among them. While most countries of the western Balkans and central and eastern Europe have performed less well, the greatest failures are seen in the former USSR, where few countries have so far succeeded in implementing effective health policies or improving population health outcomes substantially. Although neither country is consistently the best or worst in every area of policy, Sweden stands out as the country with the highest summary score and Ukraine as the country with the lowest on health policy performance.

This general pattern hides some important distinctions between countries that are in the same geographical region of Europe. Among the Nordic countries, Denmark performs distinctly less well on a number of performance indicators. In continental Europe, the Netherlands ranks first but neighbouring Belgium does least well. Among the Mediterranean countries, France does well, but Portugal and Greece do not. In the western Balkans, Slovenia stands out as a country that performs better than the others, as does the Czech Republic in central and eastern Europe. Among the countries of the former USSR, the Baltic states and Belarus do a little better than the others, while Ukraine, the Russian Federation and Armenia fill the bottom ranks, with low scores on most of the performance indicators.

Just as the list of successes of health policy is long, so is the list of failures in the 40-year period covered by this book. As noted in the previous paragraph, implementation of effective health policies has been far from universal in Europe as a whole. If all countries had achieved the age-specific mortality rates of Sweden, the country that stands out as having adopted the 'best practice' overall, far fewer deaths would have occurred in 2009: about 850,000 fewer from ischaemic heart disease, almost 600,000 fewer from cerebrovascular disease, 150,000 fewer from lung cancer and almost 120,000 fewer from cirrhosis – with substantial gains in the other areas too. When the age at which people are dying unnecessarily is taken into account, around 40% of all PYLLs in 2009 could have been saved if all countries had performed as well as Sweden. This proportion is much higher, at more than 70%, in some countries of the former USSR, with potential gains of around 90% for many specific causes of death. These are the greatest failures that this book has identified; although they represent a historical legacy that cannot be undone, the fact that some countries do decidedly better than others even while sharing the same legacy shows that better performance is feasible.

Even in countries that currently perform well, however, significant health gains are still possible. Despite the high level of life expectancy that has already been attained by many countries in western Europe, further gains are feasible if effective health policies were pursued with more determination and if implementation was more complete. In the Nordic countries, the United Kingdom, Ireland and the continental countries of western Europe, the proportion of PYLLs that could be saved if each country had achieved the age-specific mortality rates of the 'best practice' country is in the order of 30 to 50% for many specific causes of death. There were striking gaps in the health policies of many western European countries, such as those related to tobacco and alcohol control, to iodine deficiency, to child immunization, to child safety, to cancer screening and to road traffic safety. These challenges are even greater in the eastern part of the region.

The question then arises as to why some countries have been more successful in pursuing effective health policies than others. The analyses in the book have differentiated the 'will' from the 'means' to implement health policies. The many case studies reported provided clear indications that some of the differences between countries in their performance are the result of differences in 'will'. For health policies to happen, politicians must become aware that there is a problem needing to be solved and that there is a potential solution to the problem. This combination can come about in many ways and often requires the actions of a range of different individuals and organizations, taking advantage of events where necessary. However, it may also require concerted action to overcome the efforts of those who wish to block action being taken, exemplified by the actions of the tobacco industry. Although political will is important, this seemed less dependent on political ideology than on actions by highly motivated individuals. Other differences could be traced back to differences in the 'means' to implement policies, as determined by the available knowledge and information, institutional arrangements, organizational effectiveness and/or financial resources. Important differences were found, not only among countries, but also between policy sectors. For example, while European integration has been a barrier to certain measures to tackle hazardous drinking and to reduce the health-damaging effects of some foods, it has stimulated road traffic safety measures and air pollution control.

A quantitative analysis of the conditions for successful health policy shed important new light on the underlying determinants of a country's health policy. Several factors were important, many of them correlated. However, the factors that were best able to explain the observed differences in overall health policy performance were the values of a country's population, and specifically where they lay on a survival/self-expression scale, and the degree of ethnic fractionalization of a country. Both of these, as well as the other associations identified, are consistent with a large body of theory. In essence, once people have sufficient resources not to have to worry about how they will survive from day to day, they can begin to think about how they will invest in their health in the future. These views will be communicated through the democratic process or other means to their political representatives. However, those living in societies that are fragmented along ethnic lines may be less willing to invest in public goods that will benefit everyone, instead looking to mutual support within smaller groups or families. The analysis also looked at the determinants of countries' scores on specific performance indicators and found that GDP was the main predictor for nine of the indicators, survival/self-expression values for six and government effectiveness for five. Most of these associations could plausibly be interpreted as reflecting differences in 'will' or 'means' to implement health policies. Countries with a higher national income have better performance (which is intuitive as a higher national income implies more financial resources to implement effective health policies). Other factors that were studied, such as the quality of democracy and left-wing seats in government did not, or did only rarely, predict countries' scores on specific performance indicators.

This is the first ever attempt to compare quantitatively the performance of European countries in terms of their health policies. However, there have been a number of other studies using qualitative methods. These have typically focused on inputs to policy and on policy processes, and they have often been based on self-reports by policy-makers. This is quite different from the focus in this volume on the outputs of policy in the form of actual policy implementation and intermediate and final health outcomes. Although some correspondence between the results of these previous studies and this one could sometimes be seen, the results were often uncorrelated. This highlights the need for caution in relying on official documents and self-reports; there may be a large gap between intentions and the ability to implement policies on a scale that will create population-wide health impacts.

One reason why such a quantitative study has not been undertaken previously has been the lack of relevant knowledge. Our study has confirmed the existence of many major gaps in information about the policies that have been adopted by each country, the extent to which they have actually been implemented and the results that they have achieved. We were surprised to find that for most of the 11 health policy areas that this book covers there are no readily available overviews of which policies are effective and which are not. Analyses of the degree of implementation of these policies, and/or of the population health impact of these policies, were also only rarely available. This hampered our analysis. However, it does inform the development of an agenda for data collection and research that national governments, as well as the European Commission and WHO, may want to consider. Given the magnitude of the potential gains in the health of Europeans that could be achieved if the policies described in this book were implemented more widely, we believe that it is essential that more resources are devoted to regularly updated systematic analyses of the sort undertaken in this book.

We conclude that the diverging health trends in Europe are a testimony to both the successes and failures of health policy in Europe in the past decades. Despite the rich diversity of Europe, the health challenges are similar. We urge policy-makers from all of Europe to combine efforts, through mutual learning and mutual assistance, to implement what we know to be possible and thereby improve the health and well-being of their citizens in the coming decades.

Index

7622370R00221

Printed in Great Britain
by Amazon.co.uk, Ltd.,
Marston Gate.